Care Planning in Children and Young People's Nursing

Care Planning in Children and Young People's Nursing

SECOND EDITION

EDITED BY

Sonya Clarke
Senior lecturer (Education)
School of Nursing & Midwifery
Queen's University Belfast

Doris Corkin
Senior lecturer (Education)
School of Nursing & Midwifery
Queen's University Belfast

WILEY Blackwell

This second edition first published 2024
© 2024 John Wiley & Sons Ltd

Edition History
John Wiley & Sons Ltd (1e, 2012)

All rights reserved. No part of this publication may be reproduced, stored in a retrieval system, or transmitted, in any form or by any means, electronic, mechanical, photocopying, recording or otherwise, except as permitted by law. Advice on how to obtain permission to reuse material from this title is available at http://www.wiley.com/go/permissions.

The right of Sonya Clarke and Doris Corkin to be identified as the authors of the editorial material in this work has been asserted in accordance with law.

Registered Offices
John Wiley & Sons, Inc., 111 River Street, Hoboken, NJ 07030, USA
John Wiley & Sons Ltd, The Atrium, Southern Gate, Chichester, West Sussex, PO19 8SQ, UK

For details of our global editorial offices, customer services, and more information about Wiley products visit us at www.wiley.com.

Wiley also publishes its books in a variety of electronic formats and by print-on-demand. Some content that appears in standard print versions of this book may not be available in other formats.

Trademarks: Wiley and the Wiley logo are trademarks or registered trademarks of John Wiley & Sons, Inc. and/or its affiliates in the United States and other countries and may not be used without written permission. All other trademarks are the property of their respective owners. John Wiley & Sons, Inc. is not associated with any product or vendor mentioned in this book.

Limit of Liability/Disclaimer of Warranty
The contents of this work are intended to further general scientific research, understanding, and discussion only and are not intended and should not be relied upon as recommending or promoting scientific method, diagnosis, or treatment by physicians for any particular patient. In view of ongoing research, equipment modifications, changes in governmental regulations, and the constant flow of information relating to the use of medicines, equipment, and devices, the reader is urged to review and evaluate the information provided in the package insert or instructions for each medicine, equipment, or device for, among other things, any changes in the instructions or indication of usage and for added warnings and precautions. While the publisher and authors have used their best efforts in preparing this work, they make no representations or warranties with respect to the accuracy or completeness of the contents of this work and specifically disclaim all warranties, including without limitation any implied warranties of merchantability or fitness for a particular purpose. No warranty may be created or extended by sales representatives, written sales materials or promotional statements for this work. This work is sold with the understanding that the publisher is not engaged in rendering professional services. The advice and strategies contained herein may not be suitable for your situation. You should consult with a specialist where appropriate. The fact that an organization, website, or product is referred to in this work as a citation and/or potential source of further information does not mean that the publisher and authors endorse the information or services the organization, website, or product may provide or recommendations it may make. Further, readers should be aware that websites listed in this work may have changed or disappeared between when this work was written and when it is read. Neither the publisher nor authors shall be liable for any loss of profit or any other commercial damages, including but not limited to special, incidental, consequential, or other damages.

Library of Congress Cataloging-in-Publication Data

Names: Clarke, Sonya, editor. | Corkin, Doris, editor.
Title: Care planning in infants, children and young people's nursing / edited by Sonya Clarke, Senior lecturer (Education), School of Nursing & Midwifery, Queen's University Belfast, Doris Corkin, Senior lecturer (Education), School of Nursing & Midwifery, Queen's University Belfast.
Other titles: Care planning in children and young people's nursing.
Description: Second edition. | Hoboken, NJ : John Wiley & Sons, 2024. | Revised edition of: Care planning in children and young people's nursing / edited by Doris Corkin, Sonya Clarke, Lorna Liggett. 2012. | Includes bibliographical references and index.
Identifiers: LCCN 2023003578 (print) | LCCN 2023003579 (ebook) | ISBN 9781119819622 (paperback) | ISBN 9781119819639 (epdf) | ISBN 9781119819646 (epub) | ISBN 9781119819653 (ebook)
Subjects: LCSH: Pediatric nursing--Textbooks. | Nursing care plans--Textbooks.
Classification: LCC RJ245 .C368 2024 (print) | LCC RJ245 (ebook) | DDC 610.73--dc23/eng/20230602
LC record available at https://lccn.loc.gov/2023003578
LC ebook record available at https://lccn.loc.gov/2023003579

Cover Images: © Doris Corkin, SDI Productions/E+/Getty Images, Willie B. Thomas/DigitalVision/Getty Images, DC Studio/Shutterstock
Cover Design: Wiley

Set in 9.5/12pt STIXTwoText by Integra Software Services Pvt. Ltd, Pondicherry, India
Printed and bound by CPI Group (UK) Ltd, Croydon, CR0 4YY

C9781119819622_090823

Contents

Contributors	ix
Foreword	xx
Preface	xxi
Acknowledgements	xxiii

SECTION 1 Principles of Care Planning

1 Principles of Care Planning: The Nature of Care Planning and Nursing Delivery for Infants, Children, and Young People — 3
Doris Corkin and Pauline Cardwell

2 Risk Assessment and Management — 17
Sonya Clarke and Doris Corkin

3 Safeguarding to Protect Children, Young People, and Their Families — 22
Julie Brown and Sonya Clarke

4 Ethical, Legal, and Professional Implications When Planning Care for Infants, Children, and Young People (ICYP) — 33
Orla McAlinden and Sonya Clarke

5 Young People and Truth Telling — 44
Catherine Monaghan

6 Sexual Health — 51
Jim Richardson

7 Integrated Care Pathways — 55
Pauline Cardwell and Lucy Simms

8 Interprofessional Assessment and Care Planning in Critical Care — 60
Carolyn Green and Doris Corkin

9 Supporting the Planning of Care – Practice Assessor, Academic Assessor, Supervisor, and Student — 72
Nuala Devlin

10 Holistic Care – Family Partnership in Practice — 78
Erica Strudley-Brown

11	**Reflective Account** Ian and Nicola Markwell	85
12	**The Mental Health and Wellbeing of Children and Young People** Deidre O'Neill	92

SECTION 2 Care Planning – Pain Management

13	**Managing a Neonate in an Intensive Care Unit** Clare Morfoot	101
14A	**Continuous Patient- and Nurse-Controlled Opiate Analgesia and Ketamine Infusions** Sharon Douglass and Michelle Whitehouse	109
14B	**Epidural Analgesia** Sharon Douglass and Michelle Whitehouse	116

SECTION 3 Care of Children and Young Persons with Special Needs

15	**Young Person with a History of Epilepsy** Joanne Blair	123
16	**Nut Allergy – Anaphylaxis Management** Susie Wilkie	131
17	**Closed Head Injury** Carol McCormick	138
18	**Obesity** Janice Christie	149

SECTION 4 Care of Neonates and Children with Respiratory Disorders

19	**Neonatal Respiratory Distress Syndrome** Susanne Simmons	161
20	**Cystic Fibrosis** Hazel Mills and Julie Hanna	168
21	**Asthma** Barbara Maxwell, Gillian Gallagher, Katie McMullan, and Catherine Russell	175

SECTION 5: Care of Infants and Young Persons with Cardiac Conditions

22 Cardiac Catheterisation — 185
Pauline Carson

23 Infant with Cardiac Failure — 190
Pauline Carson

SECTION 6: Care Planning – Surgical Procedures

24 Tonsillectomy — 201
Jodie Kenny and Doris Corkin

25 Appendicectomy — 208
Fearghal Lewis

SECTION 7: Care of Infants and Young Persons with Orthopaedic Conditions

26 Ilizarov Frame — 217
Sonya Clarke

27 Developmental Dysplasia of the Hip — 225
Sonya Clarke

SECTION 8: Care of the Gastro-intestinal Tract in Infants and Children

28 Gastro-oesophageal Reflux — 235
Doris Corkin and Lynne Robinson

29 Cerebral Palsy and Nasogastric Tube Feeding — 241
Susie Wilkie and Sonya Clarke

30 Enteral Feeding – Gastrostomy Care — 248
Catherine Paxton

SECTION 9: Care of Children and Young Persons with Endocrine Disorders

31 Nephrotic Syndrome — 259
Janet Kelsey

32	**Newly Diagnosed Diabetic** Pauline Cardwell, Doris Corkin, and Lynne Robinson	**266**
33	**Acute Kidney Injury (AKI)** Hazel Gibson and Rosi Simpson	**273**

SECTION 10 Care of Infants and Young Persons with Skin Conditions

34	**Infant with Infected Eczema** Gilli Lewis and Debbie Rickard	**283**
35	**Burns Injury** Doris Corkin and Lydia Webb	**292**
36	**Children with Complex Needs** Julie Chambers and Doris Corkin	**300**
37	**Sickle Cell Disease** Debbie Omodele, Danielle Edge, and Doreen Crawford	**308**
38	**Transition from Children's to Adults' Services** Claire Kerr	**316**
39	**Bereavement Support** Una Hughes and Patricia McNeilly	**323**

Index **330**

Contributors

Joanne Blair
Lecturer (Education), School of Nursing & Midwifery, Queen's University Belfast, Northern Ireland: MSc in Advanced Nursing, Postgraduate Certificate in Working with People who Challenge, BSc (Hons) Specialist Practice in Nursing, Dip in Community Nursing, RNLD, CNLD

Joanne is a Registered Learning Disability Nurse. Prior to taking up her appointment within nurse education, Joanne worked in the community as a senior nurse, as part of a multidisciplinary team caring for adults with learning disabilities and a range of physical and mental-health needs. At present, Joanne is a professional lead for the learning disabilities nursing programme and is involved in teaching undergraduate and postgraduate students. Joanne works in collaboration with her colleagues to promote research-focused teaching and she has had the opportunity to present areas of her work in journal publications.

Julie Brown
Lecturer (Education), School of Nursing & Midwifery, Queen's University Belfast MSc Nursing, BSc (Hons) Biomedical Science, Registered Nurse (Child), PGCEHCP

Julie is a registered children's nurse, with a background primarily in acute children and young people's nursing and practice education. She currently co-ordinates a pre-registration children's nursing module and contributes more widely to both pre and post registration children's nursing education, simulation, and clinical skills. Her particular interests are in the promotion and development of clinical research nursing and improving the health of families in rural communities.

Pauline Cardwell
Lecturer (Education), School of Nursing and Midwifery, Queen's University, Belfast, Northern Ireland; MSc Advanced Nursing, PGCHET, BSc (Hons) Health Sciences, RN (Child DIP), RGN

Pauline has a career in nursing spanning more than 35 years commencing in 1986, across clinical and educational settings. She holds dual professional qualifications in Adult and Children's nursing, and her clinical experiences have ranged across a variety of clinical environments in acute clinical settings.

Pauline's interest and career in education began with a role as Practice Educator and progressed to a full-time role in Education from 2008. This experience has spanned teaching across a number of NMC approved curricula within pre-registration education and a varied experience relating to post-registration education in the higher educational setting.

Amongst her areas of interest within education are clinical skill development, simulated learning alongside reflection and problem-based learning. She has held a number of positions within the school, which have supported development of leadership, management, and effective teamworking skills. Additionally, Pauline has contributed to journal articles, book chapters, and supported students to develop published work and presentations across a variety of communication platforms and events.

Pauline Carson
Lecturer (Education), School of Nursing & Midwifery, Queen's University Belfast, Northern Ireland: MSc Child Health, PG Cert in Learning and Teaching in HE, BSc (Hons) Professional Development in Nursing, RN (Canada), RSCN, RGN

Pauline has both an adult and children's nursing background and has worked in both the UK and Canada. She worked within the field of children's cardiology prior to entering nurse education and is now primarily teaching within pre-registration nurse education. Areas of interest within nursing include adolescent/young people's healthcare, high dependency care and nurse education.

Sonya Clarke (Co-editor)
Senior Lecturer (Education), School of Nursing & Midwifery, Queen's University Belfast (QUB), EdD, MSc, PGCE (Higher Education), PG Cert (Pain Management), BSc (Hons) Specialist Practitioner in Orthopaedic Nursing, RN child & RGN

Sonya, a nurse for over 30 years, has experience in children's and adult nursing – her nursing career commenced in 1988. She qualified as an RGN in 1991, followed by a diploma in Children's Nursing in 1996. Clinical practice was primarily within Northern Ireland's regional elective orthopaedic unit for the adult and child until 2001, with additional nursing experience (bank position) gained as a Marie Currie nurse until 2009. Prior to her teaching position in 2003, she was employed as a Lecturer Practitioner at QUB and Musgrave Park Hospital, Belfast. Current positions within higher education include Professional Lead for a MSc pre-registration in CYP Nursing and established pathway leader within continuing professional for a short course in Orthopaedic and Fracture Trauma Nursing across the Lifespan. Sonya's teaching, research and scholarly activity reflects both children's nursing (child rights) and specialist subject area of orthopedics. Sonya was presented with the Royal College of Nursing (RCN) Award of Merit in 2020, the highest honour for service in recognition of the exceptional contribution, she has made to the RCN. She completed a Doctorate in Education in 2019, has an extensive publication history and continues to actively lead, inspire, and deliver evidenced-based education that motivates and advances nursing.

Julie Chambers
Former Community Children's Nursing Discharge Coordinator South Eastern Trust, Health & Social Care, Downpatrick, Co. Down, Northern Ireland: BSc (Hons) Specialist Practice, Teacher Practitioner, Nurse Prescribing, Asthma Diploma, D/N Cert, SCM, RSCN & SRN.

Julie commenced her nursing training in 1979 and has worked in community nursing as a District Nursing Midwifery Sister since 1986 specialising in paediatrics. She initiated the setting up of a community paediatric service with her colleague Doris Corkin in 2000. Julie made every effort to enhance and develop her practice by being a mentor to pre-and post-graduate nursing students and by contributing to and participating in international conferences, book/journal publications and presentations. She always endeavoured to ensure that all children and families were nursed to the highest standard and in 2009 was the Well Child's overall winner in the UK Community Practitioner of the Year Award. Julie retired from her former Discharge Coordinator role in 2016 but continues nursing with N I Children's HAH team, teaching assistant at QUB and Community nursing.

Janice Christie
Senior Lecturer PhD, MA, PgDip, PgCert, BSc, RN and RSCPHN

Janice Christie works as a senior lecturer at the University of Manchester. She worked for many years as a health visitor and found that working with parents and their children was challenging and rewarding. Recently through supporting the work of undergraduate, MSc, and PhD students, Janice has continued to develop her and her students' enthusiasm, knowledge, and skills in how to best meet the needs of pre-school and school age children and their parents.

Doris Corkin (Co-editor)
Senior Lecturer (Education), School of Nursing & Midwifery, Queen's University Belfast, Northern Ireland: MSc in Nursing, PG Dip Nurse Education, BSc (Hons), CCN, RN (Child Dip) ENB904 & RGN

Doris has had a privileged career in nursing, spanning more than 40 years, holding dual qualifications in Adult and Children's nursing. Specialised in neonatal for over 12 years, senior staff nurse in an acute children's medical/surgical ward for six years and was instrumental as a community nursing sister for three years, establishing a new service, before accepting current teaching position in 2003.

Her higher education teaching commitments include pre-registration and postgraduate nursing up to master's level, with specific interests in the nursing care of children and young people with critical, complex and palliation needs, encouraging parent/carer involvement across NMC approved curricula. Doris has been professional/programme lead for pre-registration year three students and continues to be a pre and postgraduate module co-ordinator, making every effort to demonstrate her clinical credibility and develop her skill set through facilitation of inter-professional education (IPE) projects, involving workshops online and blended simulated learning with third year children's nursing and fourth year medical students.

A member of various groups, Doris has held chair of the RCN CYP Specialist Care Forum and currently on steering committee of the Professional Issues Forum. Appreciates opportunity to highlight the Northern Ireland perspective and actively inspire nursing students and motivate healthcare staff in relation to life-long opportunities.

Doris was lead editor of the well-thumbed first edition of this care planning textbook published by Wiley, invited to write numerous book chapters, articles, and research papers with nursing/medical colleagues and students, and has presented her teaching and travel awards at various local and international conferences. Additionally, Doris has held a range of external examiner appointments at various universities and continues to deliver evidenced-based education that advances the field of children's nursing.

Doreen Crawford
Retired Academic, Independent Nurse Consultant, and Children's Nurse, MA Health Research, PGCE, BSc (Hons) RNT, SRN, RSCN, Fellow Higher Education Academy and Royal Society Medicine

Nurse Consultant Editor of RCNi Nursing Children and Young People Journal.

Doreen has 40 years' experience working for or in partnership with NHS, has written and edited several textbooks and has supported the development of NICE Guidelines and undertaken CQC inspections. Her specific interests were neonatal care where she sat on the Transformational Review Boards and in the care of the Highly Dependent Child.

Nuala Devlin
Lecturer (Education) Queen's University Belfast Northern Ireland: MSc Nursing (Practice Development) Postgraduate Certificate in Higher Education, NMC Practice Teacher, BSc Health Studies, Diploma in Nursing Studies RGN

The initial part of Nuala's career involved working within a nursing home in the private sector before spending time as a theatre nurse. Nuala went on to specialise in intensive care nursing, working for over a decade within a variety of different cities across the UK. On returning to Northern Ireland Nuala worked in several different nursing positions within an ICU/cardiac setting. Work roles have included ward sister, service manager, practice education facilitator and practice teacher. In 2018, Nuala accepted her current position as a Lecturer (Education) with Queen's University Belfast, with a remit that includes undergraduate and post graduate teaching. Nuala has recently been appointed as academic lead for practice within the university supplying an essential link between the university and clinical practice for both students and staff.

Sharon Douglass
Clinical Nurse Specialist in Children's Pain Management, Nottingham University Hospitals, NHS Trust. BSc (Hons) Healthcare Studies (Child Health), B72/CPAUK Children's Palliative Care, MCC-B73 managing the Care of the Child with Cancer, Specialist Practitioner Qualification in Children's Nursing, C&G Certificate in Teaching Adult Learners

Sharon qualified in Nottingham University Hospital as an RNCB in 1999, since which time she has worked on a variety of children's wards gaining valuable multi-specialty knowledge and expertise. Her main areas of interest were the Surgical High Dependency Unit and the General Surgery and gastroenterology ward. Sharon has always had an interest in Children's Pain Management, which formed the basis of her BSc Honours degree dissertation, which she undertook whilst working on the Paediatric General Surgery and Gastroenterology ward in Nottingham. Teaching is a fundamental part of Sharon's role, covering both pre and post registration students and offering education on specific modules run by the University of Nottingham. Sharon was appointed as a Clinical Nurse Specialist in Children's Pain Management in 2009 and this is where she continued to work at

Nottingham University Hospital NHS Trust. During this time, Sharon has completed specialty related qualifications such as Care of child with Cancer and Children's Palliative Care. Sharon is very passionate about End-of-Life Care for Children, Young People and their families and has developed this service liaising with community, hospice, and hospital teams. Sharon has contributed to several publishing's, helped organise conferences and presented End of Life Case Studies sharing her learning with other Health Care Professionals.

Danielle Edge
Lecturer in Child Health Nursing, University of Plymouth, England. MA Practice Education, BSc (Hons), PGCE, RN Child, fHEA

Danielle is a registered Children's nurse and has worked in higher education for the past six years as a Lecturer. During this time, she has gained an NMC teacher qualification and is a recognised fellow of HEA. She has completed her MA in practice education and shared her work around student experience and support strategies in HEI. Danielle has been a member of the CYP: Professional issues steering committee for the RCN since 2019 and was the newsletter editor for the Association of British Paediatric nurses from 2019 to 2022. Danielle's background is in general paediatrics and she has worked in the NHS, private healthcare, and overseas.

Gillian Gallagher
Paediatric Asthma/Allergy Nurse Specialist, Royal Belfast Hospital for Sick Children, BSc (Hons) Children's Nursing, RN child

Gillian qualified as a RN child in 2005 through Queens University Belfast and she began her nursing career in the Royal Belfast Hospital for Sick children working on general medical wards for six years, gaining experience in respiratory, cystic fibrosis, diabetes, and renal. In 2011, she took up her current role as Asthma/Allergy nurse specialist and helped develop the Asthma Nurse Service within the RBHSC. She was involved in the development and roll out of the Safe Asthma Discharge Pathway, which is now used regionally. Gillian holds a diploma level in Asthma and Allergy management modules and is a contributor to publications relating to safe asthma discharge and inhaler techniques. Her role is primarily to provide evidence-based education to patients and their families on the wards and through nurse-led clinics in the RBHSC. Asthma education is also provided to staff and students. A Skin Prick Testing service to aeroallergens is offered to patients at her nurse led clinics. She also works as part of the multi-disciplinary team for the DTA clinic in the RBHSC, which is a tertiary service, offering her knowledge and skills to promote the health and well-being of the child.

Hazel Gibson
Paediatric Renal Nurse Co-ordinator, Royal Belfast Hospital for Sick Children (RBHSC). RN (Child Diploma), BSc (Hons) Health Studies, ENB 136, RMN, RGN

Hazel's nursing career has included adult general and psychiatric nursing as well as adult renal care, which lead into a career move to children's renal nursing in RBHSC in 1996. Initially as a staff nurse delivering in centre haemodialysis and peritoneal dialysis, to children with acute and end-stage renal failure. Hazel took up her current post in 2003, coordinating a clinical caseload and the staff responsible for care provision for chronic and acute dialysis, also pre and post-operative transplant care. Her role involves teaching programmes regarding parental competencies for home care treatments – dialysis and albumin therapy as well as in-house training and pre and post-registration student education. Pre-transplant education and preparation for children and their carers' and link nurse for transplantation is also part of her role. Community commitments involve further educational input within schools, day nurseries, and community nursing teams, together with home visits to prepare and provide follow up support for children and their families, on home therapies and transplant preparation.

Hazel was involved in the adaptation of the haemodialysis module at Queen's University Belfast within the adult renal course, linking to a paediatric module and has presented both oral and poster presentations at local forums and national conferences. She is the lead nurse representative for Northern Ireland within the UK Paediatric Renal Nurses Group (PNNG), as well as a nurse member of UK Kidney Association (UKKA).

Carolyn Green
Ward Manager, Paediatric Intensive Care Unit, Royal Belfast Hospital for Sick Children, Northern Ireland: BSc (Hons) Biomedical Science, BSc (Hons) Children's Nursing, RSCN, PG-Dip Nursing & PGDip Developing Practice & Healthcare

Carolyn studied Biomedical Science before commencing her nursing training in 2001. After graduating, she embarked on her nursing career in the Royal Belfast Hospital for Sick Children where she worked in a surgical ward and the regional Paediatric Intensive Care Unit. For the past 14 years, Carolyn has developed her skills in caring for children requiring intensive care and the stabilisation and transport of critically ill children. Carolyn has a keen interest in the education and development of nursing staff. She has been a ward manager in PICU since 2018, a clinical educator in PICU and more recently a nurse development lead for the Royal Belfast Hospital for Sick Children.

Julie Hanna
Children's Cystic Fibrosis Nurse Specialist, Royal Belfast Hospital for Sick Children, Diploma in Children's Nursing, BSc Community and Public Health Nursing, PGcert Non-Medical Prescribing

Julie qualified as a Children's Nurse in 1996. Since qualifying, she has worked in Children's surgical, medical and Intensive Care in the Royal Belfast Hospital for Sick Children. In 2008, Julie qualified as a Health Visitor and worked for several years in Belfast, before returning to work in the hospital. As a Paediatric Cystic Fibrosis Nurse Specialist, she combines caring for children in hospital and community.

Una Hughes
Children's Nursing Services Training Coordinator, Southern Health and Social Care Trust RGN, RSCN, BSc Health Studies, PGCE for Health Professionals

Una Hughes is passionately committed to encouraging staff to further their education and provide first-rate patient care. She works closely with the Community Children's Nursing Team and the Vocational Workforce Assessment Team. She has worked in Paediatric Intensive Care and the Community Children's Nursing Team.

Janet Kelsey
Associate Professor in Health Studies (Paediatric), Plymouth University: MSc Health Psychology, BSc (Hons) Psychology, Adv Dip Ed, PGCE, RSCN, RGN & RNT

Janet has contributed to journal and book publications and presented at regional, national, and international conferences on a range of topics. She has managed both diploma and BSc child nursing programmes and teaches both acute care of the child and family and clinical skills in children's nursing. Her interests lie in the care of young people within the acute healthcare environment.

Jodie Kenny
Lead Nurse for Acute Paediatric Services, Daisy Hill Hospital, Southern Health & Social Care Trust; BSc Hons Children's Nursing

Jodie is a Registered Paediatric Nurse, specialised in Paediatric Intensive Care Nursing for over eight years, has experience in Clinical Co-ordination and has previously studied at master's level in the field of Advanced Nursing Practice for Paediatric Intensive Care before accepting her current position as Lead Nurse for Acute Paediatric Services in 2020.

Jodie has a wealth of experience and clinical expertise in critical care nursing and leads on several Trust priorities, key objectives, strategic goals to enhance service provision as well as innovative workforce planning, responding to, and influencing changes to healthcare policy and practice and quality care improvement initiatives. Jodie has numerous journal publications and is committed to healthcare service improvement and meeting the needs and expectations of service users and the public.

Claire Kerr
Reader, School of Nursing and Midwifery, Queen's University Belfast, Northern Ireland. PhD; BSc (Hons) Physiotherapy; PG Cert in Higher Education and Teaching

Claire leads a programme of clinical and epidemiological research into childhood disability at Queen's University Belfast (QUB). She is a Chartered Physiotherapist and has worked in clinical and academic settings in the UK, Ireland and Australia. Claire contributes to undergraduate and post-registration nursing programmes in QUB, with particular focus on evidence based healthcare, transition from paediatric to adult healthcare services, and orthopaedic and musculoskeletal practice. Claire is co-manager of the Northern Ireland Cerebral Palsy Register, contributing to the Surveillance of Cerebral Palsy in Europe group. She supervises MSc and PhD students, has co-authored over 50 papers in high quality peer-reviewed journals and presents frequently at national and international conferences.

Fearghal Lewis
Lecturer (Education), School of Nursing & Midwifery, Queen's University Belfast (QUB), MSc. Advanced Nursing Practice, PGCHET, BSc (Hons) Children's Nursing, BSc (Hons) Adult Nursing Science and RN

Having graduated from QUB with a BSc in Adult Nursing in 2008, he took up his first nursing post in a rural coronary care unit, but it was perioperative care where he would spend the next 12.5 years. In 2014, he completed the MSc. in Advanced Nursing Practice and in 2017 returned to QUB for a third time to carry out his BSc. in Children's Nursing. In 2018, he took up his Charge Nurse position, overseeing the delivery of over 2000 perioperative day cases per year in the award-winning Daisy Hill Hospital, Paediatric Theatre. As COVID-19 gripped our health service, the Paediatric Theatre ceased operating overnight and an opportunity to move into further education was obtained in 2020. Since joining the QUB children's and young people (CYP) team, he teaches, coordinates the final-year undergraduate student programs, and is the lead for the post-graduate courses in perioperative nursing. In 2022, he was appointed lead of the paediatric specialist interest group for the Association of Perioperative Practice (AfPP) and is keen to enhance and improve the quality of care provided to CYP within the perioperative environment.

Gilli Lewis
Nurse Practitioner Intern for Children and Youth with Diabetes, Capital & Coast District Health Board Wellington, New Zealand: MNS (Master of Nursing Science), MPH (Masters in Public Health), PG Diploma in Higher Education, PG Diploma in Child Health, BN (Bachelor of Nursing), PG Cert Advanced Diabetes Care, PG Diploma in Asthma Care

In 1993, Gilli qualified as a nurse from the University of Southampton and headed to New Zealand where she spent five years working in Asthma and Allergy research at the University of Otago. During this time, she provided nursing support to the annual Asthma NZ camps in Wellington. She worked on a children's ward for three years, in New Zealand and in Belfast, Northern Ireland. She taught children's nursing at Queen's University Belfast for five years, and there set up Asthma UK camps, which became an annual placement for student nurses. Many of the children at this camp suffered from severe eczema as well as asthma.

In 2005, Gilli returned to New Zealand and taught children's nursing at Massey University, before becoming the Child Health Nurse Lecturer within the Professional Development Unit at Capital & Coast District Health Board. For the last ten years, she has worked as a Clinical Nurse Specialist in Paediatric Diabetes, become a Nurse prescriber and this year became a Nurse Practitioner Intern – an extended advanced nursing role, in the care of Children and Young Adults with Diabetes.

Gilli has been the facilitator for the New Zealand Child and Youth Clinical Network for paediatric diabetes for the past three years. The Ministry of Heath commissioned this group of experts to develop evidence-based national resources for whānau, health professionals working in this field, in order to improve outcomes for all New Zealand children and youth. She is now recognised as a leader in the field of paediatric diabetes nursing across NZ.

Nicola Markwell
Parent, RGN

Nicola commenced her nurse training in 1986 and qualified as a Registered General Nurse in December 1989. She took up a staffing post in the diabetic unit until 1994 and then transferred to the acute stroke unit where she worked until 2000, when Ryan was born. Since then, she has given up her nursing career to look after Ryan on a full-time basis. During this time, she has become involved in assisting in a Queens University course for children's nurses, by presenting on the challenges of caring for a child with complex needs in the community.

Barbara Maxwell
Children's Nurse, Allen Ward, Royal Belfast Hospital for Sick Children, Northern Ireland: Cert in care of child with CF, Asthma Dip, RSCN, RGN, Non-medical prescriber

Barbara Maxwell is the lead respiratory nurse at the Royal Belfast Hospital for Sick Children. Barbara's role includes caring for children with complex respiratory conditions such as difficult-to-treat asthma, long-term/non-invasive ventilation, tracheostomy management and sleep disorders.

Orla McAlinden
Occupational Health Nurse, Belfast Health and Social Care Trust, RN Child, RN Adult BSc (Hons) Nursing, ENB 415, M.Phil (Medical Ethics and Law)

Orla is a Registered Nurse for Adults and for Children & Young people and has qualifications and expertise in Children's Intensive Care nursing. She worked for 23 years as a Lecturer in Queen's University Belfast (QUB) and currently works in clinical practice with children and adolescents who have mental health problems (CAMHS). Orla also works in the area of Prison healthcare and in Occupational Health. Orla's specialist qualifications include neonatal intensive care, infant mental health, and she holds an M.Phil. in Medical Ethics and Law from Queens University Belfast.

Katie McMullan
Children's Nurse, Royal Belfast Hospital for Sick Children BSc (Hons) Children's Nursing, RN child

Katie has been qualified seven years after training in Queen's University Belfast and graduating with a Bsc Hons in Paediatric Nursing. She started her career in Great Ormond Street, working on a specialist respiratory ward. After one year, she moved to Newcastle upon Tyne where she spent a year in A&E before relocating to Worcester. In Worcester, she worked in a district general hospital Children's ward. In 2019, she moved back to Belfast to work in the regional Children's hospital, RBHSC. After two years on Allen (general medical ward), she undertook the Asthma Nurse Specialist role which includes nurse led clinics, consultant clinics and education for health professionals, children and their families. She is currently waiting to start Advancing Paediatric Asthma Care Course for further development.

Carol McCormick
Ward Manager, Paediatric Intensive Care, Royal Belfast Hospital for Sick Children, Northern Ireland: Paediatric Intensive Care Course, RSCN & RGN

Carol has experience in adult critical care, thoracic and vascular surgery. She has also worked in a variety of specialties within paediatrics. However, critical care is where she spent many years of her nursing career and what she finds most challenging and rewarding. Carol has a special interest in the transfer and retrieval of a critically ill child and is currently developing her clinical skills in this area following completion of the relevant short courses.

Patricia McNeilly
Senior Lecturer Children's Nursing, Queen's University Belfast; Associate Professor Mohammad Bin Rasheed University PhD, MSc Nursing, MSc Social Research Methods, BSc, PG cert in Education

Patricia worked for many years as a children's nurse in both the acute hospital and community setting and held a specialist post as a children's palliative care in the community prior to commencing her career in nurse education in 2003. She has a wide teaching and publication portfolio with a special interest in disabled children and those with complex and palliative care needs.

Hazel Mills
Cystic Fibrosis (CF) Nurse Specialist, Royal Belfast Hospital Sick Children, Northern Ireland: Advanced Diploma in Health Care at QUB, Management of CF Patients Course, (Brompton, London), RSCN & RGN

Hazel has over 22 years' experience working with CF patients. Currently she works as part of the multidisciplinary team facilitating the provision of a high standard of hospital and domiciliary care to children and adults with CF in Northern Ireland. This involves developing clinical policies and providing expert advice and support to patients and their families. Before specialising in CF, Hazel gained experience nursing patients in adult neurosurgery and paediatric general surgery and cardiology.

Catherine Monaghan
Senior Lecturer (Education), School of Nursing and Midwifery, Queen's University Belfast: EdD, MSc, BSc, PGCHET, RGN, RMN, FHEA

Catherine's research interests include international students' experience when studying at a host university, dementia care and ethical dilemmas in clinical practice. Catherine is a member of the School International Committee, the Equality, Diversity, and Inclusion Steering Group and the School Research Committee. Catherine has presented her work at regional, national, and international conferences and contributed to journal publications. She is also a peer reviewer for two nursing journals. Catherine teaches on a range of topics, which address: Developing Leadership and Professionalism, Specialist and Complex Care, Evidence Based Nursing, and Community and Integrated Care.

Clare Morfoot
Senior Lecturer, School of Sport and Health Sciences, University of Brighton, Brighton, BN1 9PH: Fellow of the Higher Education Academy, MSc Clinical Studies & Education, Postgraduate Certificate in Health & Social Care Education, BSc (Hons) Anatomy & Developmental Biology, ENB 405 (Neonatal Pathway), RN (Adult) & Dip Nursing Studies

Clare completed a degree in Anatomy & Developmental Biology at University College London prior to qualifying as an adult nurse from St Bartholomew's Hospital & City University, London in 1997. Clare worked in adult oncology and then specialised in neonatology, nursing in neonatal intensive care for twenty-one years. Clare is a Senior Lecturer at the University of Brighton, within the School of Sport and Health Sciences, where she teaches pre and post registration healthcare students.

Debbie Omodele
Children's Haemoglobinopathy Nurse Specialist, Barking, Havering and Redbridge University Hospital Trust, RSCN

Debbie is a children's nurse with over 15 years of experience and now specialises in haemoglobinopathies (HBO). Her interest in HBO soon began after her first job on a medical ward that provided care for patients with sickle cell disease. Soon after, she took a post as a community specialist nurse dedicated to children and adults with sickle cell and thalassaemia disorder. During this time, her school project was chosen for development as part of the RCN Celebrating Nursing Practice. She has been instrumental in the creation of a sickle cell crisis emergency department passport for her current trust, which aims to improve prompt and effective pain management. Debbie continues to drive forward the transition programme for teenagers to facilitate a smooth and seamless transfer of care to adult services. Debbie facilitates lectures at London Southbank University for pre/post registration students (Child branch and SCPHN) in the care and management of children with HBO and facilitates teaching sessions for primary and secondary school staff on sickle cell disease. She is an active volunteer with the Sickle Cell Society Charity and is the creator of an educational podcast Genes Triggered.

Deidre O'Neil
Lecturer (Education), School of Nursing & Midwifery, Queen's University Belfast, Northern Ireland. Associate Professor in Health Studies (Paediatric), Plymouth University: MSc Family Therapy Specialist Practitioner CAMH BSc (Hons) Nursing RMN Advanced Diploma in Executive and Life Coaching

Deirdre has contributed to journal publications and presented at regional, national, and international conferences on a range of topics. She currently is Year Lead for the BSc Undergraduate year two nursing programmes and teaches and co-ordinates both undergraduate and postgraduate modules. She is the lead for trauma informed practice education for undergraduate nursing and is part of the coaching community in Queen's University Belfast. Her areas of interest are early intervention and prevention of mental ill health and wellbeing.

Jim Richardson
Retired, PhD, PGCE, BA, RSCN, RGN

Jim Richardson has been a children's nurse and children's nurse educator for the last 40 years. His latest post was at Kingston University and St George's, University of London.

Debbie Rickard
Child Health Nurse Practitioner, Capital & Coast District Health Board Wellington, New Zealand: MN (Child & Family, Hons), Cert in Community Child Health, Cert in Allergy Nursing, BN & RN (comp)

Debbie has been nursing in child health for 28 years. Along with three years acute paediatric nursing, 15 years community nursing with 10 of these years including team management and leadership. In 2012, Debbie registered as a Nurse Practitioner. Debbie's interest in working with children and their families has a focus on empowering those living with chronic and/or complex conditions.

Debbie was awarded the Margaret May Blackwell Travel Study Fellowship, which enabled her to visit child health services in the United Kingdom and Australia in 1999. This experience was pivotal in consolidating her vision for improved outcomes for children and families through proactive nursing services. Debbie established the first Nurse Eczema Clinics in New Zealand, which has provided a template for nursing services around the country, adapted to meet the needs of the community they serve. This includes providing education and support to clinicians across health sectors with a multi-disciplinary approach.

Debbie assisted in setting up the Paediatric Society New Zealand (PSNZ) Eczema Clinical Network, was co-clinical lead for six years and member of the Clinical Reference Group for eight years. Debbie is presently a member of the PSNZ Council, continues as a member of the Eczema Clinical Network and Allergy Special Interest Group. Debbie is a clinical expert advisor for the Wellington region clinical pathways including eczema.

Lynne Robinson
Teaching Assistant, School of Nursing and Midwifery, Queen's University Belfast, Northern Ireland; Diploma in Advanced Standing Children's Nursing, BSc (Hons) in Nursing Sciences

Lynne has a career in nursing spanning over 16 years commencing in 2006, across clinical and educational settings. She holds dual professional qualifications in Adult and Children's nursing and her clinical experiences have ranged across a variety of clinical settings.

Lynne's interest and passion for education began with working alongside nursing and midwifery students in the clinical settings and subsequently when she joined the teaching team at Queen's, part-time teaching on areas of interest within the children's nursing curriculum. This progressed to a full-time role in education as a teaching assistant in January 2020. She is currently working on completing her PGCHET and has continued to develop her teaching range and activities across the pre-registration curricula and post-graduate courses.

Amongst her areas of interest within education are clinical skills, simulated learning, and developing educational materials to support student learning. She continues to work in clinical practice to maintain her clinical currency to support her educational knowledge and passion for nursing.

Catherine Russell
Children's Nurse, Royal Belfast Hospital for Sick Children, DipHE Nursing (Children's accredited)

Catherine is currently employed as a Paediatric Asthma/Allergy Nurse Specialist Nurse at the Royal Belfast Hospital for Sick Children for the past five years. After first qualifying as a RCN in 2000, she started work as a staff nurse in the RBHSC, in Infant surgical unit and Medical wards. She is now working as a haemodialysis nurse since six years. Catherine is experienced in working in acute and ambulatory areas, in A&E, and as Deputy Sister of Outpatient department. She has undertaken and completed postgraduate study through Queens University, and holds a postgraduate diploma in Asthma management. Contributor to publications relating to inhaler technique, Safe Asthma Discharge pathway and spirometry in children. Her role is primarily that of providing education for patients and their caregivers, staff, and students, relating to the self-management of chronic condition of asthma. She is working as part of multi-disciplinary team at a tertiary service severe asthma clinic.

Susanne Simmons
Principal Lecturer, University of Brighton, PhD RN (Child)/RN (Adult), PhD, SFHEA

Susanne is a Registered Sick Children and Adult Nurse. She is currently working at the University of Brighton as a Principal Lecturer in Child Health and is course leader for the Post Graduate Certificate Clinical Practice (Neonatal Care) degree. Prior to entering higher education Susanne held a neonatal Lecturer/Practitioner role for three years. In 2012, she was a member of the national task and finish group, which developed the knowledge required for a national core neonatal curriculum for neonatal nurse education (BAPM/RCN 2012). Also in 2012, Susanne and a colleague were successful in applying for a £30,000 Department for International Development grant to develop the first Paediatric Nursing course in Zambia. The course was validated in 2014 and has successfully been delivered in country every year. During 2020, Susanne was part of the trailblazer group for the Enhanced Clinical Practitioner Apprenticeship Standard. Susanne completed a PhD in 2019 entitled Moratorial fathering: enduring sustained uncertainty in the transition to premature fatherhood. The grounded theory from this work focuses on the sociological response to event familiarity and draws on Uncertainty in Illness theory.

Rosi Simpson
Paediatric Renal Nurse, Royal Belfast Hospital for Sick Children, Northern Ireland. RGN, RSCN, ENB 147

Rosi trained in both adult and children's nursing at the Ulster Hospital, Dundonald. After working in the Isle of Man, she returned to initially work in the regional Cardiac Surgery Intensive Care Unit, before moving to the Royal Belfast Hospital for Sick Children. She completed her ENB 147 Paediatric Nephro-Urology Course at the University of Central England and Birmingham Children's Hospital before taking up her current position. Her role includes providing clinical care for pre dialysis, dialysis and post-transplant children and families, supporting the role of Renal Nurse Co-ordinator, and is involved in parental teaching programmes and in house training. She is a member of PNNG and is the Northern Ireland Educational representative for this group.

Lucy Simms
Teaching Assistant at Queen's University Belfast School of Nursing and Midwifery. BSc (Hons) Children's Nursing, Registered Children's Nurse

Lucy is a children's registered nurse with a background mainly in Paediatric Intensive Care nursing. Now involved in education, she teaches at Undergraduate and Postgraduate level, teaching in a variety of modules alongside clinical skills and simulation.

Erica Strudley-Brown
Senior Fellow University of Worcester, Vice President of Acorns Children's Hospices, M.Ed, M.A. Dip Ed. (SEN), FRSA

Erica is a Senior Fellow at University of Worcester, Vice President of Acorns Children's Hospices, and a Professional Adviser to SOFT UK for families of a baby with Trisomy. She is Trustee of The Myriad Centre in Worcester a charity caring for young adults with complex needs. Erica has longstanding experience as a senior manager and Head Teacher in schools and she was Head of Special Education at Oxford Brookes University. Erica has lectured and published nationally and internationally. She is a Fellow of the Royal Society of Arts.

Erica works tirelessly to enhance the quality-of-life experience for disabled children and young people and those with life-limiting or life-threatening conditions and their families. She has made local, national, and international contributions to the development of education, care, and support for children, young people and adults undergoing and recovering from adverse life experience, including family breakdown, imprisonment, and bereavement.

Michelle Whitehouse
Clinical Nurse Specialist in Children and Young People's Pain Management, Nottingham Children's Hospital. Independent Prescriber, MSc in Pain Management, BSc (Hons) Advanced Nursing Practice, RSCN, RGN

Michelle qualified as an RGN in Chichester in 1989 and then went on to train as a children's nurse at Great Ormond Street hospital in 1992. After working in London for a brief time, she moved to Nottingham in 1995 to specialise in both paediatric high dependency and intensive care settings within Nottingham. Michelle has always had an interest in children's pain management, which formed the basis of her BSc Honours degree dissertation, which she undertook whilst working on PICU in Nottingham. During this time, Michelle also undertook the role of health lecturer – practitioner in the University of Nottingham, working with undergraduate master's degree child branch student nurses.

Michelle was appointed as a Clinical Nurse Specialist in Children and Young People's pain management in 2005 and continues to work in this role in the Nottingham Children's Hospital at the Nottingham University Hospitals NHS trust. In this time, Michelle has completed MSc in pain Management and additional courses in Pain Management, Cancer and Palliative care and Transition, and has a special interest in complex pain management. Michelle has presented at several conferences and published articles related to children and young people's pain management, non-medical prescribing and related topics.

Susie Willkie
Lecturer (Education), School of Nursing & Midwifery, Queen's University Belfast MSc, BSc, RN child

Susie is a new lecturer within higher education; she is a registered children's nurse with a special interest and background in neurodevelopmental disability and complex needs within palliative care. She holds an MSc in caring for children and young people with complex health needs. Susie's background includes caring for CYP in Scotland and Northern Ireland plus nurse reviewer in safeguarding.

Lydia Webb
Children's Nurse, Royal Belfast Hospital for Sick Children (RBHSC), Belfast. BSc Children's and General (Integrated) Nursing

Since graduating in January 2015, Lydia has worked in a variety of areas within the clinical setting in Dublin, Brisbane, and Belfast. Even though her travels have taken her far, her heart has never left her first workplace – St Anne's Ward, OLCHC, Dublin – a burns and plastics specialist unit. She currently works in Neurology and Neurosurgery in RBHSC but keeps up to date in burns management and hopes to specialise in burns in some capacity in the future.

Foreword

Planning and delivering high quality, expert care to infants, children, and young people is at the heart of nursing infants, children, and young people. In the first edition of their book, Sonya Clarke and Doris Corkin created an excellent resource for guiding nurses to acquire knowledge, reflect on their practice, appreciate key evidence, and develop their skills in care planning. In this second edition they build on their previous success but add breadth and depth to the content. Crucially in this edition, they incorporate the voice of children and young people as well as parents; this enhances the child and family-centred perspective evident throughout the chapters. This second edition presents a comprehensive and innovative exploration of care planning that addresses the key principles. It also uses detailed case scenarios to stimulate discussion and promote confidence and competence in planning care for infants, children, young people, and their families.

Nursing infants, children, and young people requires commitment, knowledge, and skills, and, as nurses, we are privileged to be part of their lives. Every act of nursing care impacts not only on us but also on the infants, children, young people, and their families and our colleagues. What we do, even in a seemingly mundane situation, can have short and long-term consequences for the child, so we need to make sure that we plan care in a way that enhances their well-being and experience. We need to make every act within our nursing care count; this requires multiple acts of connection and skilled communication. We need to tailor our care to each child's individual context and needs; this requires us to listen and act on their concerns, perspectives and wishes. As nurses working with infants, children, and young people our work is made both more complex and rewarding as we also must consider the needs and concerns of their parents and weave these into child/person and family-centred care.

Nursing is a complex choreography and planning care is core to ensuring that our practice is the best it possibly can be. To do this well we need to draw on technical, theoretical, conceptual, and experiential knowledge as well as a portfolio of skills and personal and professional attributes.

This book is an indispensable resource for nursing students, nurse educators, practitioners, researchers, and carers. In this book the editors and contributors bring their extensive knowledge, experience, and expertise together, offering a clear, accessible, and informative resource for planning the care of infants, children, and young people. Each one of the 39 chapters is written by experts and leaders within their field. Each chapter informs, challenges, and promotes reflection and self-directed learning. The content helps to shape the readers' understanding and appreciation of the topics addressed.

This book will be a wonderful companion across years of life-long learning.

Bernie Carter PhD, BSc, SRN, RSCN.
Fellow of the Royal College of Nursing
Professor of Children's Nursing,
Edge Hill University, UK.

Preface

Welcome to the second edition of Care Planning in Children and Young People's Nursing. The editors and contributing authors address a selection of the most common concerns that arise when planning care for infants, children, and young people within the hospital and community setting. Discussion within each chapter and scenario will highlight that effective care planning needs to be individualised, yet collaborative, negotiated in partnership with the child or young person and their family to meet their many needs. It is hoped the title provides a clear, detailed, and comprehensive insight into children's nursing and that this text is appropriate for practitioners throughout the world.

This textbook is primarily aimed at the field of children's nursing. It is developed to support pre-registration programs at both undergraduate and postgraduate, which leads to registration with the Nursing and Midwifery Council (NMC) as a children's nurse. It also aims to meet the continuing professional development educational needs for those who continue the path of lifelong learning and those recently qualified as a children's nurse. It should also be an invaluable resource for the registered nurse (RN), especially when undertaking the valuable role of student support and assessment – practice supervisor and practice assessor. This text is richly designed with diagrams and photographs to inform the practice of care planning through the report of current research, best available evidence, policy, and education, which reflects both the uniqueness and diversity of contemporary children's nursing. The overall intention is that this second book will again become a core text within children's nursing curricula and serve as a guide when teaching the theoretical foundation and clinical skill of care planning at each stage of the process. Furthermore, it will become an innovative resource for nursing students, educators, practitioners, researchers, and carers.

Chapters 1–12 explore central aspects in the rapidly changing field of children's nursing. Key principles are addressed to facilitate children's nurses with the understanding and knowledge that will underpin their care delivery. A new chapter (Chapter 12) on mental health has been developed and added to this section of the book.

The scenarios outlined in Chapters 13–38 provide the link between theory and practice, whilst highlighting the implications for good practice. This section includes the addition of new chapters on Holprosencephaly and Pompe Disease and Transition from Children's to Adult Healthcare Services.

Proposed questions follow the individual scenarios, offering lists of potential responses with limited rationale; it is therefore recommended that the nursing student/healthcare professional should explore the issues through further reading. Answers are not meant to be definitive or restrictive, and may be amended to facilitate changing circumstances at any time. These scenarios will also help develop the fundamental skills of writing competent focused care plans for infants, children, and young people. Throughout the scenarios a family-centred partnership has been incorporated within a multidisciplinary and interagency framework – it is however contemplative of the child and young person's right to be involved in all matters that affect them and therefore, first and foremost person centered! A collective global approach to care planning, whereby the nursing process and a model/model of nursing have been utilised, demonstrates the art and science of individualised care plans. The activities within the scenario chapters are designed to encourage self-directed learning, assimilation of information and searching of literature to stimulate the enquiring mind.

The editors have drawn together a wealth of expertise locally, nationally, and internationally from a wide variety of practitioners/nurse specialists, academics, and parents and we would like to thank them for their enthusiasm and commitment. Authors have reflected upon their personal/professional experience and in-depth knowledge, whilst respecting confidentiality, to explore prominent issues that arise when caring for infants, children, and young people with a range of conditions some of which could be life-threatening or indeed life-limiting. Outstanding features within this book include updated contributions from parents and a young person who have shared their 'lived experiences', therefore taking cognisance of the Nursing and Midwifery Council stance on service user involvement. We hope you enjoy the book.

Sonya Clarke
Doris Corkin

Acknowledgements

Having reflected upon the Queen's University Belfast philosophy, which is to 'lead, inspire and deliver', the editors would like to take this opportunity to acknowledge the support from Head of School, Professor Donna Fitzimmons, who has encouraged our learning trajectory.

We would also like to thank all existing and new contributors for agreeing to share their expertise, their dedication and for their patience during the book's journey to publication.

Finally, we also Wiley Blackwell and their team for their editorial assistance and patience throughout this timely editing process.

Sonya Clarke
Doris Corkin

Principles of Care Planning

SECTION 1

Principles of Care Planning: The Nature of Care Planning and Nursing Delivery for Infants, Children, and Young People

CHAPTER 1

Doris Corkin and Pauline Cardwell

(Contribution from Lisa Hughes)

INTRODUCTION

Care planning is a continuous concept that requires ongoing review and adjustment, while children and young people's nursing is a human activity that must be founded on a continuity of care and compassion. The COVID-19 pandemic has made its impact on the family across the globe with many healthcare staff creating new ways of working.

As healthcare professionals, we are accountable for our individual practice. Therefore, we must strive to deliver high quality care, acknowledging evidence-based practice and recognising finite resources within contemporary healthcare systems. In order to achieve success, care planning and delivery of individualised care must encompass effective interdisciplinary and multiprofessional collaboration (Corkin et al. 2012).

Within this second edition, the children and young person's nurse will be provided with an overview of the nursing process, its components, and how these assist in organising and prioritising care delivery to the child and family. Philosophical perspectives of care will also be discussed and how this impacts on care delivery in the clinical setting. In conjunction with these aspects of care planning, several models of nursing will be explored, and their contribution in the planning and delivery of care will be illustrated within the timely updated scenarios in the second section of this book.

SERVICE USER – THE CHILD AND YOUNG PERSON

The involvement of children, young people, and their parents as service users and carers is essential and recognition of their overall contribution to the care planning process. Nurses can achieve this by placing the child, young person, and/or parent at the centre of decision-making, a fundamental part of nursing, actively seeking out their wishes and supporting them to have a voice heard (DoH 2012). Open and timely communication is vital to improve experiences. Governmental policies have identified the importance of involving parents in the care of their children and identified this as a major theme in the development of services (Audit Commission 1993; DH 1991, 1996). Chapter 5 has incorporated views from a young person perspective, also Chapters 11 and 36, alongside the parents' journey.

EQUALITY, DIVERSITY, AND INCLUSION

All individuals, including academic and professional healthcare staff and students have a responsibility to treat all patients and colleagues fairly, with dignity and respect and act in accordance with their Trust Employer and University Equality and Diversity Policies (The Equality Act 2010; NMC 2018a). Equality and inclusion requires recognising, valuing and engaging with diversity. Important to have an awareness of the issues that may be sensitive to others, whilst respecting one's own beliefs and values. Areas that should be considered include age, disability, race, religion/belief, gender, gender reassignment, and sexual orientation. According to Stonehouse (2021), diversity recognizes and values our differences as individuals. Common needs tend to unite us, including the need for good health and a social care service.

Care Planning in Children and Young People's Nursing, Second Edition. Edited by Sonya Clarke and Doris Corkin.
© 2024 John Wiley & Sons Ltd. Published 2024 by John Wiley & Sons Ltd.

NURSING PROCESS—WHAT IS THE NURSING PROCESS?

The nursing process is a logical, structured approach, which promotes the nurse's critical thinking in a dynamic manner. This process is used to identify and deliver individualised family-centred care, supported by nursing models and philosophies. Yura and Walsh (1978) identified this process, consisting of four interrelated stages (see Figure 1.1):

- Assess
- Plan
- Implement
- Evaluate

During 2011, Castledine acknowledged the evolvement of the nursing process to be a methodical way of thinking that guides care delivery; whilst focusing on the patient the nurse should base best practice on available evidence with artistic interpretation.

More recently, however, this process has sometimes included a fifth stage relating to 'nursing diagnosis'. For example, a six-week-old infant has been brought to the hospital with a history of breathlessness and poor colour, especially during feeds, who tires easily and the weight gain is poor. Upon examination, heart rate and respiratory rate are both increased and this may lead the nurse to consider a possible cardiac related diagnosis. In utilising the nursing process, a problem-solving approach is applied to the management of individualised patient care. The application of the process is continuous and cyclical in nature and commences with the assessment stage.

ASSESSMENT

This important stage of the care planning process aims to collect and record information pertaining to the health status of the individual child and its effect on the family unit. This phase of the nursing process should provide a comprehensive insight into the needs of the child and their impact on the integrity of the family. The children's nurse must consider not only the physical needs of the child but address the social, emotional, and spiritual needs of the child and entire family. In order to achieve a comprehensive assessment, the children's nurse must utilise a range of proficiencies, including theoretical knowledge and interpersonal skills. Matousova-Done and Gates (2006) highlight the need to both observe and listen to the child and family, utilising verbal and non-verbal communication with the use of appropriate questioning skills to ensure an accurate nursing assessment.

A precise and comprehensive assessment is vital to identify the problems which are currently encroaching on the child's health status and ultimately will ensure safe, effective, and efficient nursing care for the child. This stage of the process links closely with the discrete fifth stage identified earlier as nursing diagnosis, which is supported by an accurate and comprehensive assessment of the child's health needs. During the assessment stage the children's nurse is also involved in analysing and interpreting the information collected, thus contributing to the formulation of a care plan.

A very good example of assessment is the ABCDE (airway, breathing, circulation, disability, exposure) systematic approach to assessing the acutely ill child, as recommended by the Resuscitation

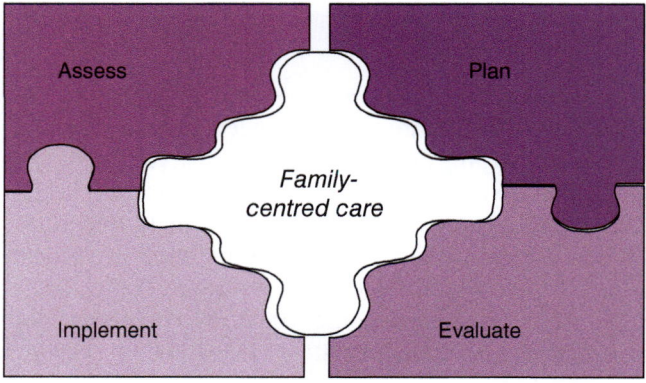

FIGURE 1.1 The nursing process.

Council UK (2021). This approach aims to enable healthcare staff to recognise when they need additional support from the interprofessional team (see Chapter 8). Furthermore, this systematic process helps guide the healthcare professional in planning the frequency of ongoing assessment, especially in the paediatric intensive care setting (see Chapter 17).

PLANNING

During the essential second stage of the process, a plan of care is developed aimed at addressing the problems identified in the assessment phase. This phase of the process involves cognitive and written elements in identifying goals to meet the child's needs. The children's nurse develops mutually agreed goals which endeavour to address the child's problems through the provision of nursing care. These goals are then further developed within the plan, in a sequence of interventions aimed at resolving, controlling or preventing escalation of the problem. In creating these goals, Wright (2005) proposes they should be SMART: specific, measurable, achievable/agreed, realistic, and time-limited. The care plan is developed to guide the nursing interventions in a timely manner to meet the needs of the child and family.

The children's nurse must be able to clearly articulate and document priorities of care, tailored to meeting the individual needs of the child and family, and easily understood by all members of the interdisciplinary team (Cardwell et al. 2011). Effective communication with the child and family are integral to this stage of the nursing process, as the children's nurse must work collaboratively to ensure the care plan is dynamic in meeting the needs of the child and family. In developing the care plan the children's nurse must engage in developing a partnership with the child and family in which they are active partners in the decision-making processes and their involvement in care provision is recognised. This partnership requires empowerment and negotiated involvement of the child and family, which requires skilled children's nurses who are able to ensure children and their families are at the centre of effective care planning (Corlett & Twycross 2006). Having identified, agreed, and set short- and long-term goals specific to the child's needs, these must be regularly evaluated during implementation to ensure they remain responsive to the individual's requirements.

IMPLEMENTATION

This penultimate stage of the nursing process relates to the delivery of care, which has been planned based on the needs of the child and family. Nursing interventions should aim to achieve the goals identified in the care plan and these should clearly identify the actions to be undertaken by the children's nurse. The children's nurse must possess the knowledge, skills, and abilities to deliver the care to the child and assess the appropriateness of planned interventions (Alfaro-LeFevre 2006). Effective communication with the child and family is central to the success of implementing the care plan, which may require adjustment in response to changing needs.

The cooperation and involvement of the child and family is a pre-requisite in this phase of the nursing process. Children and their families must be given choices and involved in decisions regarding nursing interventions, and their participation will personalise their own care implementation. All goals set must be clear and agreed by the child, family, and other carers, including health professionals. Identifiable goals should be achievable, within a realistic timeframe for those involved in care delivery, whilst recognising their continued appropriateness for the child.

EVALUATION

The fourth and final stage of the nursing process requires the children's nurse to consider the impact of the preceding three stages on the child's care trajectory. However, it is essential that the children's nurse continually evaluates the child's response to interventions and modifies planned care to meet the individual's needs and their response to previously identified goals. Overall, this evaluation process aims to recognise changes in the child's condition and identify the need for modification. Analysis of the care delivered by the children's nurse requires critical thinking in order to consider its effectiveness and other possible required interventions to meet the changing needs of the child. The frequency of evaluation may vary depending on the acuity of the child's condition.

This evaluative stage of the nursing process links closely with the assessment phase of the cycle, assessing the attainment of previously identified priorities of care and goals (Heath 2005). Documentation and reporting in this phase of the nursing process is critical in accurately measuring and recording the child's response to planned interventions and to support the continuity of care delivery. Furthermore, this assists in information sharing between healthcare professionals and identification of progress towards goal attainment and also the continued relevance of previously identified goals.

NURSING DIAGNOSES

The North American Nursing Diagnosis Association (NANDA International) is the clearing house for nursing diagnosis work both within the United States of America and internationally (Carpenito-Moyet 2010). This association was initially established in 1973, and later recognised worldwide as NANDA-I in 1982 and is committed to developing the nursing contribution to patient care through 'nursing diagnoses' which informs the creation of care plans (NANDA International 2008). Those care plans approved by NANDA International are rigorously tested and refined in line with current best practice and evidence-based guidelines in clinical settings. Within the NANDA International system, five levels of nursing diagnoses are identified:

- Actual
- Risk
- Possible
- Syndrome
- Wellness

WHAT IS A NURSING DIAGNOSIS?

This is a professional judgement relating to the health problems of the individual or family, which is used to identify appropriate goals and interventions in nursing plans of care, based on a holistic nursing assessment (see Chapter 35).

NURSING PROCESS IN PRACTICE

Overall, this nursing process provides a flexible framework to organise and deliver care of a high standard to the child and family in a holistic manner (NMC 2018a). This facilitates recognition of the individual's contribution, their consent to care, whilst acknowledging organisational quality initiatives, such as policies, procedures, and clinical audit (Holland & Jenkins 2019). This nursing process framework assists the children's nurse in documenting care assessment, planning, implementation, and evaluation, whilst recognising the legal responsibility and professional accountability aspects of accurate record keeping.

Children's nursing is a unique part of the nursing paradigm, with the child and young person's nurse influencing policy and practice (Hollis et al. 2016). In order to apply the nursing process, the children's nurse requires knowledge, skills, and attributes which will only develop over time with practice and experience. Therefore, the nursing student will initially require direct supervision and clinical support (see Chapter 9) in applying the nursing process to their clinical practice, ensuring that care planning and delivery is safe, competent, and effective in meeting the child's and family's needs (NMC 2018b).

PLANNING OF CARE – WHAT IS A CARE PLAN?

A care plan is a comprehensive record (handwritten, pre-printed, or electronic) of essential information which is created following discussions between the child, family, and the children's nurse, detailing priorities of care aimed at meeting the individual's needs (Cardwell et al. 2011). This record consists of a table featuring problem identification, patient goals, and nursing intervention, alongside day-to-day living activities affected (see Appendix 1). This is a legal document which is managed and stored in accordance with legislative and professional guidelines, whilst still being accessible to the individual patient and other healthcare professionals with responsibility for care delivery, whether in the hospital or community setting (NMC 2009).

ACTIVITY 1.1

Look at these practice-based questions.

1. Identify which care planning documentation is currently being used in your clinical placement:
   a. Hospital
   b. Community

2. Discuss with your **practice assessor/supervisor** which nursing model is being utilised to support care delivery:
   a. Has the model been adapted for children's nursing?
   b. How does the model ensure individualised care of the child and family?

In addition to the framework provided by the nursing process, care plans are normally developed with the support of a nursing model, which assists in managing and enhancing effective, high quality care delivery. The development of nursing models attempts to link nursing theory to clinical practice and indirectly informs the growing body of nursing knowledge. Various models of nursing are available and utilised, for example Roper et al. (1985), Casey (1988, 1995), Mead (McClune & Franklin 1987), Orem (1995), and Neuman's system model (Neuman & Fawcett 2002), as well as chapters within this book that demonstrate the application of these models to clinical practice. These models are flexible structures that can be easily adapted to incorporate elements from other models in order to address individual care needs, encouraging the children's nurse to think creatively about the holistic care of the infant, child, or young person and their family.

Increasingly, evidence-based practice is advocated globally as effectively delivering quality care, and thus must be integrated within care plans for the individual (Parsley & Corrigan 1999). The children's nurse must be able to appraise nursing research critically and use this up-to-date knowledge to underpin their clinical judgement and practice, and promote efficiency within healthcare systems. Whilst aiming to provide contemporary high quality care, the children's nurse should reflect upon his/her knowledge and experiential learning, which are key requisites to ensuring best practice as identified in professional regulatory guidelines (NMC 2018a).

The nursing care plan is also supportive of engaging and sustaining interdisciplinary collaboration with the child, family and other health professionals involved in their care. Children's nurses do not work in isolation; instead, care delivery is organised around a team approach and in collaboration with other members of the multiprofessional team. More recently, integrated care pathways have evolved, supporting the development of a multiprofessional document, to which the nursing care plan is integral. These multiprofessional documents are supported by clinical governance and quality agendas within healthcare organisations in delivering effective outcomes (DH 1998).

ACTIVITY 1.2

Using the template below, identify concepts related to care planning. We have given you some ideas for the first letter of each word.

Child-centred care
A_____
R_____
E_____

Process guided by model(s) of care
L_____
A_____
N_____

PHILOSOPHY OF CARE	This aspect of professional practice relates to the expectation of service users and nursing staff in a particular clinical environment of how care and services will be organised and delivered. A philosophy of care helps nurses to define their role and guide practice, within a growing diversity of roles in the clinical environment. Children's nursing, as a distinct field of practice, may relate to a philosophy of care that recognises the individuality of each child and their family, understanding their unique needs in relation to healthcare provision and ensuring their involvement in decisions about their care. The child's needs must be paramount, whether physical, psychological, social, cultural, or spiritual, as well as those of their family, and these should be embedded in the philosophy of care within the clinical environment (RCN 2003).

ACTIVITY 1.3

Seek out the philosophy of care in your clinical placement:

- Enquire from ward manager how this ward philosophy was created.
- Does it identify what children and their families can expect from the service?

WHAT ARE NURSING MODELS?	Nursing models, which are also known as grand theories, attempt to illustrate the theory of nursing practice and facilitate the children's nurse to organise and deliver care. When applied to practice these models of care influence the performance of the nurse and the experience for the child and family (Pearson et al. 2005). The construction and application of nursing models support the development of nursing practice, whilst recognising the values, beliefs and culture of the individual and the changing clinical environment.

Since early work by Fawcett in 1984, numerous nursing models identify the four components of a model as:

- The person
- Their environment
- Health
- Nursing

Care is organised and delivered around identified deficits relating to these components. The development of nursing models, aims to enhance the delivery of family-centred care whilst facilitating the experienced children's nurse to practice autonomously. Through engagement with the child and family the children's nurse is able to identify needs and create a plan of care for the individual and their family, when employing the nursing process in conjunction with a model/s of care.

ROPER, LOGAN, AND TIERNEY – THE 12 ACTIVITIES OF LIVING MODEL

This conceptual model of nursing was devised by three United Kingdom-based nurses and is widely recognised both nationally and internationally. The model is practice orientated whilst incorporating a theoretical framework for care delivery. The model relates to the lifespan of the individual, identifying twelve activities of living (see Table 1.1), which are considered in relation to the continuum of dependence to independence throughout life, appreciating aspects of age, environment, and circumstances which may impinge on this continuum. Each activity of living is influenced by five identified factors, which are biological, psychological, socio-cultural, environmental, and politico-economic (Roper et al. 1985). This model is used in conjunction with the nursing process to identify actual and potential problems for the individual and how nursing care can advance the patient along the dependence to independence continuum. This model of care will be utilised in subsequent chapters such as Chapter 22, illustrating its application in care planning.

Table 1.1 An adaptation of the Roper, Logan, and Tierney Model of Nursing (1985).

1. Maintaining a safe environment	2. Communication	3. Breathing	4. Eating and drinking
• Risk management • Medications • Infectious diseases	• Difficulties with hearing, sight or speech • Cognitive disability • Interpreter services required	• Respiratory problems • Cardiac conditions • Compromised airway	• Special diets • Alternative feeding methods • Swallowing difficulties
5. Elimination	**6. Personal cleansing and dressing**	**7. Controlling body temperature**	**8. Mobilising**
• Altered function of bowel/bladder • Infections • Structural anomalies	• Level of dependence • Skin integrity • Personal preferences	• Abnormal body temperature • Regulatory disorders • Environmental factors	• Level of independence • Mobilising disabilities • Use of aids
9. Working and playing	**10. Expressing sexuality**	**11. Sleeping**	**12. Dying**
• Relevant to age • Effects of hospitalisation/illness • Hobbies/interests	• Stage of development • Altered body image • Sexual preferences	• Altered sleep patterns • Sleeping aids • Environmental factors	• Relevance to illness • Fear of dying • Spiritual needs

CHILD AND FAMILY-CENTRED CARE

Both child- and family-centred care approaches have evolved, as central tenets of children's nursing and other health professionals' practice and viewed as multifaceted concepts that have been reframed during recent years (Coleman 2010; Coyne et al. 2016; Ford et al. 2018). Various attributes of family-centred care are identified in the nursing literature, and include collaborative working, partnerships, respect and involvement of family, negotiation, empowerment/engagement, and provision of a family friendly environment (see Figure 1.2). Whilst there is no clear definition, this concept of family-centred care (FCC) has continued to grow and develop a body of evidence to support its utilisation in contemporary children's nursing practice, since the earlier work of Casey (1988, 1995). The evolvement of the concept FCC and its theoretical underpinnings can be sourced in early work by psychologists Bowlby (1953) and Robertson (1958) who recognised the damaging effects of maternal deprivation and separation caused by hospitalisation on children. These important findings were later endorsed and supported in the findings and recommendations presented by the Platt Report (Ministry of Health 1959).

The development of a national association by parents in 1961 (National Association for the Welfare of Sick Children in Hospital (NAWCH): https://register-of-charities.charitycommission.gov.uk/charity-details/?regid=296295&subid=0) gave parents a voice to demand services which recognised them as central caregivers to their children. This further supported and challenged the need for healthcare delivery for children and their families, to change from a medically dominated service to a service responsive to the needs of children and their families, which provided facilities for parents to remain with their hospitalised child. Recognising and supporting the family as central care providers alongside children's nurses, requires respect for the integrity of the family unit, whatever its structure, with the provision of services which are responsive to the needs of the child and family (United Nations (UN) 1989; Department of Health (DH) 2003). The notion of children, families, and children's nurses as partners in care delivery is integral to achieving the best plan of care and promotes functioning at the highest possible level (Gance-Cleveland 2006). Indeed, Shields et al. (2006) suggest FCC aims to plan and deliver care not just to the child but to the family as a whole, and all family members are recognised as care recipients. An example of how family-centred care can be enhanced in practice is encouraging the presence of parents at the bedside, during a ward round (Montgomery et al. 2016). Optimising the health and safety of hospitalized children.

Further progress has led to the demand for service users, including parents and children, to have a greater voice in shaping future services as identified in more recent literature (DHPSSPS 2005; Noyes 2000). Conversely, Bradshaw et al. (2000/2001) suggest delivering FCC is challenging

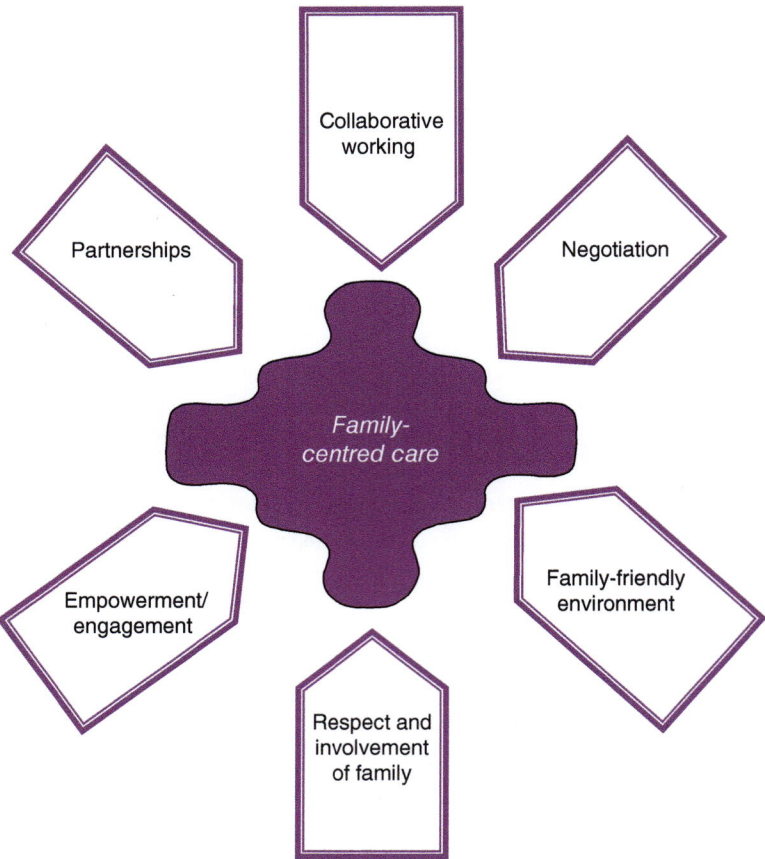

FIGURE 1.2 Attributes of family-centred care.

and demanding, requiring the children's nurse to possess a range of complex skills to ensure its implementation in practice is effective, whilst proposing the theory of FCC has advanced ahead of clinical practice to the detriment of its operationalisation. The lack of a nursing model to support the implementation of this concept in children's nursing is identified by Coleman (2002) as a contributory factor in the difficult translation of the concept from theory to clinical practice.

The lack of involvement of children and their families in the decision-making process regarding their care provision, as perceived by children and their parents, has been identified within nursing literature (Noyes 2000). To address this issue children's nursing must relinquish power in relation to the service they provide and embrace children, young people and their parents as partners in care provision. Family involvement in the design and development of services to meet their individual needs is vital in ensuring an equitable service irrespective of regional, cultural, or socio-economical status.

ACTIVITY 1.4

The nurse plays a vital role in 'Family Nursing' – reflect upon how it has evolved, as a clinical competence, then consider the following:

(a) *Partnerships with Families – across the Lifespan (infant, child, and young person)
Read research: Bannerman et al. (2021) see reference end of this chapter

(b) *Impact of the COVID-19 pandemic on Nurse and Family – important considerations
Needs of the family must be explored if we are to make a difference in health outcomes!

Other frameworks such as 'Me and My Family' a regional document for person-centred assessment and planning of care, is specific to Northern Ireland across the Health and Social Care Trusts. Also during 2014 the Chief Nursing Officer recruited the help of the Northern Ireland

Practice and Education Council for Nursing, to undertake a project in relation to helping nurses and midwives record the care they planned, for example within the Neonatal care setting. The PACE framework was produced (NIPEC 2017) followed by user friendly leaflet – also see children's resources at https://nipec.hscni.net:

PACE = Person centred, Assessment, Plan of Care, Evaluation.

> ### ACTIVITY 1.5
>
> **'Test your knowledge' preparing children and young people for hospital – link to valuable resources: animation and information sheets**
>
> https://www.edgehill.ac.uk/childrencomingtohospital

THE MEAD MODEL

This model was developed for the intensive care setting and for practical use at the bedside. Mead's framework was adapted from the Roper et al. (1985) nursing model, with which it shares some of its attributes. In addition to knowledge and experience of the intensive care environment, the nurse must be familiar with Roper's model, to ensure care planned is delivered in an effective manner. This adapted model identifies the individuality, lifespan (age), dependence/independence, and needs of the patient as the aspects to be assessed when planning care. Factors which impact on the health and wellbeing of the individual are similar to those identified by Roper et al., namely physical, psychological, environmental, socio-cultural, and politico-economical. Additionally, within the dependent/independent continuum on the nurse, Mead (McClune & Franklin 1987) identifies five stages:

1. Total dependence
2. Intervention
3. Intervention with some prevention
4. Prevention
5. Total independence

Each patient is continuously evaluated within the continuum in relation to the five factors highlighted above, identifying appropriate goals for the patient and progression towards independence, with cognisance of the patient's lifespan position. In conjunction with the nursing process the nurse is able to devise a plan of care unique to the needs of the individual patient. In devising a care plan, physical care needs are subdivided into elements specific to the intensive care environment. These include: respiratory, cardiovascular, pain sedation, neurology, nutrition, elimination, skin care, mobility, psychological and social/cultural, and circumstantial (Viney 1996). To illustrate the stages on the dependence/independence continuum, which are relevant to the neurology element as identified in the Mead model, see Table 1.2 which is linked to care planning in Chapter 16.

Table 1.2 Stages on the neurology dependence/independence continuum.

Criteria for stages on neurology continuum
1. Unstable neurological state, requiring continuous monitoring.
2. Potentially unstable neurological state, requiring frequent monitoring.
3. Potentially unstable neurological state, requiring monitoring.
4. Stable neurological state, requiring monitoring to detect/prevent deterioration.
5. No assistance required to maintain neurological state.

OREM'S SELF-CARE MODEL

The self-care model of nursing was developed by Dorothea Orem (between 1959 and 2001) with the aim of helping the patient and family achieve self-care (Walsh 1998). The Orem model is based on the premise that individuals have self-care needs which they themselves have an ability and right to meet except when their ability to do so has been compromised (Pearson et al. 2005). When undertaking a comprehensive assessment this, self-care model identifies what care the patient or family can do for themselves (Nevin et al. 2010). The model has three key concepts: self-care, self-care deficit and nursing systems. Self-care concerns the various activities individuals carry out on their own behalf in maintaining life, health, and wellbeing, which Orem (1995) categorises as universal self-care requisites, developmental self-care requisites, and health deviation self-care requisites (Table 1.3), and also identifies actions for meeting the universal self-care requisites. According to Orem the person best placed to meet these requisites is the individual themselves, whom she calls the self-care agent. In the case of an infant and child this would be the parents; Orem identifies this as dependent care (Orem 1995). When in an individual or, in the case of a child, a parent demand for self-care is greater than the individual or parent's ability to meet it then a self-care deficit occurs and nursing may then be required.

Orem (1991) identifies four goals of nursing:

- Reducing the self-care demand to a level whereby the individual or parent is able to meet the demand independently.
- Increasing the individual or parent's capacity or ability to meet the demand independently.
- Enabling the individual or parents (or significant others) to give dependent care when self-care is impossible for the individual or parent.
- The nurse meets the individual or parent's self-care demand directly.
- Orem (1995) also refers to the role of the nurse within nursing systems, which are carried out on one of three levels:
- Total compensatory system – the nurse provides all the patient care.

Table 1.3 Self-care requisites (Orem 1995).

Universal self-care requisites
Universal self-care requisites are associated with the maintenance of human functioning and serve as a framework for assessment (Cutliff et al. 2010): • The maintenance of sufficient intake of air. • The maintenance of sufficient intake of water. • The maintenance of sufficient intake of food. • The provision of care associated with elimination processes and excrements. • The maintenance of a balance between activity and rest. • The maintenance of a balance between solitude and social interaction. • The prevention of hazards to human life, human functioning, and human wellbeing. • The promotion of human functioning and development within social groups in accordance with human potential, known human limitations, and the human desire to be 'normal'. Orem calls this 'normalcy' (see Chapter 21).
Developmental self-care requisites
Developmental self-care requisites are related to developmental processes throughout the life cycle and can include physical, social or psychological changes, that is, adolescence or social life changes such as bereavement.
Health deviation self-care requisites
Arise out of ill health or injury and are associated with the effect and changes of disease or trauma on the individual.

- Partial compensatory system – nurse assists with care of patient.
- Educative/supportive system – patient has control over their health.

Although the children's nurse may find this self-care theory process time consuming, the overall aim is that the young person or parent is able to meet most of their needs with supportive education. Therefore, the nurse's role is one of teaching and supporting in order to meet the self-care need.

NEUMAN'S SYSTEMS MODEL

Betty Neuman, an American nurse devised this theoretical model of nursing which places great emphasis on prevention (primary, secondary, and tertiary), interventions and a systems approach to holistic wellness (Neuman & Young 1972). The overall focus of this model is the total wellness of the person in attaining and maintaining health to a maximum level. Neuman's model identifies three types of stressors (intrapersonal, interpersonal, and extrapersonal) that act on five individual variables, namely physiological, psychological, socio – cultural, spiritual, and developmental aspects, which interrelate with each other. This model is easily adapted to the community setting where the wider contextual (environmental) factors affecting individual health need consideration, and are fundamental to service provision. When used in conjunction with the nursing process this model aims to support the stability of the person. For further discussion, please see Chapter 17.

ADVANCED CARE PLANNING

End of life treatment tends to be discussed following the initiation of advanced care planning, which gives parents the opportunity to discuss decisions and their wishes, though parents of life-threatened children have reported that discussions were not always aligned to the dynamics of their family life (Carr et al. 2022). When caring for children with life-limiting conditions, parents will need time and help to accept the end of their child's life is near. A trusting relationship has been identified within research as necessary for parents to participate within these palliative care planning discussions (Mitchell et al. 2020).

SUMMARY

The authors of this first chapter have shared accessible and flexible education, by attempting to outline some of the nursing models in contemporary practice within children's nursing, which will be applied to clinically based care planning scenarios within this book. These nursing models have been summarised in Chapters 1–10 and then analysed within care planning scenarios (Chapters 12 – 39) with emphasis on assessing the individual needs of infants, children, and young people. The children's nurse has also been introduced to several reflective activities and online resources. An appreciation of the PACE framework (NIPEC 2017), other nursing models such as the Nottingham model (Smith 1995) and their application in clinical practice, is encouraged, to help enhance knowledge and a deeper understanding of care planning.

CARE OF THE CHILD AND FAMILY DURING ILLNESS: STUDENT/STAFF NURSE PERSPECTIVE

Scenario

Ollie Love (a pseudonym), aged four months, was taken this afternoon to his GP by his parents, with a history of being unwell for the past 24 hours with a troublesome cough and difficulty with breathing. The GP diagnosed Ollie as suffering from croup, so he was quickly referred to the children's medical ward for admission and further management. On arrival at hospital, Ollie was accompanied by his six-year-old sister and anxious parents. Whilst establishing Ollie's clinical observations the children's nurse noted sudden deterioration in his condition.

Proposed care plan

Using the care plan sheets provided, *two* key activities of living (A/L) requiring *immediate* attention were selected by the nursing student and goals identified. A plan of care for Ollie and his family was constructed, supported with rationale, relating to the nursing process and Roper et al. (1985) model of nursing, incorporating a family-centred approach to care and reference to literature.

Sample care plan

Child's Name: Ollie Love DOB: **8th April 2022**

(Continued)

Date and time	A/L No	Potential/ actual problems	Nursing objectives/ outcomes/ goals	Nursing care plan (actions with rationale)	Review dates	Nurse's signature
03/08/22 16.00 h	No.3	Ollie has been admitted to the ward with a troublesome cough and difficulty with his breathing – differential diagnosis is croup.	Ensure Ollie is nursed safely and effectively to maintain patency of his airway, relieve cough, and return breathing pattern to within normal limits.	Approach Ollie and his family in a calm and friendly manner; introduce them to the ward, try to reassure parents and keep them informed. **Gain consent for nursing intervention.** Nurse Ollie upright, prop with pillows to increase his lung capacity and beside working oxygen and suction in case of an emergency situation. If Ollie is unsettled his mum may nurse him on her lap, though handling should be avoided. Use the ABC approach (Resuscitation Council UK 2021). Assess Oliver's respiratory function – initially assess patency of his airway using look, listen, and feel approach; gently check for any obstruction or signs of inflammation and distress. Next assess Ollie's breathing – record and monitor his respiratory rate, rhythm and depth of breaths; note respiratory effort, e.g. if indrawing, nasal flaring or tracheal tug. Important to assess Ollie's cough, recording frequency and effects it has on Ollie's breathing (Holland et al. 2018). Check Ollie's oxygen saturations – if less than 92% consult doctor and administer humidified oxygen at a rate of 5 litres per minute initially, record response and adjust accordingly (BNFC 2020–2021). Assess Ollie's circulation – check and monitor his capillary refill time. Note any signs of cyanosis, e.g. mottled skin appearance and check body temperature. Record and report accordingly (NMC 2009). Administer medication (e.g. adrenaline or steroid via nebuliser) as prescribed by doctor and as per ward policy – check against six rights of administration (Olsen et al. 2010) and medicine guidelines. Carry out oral and nasal hygiene as and when required – should Ollie produce secretions obtain a specimen and send to laboratory for culture and sensitivity.		Staff Nurse Lisa Hughes Staff Nurse Lisa Hughes Staff Nurse Lisa Hughes
03/08/2022 16.00 h	No.2	Ollie's parents are very anxious about his condition.	Ensure Ollie's parents are well informed about his condition, in order to reduce their fears and anxieties.	Welcome Ollie and his parents to the ward. Introduce Ollie and his parents to their primary nurse who will show them the facilities available and inform them of visiting times for extended family. Accompany doctor when he explains to parents the effects croup will have on Ollie and be aware that his parents may want answers to questions. Provide Ollie's parents with both written and verbal information on croup – encourage parents to participate in Ollie's care. Establish a therapeutic relationship with Ollie and his parents, work in partnership to help meet holistic needs (Casey 1995). Ollie is in the sensorimotor stage of development, so the children's nurse needs to be aware of his needs throughout hospitalisation (Bee & Boyd 2013). Contact play therapist who can provide suitable toys for Ollie during his stay in hospital. Complete a detailed history from Ollie's parents, in order to accurately assess and develop a plan of care and aid diagnosis.		Staff Nurse Lisa Hughes

REFERENCES

Alfaro-LeFevre, R. (2006) *Applying Nursing Process–a Tool for Critical Thinking*, 6th edn. Philadelphia: Lippincott Williams and Wilkins.

Audit Commission (1993) *Children First: A Study of Hospital Services*. London: HMSO.

Bannerman, K., Aitken, L., Donnelly, P. & Kidson, C. (2021) Research: Parental perceptions of the impact of COVID-19 restrictions on family-centred care at a paediatric intensive care unit. *British Journal of Child Health*, **2**(4), 195–200.

Bee, H. & Boyd, D. (2013) *The Developing Child*, 13th edn. Pearson.

BNF for Children (2020–2021) *BNF for Children*. London: BMJ Publishing Group.

Bowlby, J. (1953) *Child Care and the Growth of Love*. Harmondsworth: Penguin.

Bradshaw, M., Coleman, V., Cutts, S., Guest, C. & Twigg, J. (2000/2001) Family-centred care: A step too far? *Paediatric Nursing*, **12**(10), 6–7.

Cardwell, P., Corkin, D., McCartan, R., McCulloch, A. & Mullan, C. (2011) Is Care Planning still relevant in the 21st Century? *British Journal of Nursing*, **20**(21), 1378–1382.

Carpenito-Moyet, L.J. (2010) *Nursing Diagnosis: Application to Clinical Practice*, 13th edn. Philadelphia: Wolters Kluwer/Lippincott Williams & Wilkins.

Carr, K., Hasson, F., McIlfatrick, S., & Downing, J. (2022) Parents' experiences of initiation of paediatric advance care planning discussions: A qualitative study. *European Journal of Pediatrics*, **181**, 1185–1196.

Casey, A. (1988) A partnership with child and family. *Senior Nurse*, **8**(4), 8–9.

Casey, A. (1995) Partnership nursing: Influences on involvement of informal carers. *Journal of Advanced Nursing*, **22**, 1058–1062.

Coleman, V. (2002) The evolving concept of family-centred care, Chapter 1. In: Smith, L., Coleman, V. & Bradshaw, M. (eds). *Family-centred Care–Concept, Theory and Practice*. Basingstoke: Palgrave.

Coleman, V. (2010) The evolving concept of child and family-centred healthcare, Chapter 1. In: Smith, L. & Coleman, V. *Child and Family-centred Healthcare–Concept, Theory and Practice*, 2nd edn. Basingstoke: Palgrave Macmillan.

Corkin, D., Clarke, S. & Liggett, L. (2012) *Care Planning in Children and Young People's Nursing*, 1st edn. Wiley-Blackwell.

Corlett, J. & Twycross, A. (2006) Negotiation of parental roles within family-centred care: A review of the research. *Journal of Clinical Nursing*, **15**(10), 1308–1316.

Coyne, I., Hallstorm, I. & Soderback, M. (2016) Reframing the focus from a family-centred to a child-centred care approach for children's healthcare. *Child Health Care*, **20**(4), 494–502.

Cutliff, J., McKenna, H. & Hyrkas, K. (2010) *Nursing Models Application to Practice*. London: Quay Books.

Department of Health (1991) *Welfare of Children and Young People in Hospital*. London: HMSO.

Department of Health (1996) *The Patient's Charter: Services for Children and Young People*. London: DH.

Department of Health (1998) *A First Class Service: Quality in the New NHS*. London: The Stationery Office.

Department of Health (2003) *Getting the Right Start: The National Service Framework for Children, Young People and Maternity Services–Standard for Hospital Services*. London: DH.

Department of Health (2012) *Liberating the NHS: No Decision about Me, without Me*. London: The Stationery Office.

Department of Health, Social Services and Public Safety (DHSSPS) (2005) *A Healthier Future: A Twenty-year Vision for Health and Wellbeing in Northern Ireland 2005–2025*. Belfast: DHSSPS.

Equality Act (2010) Guidance. www.gov.uk/guidance/equality-act-2010-guidance [Last Accessed 4th August 2022].

Ford, K., Dickinson, A., Water, T., Campbell, S., Bray, L. & Carter, B. (2018) Child centred care: Challenging assumptions and repositioning children and young people. *Journal of Pediatric Nursing*, **43**, e39–e43.

Gance-Cleveland, B. (2006) Family-centred care, decreasing health disparities. *Journal of Specialist Pediatric Nurses*, **11**(1), 72–76.

Heath, H.B.M. (2005) *Potter and Perry's Foundations in Nursing Theory and Practice*. London: Mosby.

Holland, K. & Jenkins, J. (2019) *Applying the Roper-Logan-Tierney Model in Practice*, 3rd edn. Elsevier.

Hollis, R., Corkin, D., Crawford, D. & Rigby, L. (2016) RCN G613 Children's nurses: Influencing policy and practice. *Archives of Disease in Childhood*, **101**, A364-2-A365.

Matousova-Done, Z. & Gates, B. (2006) The nature of care planning and delivery in intellectual disability nursing, Chapter 1. In: *Care Planning and Delivery in Intellectual Disability Nursing*. Oxford: Blackwell Publishing.

McClune, B. & Franklin, K. (1987) The Mead model for nursing–adapted from the Roper/Logan/Tierney model for nursing. *Intensive Care Nursing*, **3**(3), 97–105, cited in Viney, C. (1996) *Nursing the Critically Ill*. Edinburgh: Baillière Tindall.

Ministry of Health and Central Health Services Council (1959) *The Welfare of Children in Hospital–Platt Report*. London: HMSO.

Mitchell, S., Bennett, K., Morris, A., Slowther, A.M., Coad, J. & Dale, J. (2020) Achieving beneficial outcomes for children with life-limiting and life-threatening conditions receiving palliative care and their families: A realist review. *Palliative Medicine*, **34**, 387–402.

Montgomery, L., Benzies, K. & Barnard, C. (2016) Effects of an educational workshop on pediatric nurses' attitudes and beliefs about family-centred bedside rounds. *Journal of Pediatric Nursing*, **31**, e73–e82.

Neuman, B. & Young, R.J. (1972) A model for teaching person approach to patient problems. *Nursing Research*, **21**(3), 264.

Nevin, M., Mulkerrins, J. & Driffield, A. (2010) Essential skills. In: Coyne, I., Neill, F. & Timmins, F. (eds). *Clinical Skills in Children's Nursing*. Oxford: Oxford University Press.

Newman, B. & Fawcett, J. (2002) *The Neuman Systems Model*, 4th edn. Upper Saddle River, NJ.

North American Nursing Diagnosis Association International (NANDA-I) (2008) *Nursing Diagnoses: Definitions and Classification, 2009–2011 Edition*. Indianapolis: Wiley-Blackwell.

Northern Ireland Practice and Education Council for Nursing and Midwifery (2017) Recording care – PACE care planning. NIPEC. https://nipec.hscni.net. [Accessed 10 March 2023]

Noyes, J. (2000) Are nurses respecting and upholding the rights of children and young people in their care? *Paediatric Nursing*, **12**(2), 23–27.

Nursing and Midwifery Council (2009) *Record Keeping: Guidance for Nurses and Midwives*. London: NMC.

Nursing & Midwifery Council (2018b) *Standards Framework for Nursing and Midwifery Education*. London: NMC.

Nursing and Midwifery Council (2018a) *The Code: Professional Standards of Practice and Behaviour for Nurses, Midwives and Nursing Associates*. London: NMC.

Olsen, J., Giangrasso, A., Shrimpton, D., & Cunningham, S. (2010) *Dosage Calculations for Nurses*. Harlow: Pearson Higher Education.

Orem, D.E. (1991) *Nursing: Concepts of Practice*, 4th edn. St Louis: Mosby.

Orem, D.E. (1995) *Nursing: Concepts of Practice*, 5th edn. St Louis: Mosby.

Parsley, K. & Corrigan, P. (1999) *Quality Improvement in Healthcare–Putting Evidence into Practice*, 2nd edn. Cheltenham: Stanley Thornes.

Pearson, A., Vaughan, B. & FitzGerald, M. (2005) *Nursing Models for Practice*, 3rd edn. Edinburgh: Butterworth Heinemann.

Resuscitation Council (UK) (2021) *Resuscitation Guidelines*. London: RCUK.

Robertson, J. (1958) *Going to Hospital with Mother*. London: Tavistock.

Roper, N., Logan, W. & Tierney, A. (1985) *The Elements of Nursing*, 2nd edn. Edinburgh: Churchill Livingstone.

Royal College of Nursing (2003) *Children and Young Peoples Nursing: A Philosophy of Care, Guidance for Nursing Staff*. London: RCN.

Shields, L., Pratt, J. & Hunter, J. (2006) Family-centred care: A review of qualitative studies. *Journal of Clinical Nursing*, **15**, 1317–1323.

Smith, F. (1995) *Children's Nursing in Practice: The Nottingham Model*. Oxford: Blackwell Science.

Stonehouse, D.P. (2021) Understanding nurses' responsibilities in promoting equality and diversity. *Nursing Standard*, **36**(6), 27–33.

United Nations (1989) *The Declaration of the Rights of the Child*. New York: United Nations.

Viney, C. (1996) *Nursing the Critically Ill*. Edinburgh: Ballière Tindall.

Walsh, M. (1998) *Models and Critical Pathways in Clinical Nursing. Conceptual Frameworks for Care Planning*, 2nd edn. Edinburgh: Baillière Tindall.

Wright, K. (2005) Care Planning: An easy guide for nurses. *Nursing and Residential Care*, **7**, 71–73.

Yura, D. & Walsh, M.B. (1978) *The Nursing Process: Assessing, Planning, Implementing and Evaluating*. New York: Appleton Century Crofts.

Risk Assessment and Management

Sonya Clarke and Doris Corkin

CHAPTER 2

INTRODUCTION

Risk assessment and management is everybody's business; it is a major component of daily living and nursing practice. In 2019, Boholm proposed an everyday meaning of the word 'risk', where it relates to the presence of two conceptual elements: uncertainty (or potentiality) and adversity. As healthcare professionals, we come across difficult and challenging moments that are often unexpected each and every day, as patient care is individual and unpredictable on occasions. Therefore, when the unexpected happens, making time to learn from the experience is essential, as learning after the event may be the single most powerful insight into any healthcare organisation.

RISK ASSESSMENT

Risk assessment is simply *an assessment or calculation of risk or potential risk of an issue which cannot be easily rectified* (Stower 2000, p. 42). In 2020, the Royal College of Nursing (RCN) placed the spotlight on risk assessment. RCN safety representative, Neil Thompson reports, *If an effective risk assessment hasn't been carried out, how can the employer know that what you're doing is safe for you, your colleagues and your patients?* Neil further suggests, *in an ideal world, where the workplace also has sufficient people with time release to carry out health and safety duties, there would be a much more regular programme of risk assessment in place.* Assessing risk factors and establishing that a patient is at risk should be part of the initial assessment and care planning for any patient who is entering the healthcare system. As children's nurses our behaviours become as important as our technical skill and knowledge when serving the best interests of sick children, their families, and our colleagues. Nurses monitor risk each time they meet patients; it may be through experience and intuition or through application of a valid and reliable risk assessment tool. Indeed, a student or staff nurse can often walk onto a ward and know when something is 'just not right'; such an emotion can be described as a 'gut feeling'. We must, however, question the weight that the nursing profession gives to a decision based on intuition, as opposed to those who follow best practice, national standards, or clinical guidelines.

MAIN SOURCES OF RISK

- Poor communication pathways
- Lack of clear up-to-date policies/procedures/guidelines
- Poorly defined responsibilities
- Staff working beyond their level of competence (Bowden 1996).

Nonetheless, a *Nursing Times* reporter (Lomas 2009) on behalf of Professor Peter Griffiths warns that risk assessment tools are not always backed by evidence. He has suggested that: 'tools should be used as a baseline, but they also need to be reused when it is clinically indicated or in line with 'NICE' guidelines – NICE | The National Institute for Health and Care Excellence . It must not be a paper filing exercise.'

An article by Griffiths and Jull (2010) concludes that formal assessment tools may or may not have a place within risk assessment with good clinical judgement and appropriate intervention but does not advocate the 'use of a tool' as the vital indicator to produce the absence of a pressure ulcer.

Studies published in the early 1990s found that nurses base decision making on experience (Luker & Kendrick 1992), with intuition being described as the process of instant understanding of a situation (Miller 1993). There is limited empirical evidence that examines how risk is actually assessed within clinical practices. Trenoweth's limited small study in 2003 suggests that in a crisis situation risk assessment may be based on intuition. Even though risk assessment has been around for decades we are often unaware of how 'we do it' and most often do not realise we are undertaking 'risk assessment.' Brunton (2005) suggests that the method for making a decision regarding risk is situation dependent, where the nurse will in the first instance use a risk assessment tool to aid in a scientific manner. The tool's high inter-rater reliability may reduce the risk to patients from an individual nurse's lack of experience and ability. They may be of comfort to the nurse, but if time consuming, they may not always be practical for every patient/nurse contact.

Healthcare professionals undertake risk assessments to identify problem areas so that risk management measures can be put in place to make a situation as safe as possible for all concerned.

Risk assessments are carried out daily, sometimes without nurses even realising it, such as checking the emergency trolley every morning. NICE (2015) clinical guidance (CG179) on pressure ulcer prevention and management in neonates, infants, children, and young people offer guidance around the key areas – skin assessment, repositioning, skin massage, nutritional supplements, hydration, pressure redistribution, devices, and barrier creams. For further information go to 1 Recommendations | Pressure ulcers: prevention and management | Guidance | NICE. Similarly, Liversedge (2019) concur, and report the steps which exist that nurses can take to minimise the risk of skin damage, including regular skin assessments, pressure relief where possible, and the removal of medical devices when they are no longer necessary. Renowned risk assessment tools such as Waterlow (1997), Braden and Bergstrom (1987), and Norton et al. (1962) are used to predict a patient's high-profile areas such as patient falls, malnutrition, moving and handling, and pressure ulcers. Such tools have been widely used by nurses in clinical practice for many years. A recent tool developed for CYP, is the Adapted Glamorgan Pressure Ulcer Risk Assessment Scale – Suitable for use from Birth-18yrs: December 2020 (healthcareimprovementscotland.org).

Sadly, nurses can be put in difficult situations when staffing levels are stretched. For example, the moving and handling of patients continues to cause nursing staff to have back injuries, and to suffer severe pain for weeks and ongoing pain for years.

CATEGORIES OF RISK

- Risks for the nurse (Chadwick & Tadd 1992)
- Risks for the child and parents
- Risks arising from research (Coyne 1998)

More tools are currently being developed for the child and young person, as highlighted by Willock et al. (2007), who have found the Glamorgan scale for pressure ulcer prevention in children may give a more accurate estimate of risk than other scales. The study notes nurses should examine and try to resolve the individual problems that contribute to the 'total risk'. In summary, the Glamorgan scale appears to be the first paediatric pressure ulcer risk assessment scale developed statistically using patient data. Anthony et al. in 2010 completed a comparison of Braden Q, Garvin, and Glamorgan risk assessment scales in children – they reported the Glamorgan scale to be the most valid of the three children's risk assessment scales. Anthony et al. (2010, p. 98) further report, 'Mobility alone may be as effective as employing the more complex risk assessment scale.'

However, it is important to note no risk assessment tool is 100% accurate. If a paediatric risk assessment scale is employed to predict risk, then unless it is valid, it may identify children who are not at risk and waste resources or fail to identify children at risk possibly resulting in adverse health outcomes (Anthony et al. 2010).

Shields and Clarke (2010) previously explored 'reducing the risk' through the use of a validated tool for children. The paper suggests that children who require orthopaedic surgery or have casts or fixation devices applied will require ongoing neurovascular monitoring as they will have a restriction of movement. The Royal College of Nursing and British Orthopaedic Association jointly developed consensus guidance around peripheral neurovascular observations for acute limb compartment syndrome (RCN 2022). The guidance underpinned by a systematic review (Ali et al. 2014) developed clinical guidance (RCN 2022) and an observation chart designed to help monitor patients who may have or be at risk of developing acute limb compartment syndrome. Pain out of proportion to the injury/treatment and pain on passive movement of the muscles of the involved compartment are the key clinical findings (RCN 2022). Access the tool at Acute limb compartment syndrome observation chart | Royal College of Nursing (rcn.org.uk).

Brunton (2005) alternatively suggests that nurses should use 'decision trees' which assess risk using a systematic approach. The decision trees can be presented as a flow chart or algorithm. Good examples of decision-making trees are generated by the NHS National Patient Safety Agency, which aims to reduce risks to patients receiving NHS care and improve safety. NPSA developed *How to Confirm the Correct Position of Nasogastric Feeding Tubes* for the adult, child, and infant in 2005 and further safety alert, reference number: NHS/PSA/RE/2016/006 in 2016 (view via Activity 2.1).

ACTIVITY 2.1

View decision making trees at:

https://www.ahrq.gov/downloads/pub/advances/vol4/meadows.pdf [Accessed 10 March 2023]
Patient_Safety_Alert_Stage_2_-_NG_tube_resource_set.pdf (england.nhs.uk)

Back in 1994, Ainsworth and Wilson recognised that tools are based around the probable outcomes of specifications, which should be evidenced based. A significant advantage of the decision tree is that they are seen to offer choices, highlight the strengths and weakness of those choices, and give evidence of them (Monkey-Poole 1998). Strategies such as clinical assessment tools and decision trees involve employing formal methods to assess risk. However, the majority of risk assessments carried out by nurses are based on decisions made by the individual nurse (Doyle & Dolan 2002).

A key risk assessment tool is the paediatric early warning score (PEWS) system which is used to record clinical observations systematically to help healthcare staff identify children at risk of deterioration, and prompt increased monitoring and escalation to staff with appropriate skills in emergency and critical care. A recent scoping review by Ball et al. in 2021 found some evidence that PEW scores and systems have benefits beyond clinical outcomes, such as improvements in situational awareness, staff empowerment, communication, and recognition of deterioration.

RISK MANAGEMENT

Risk management is linked with clinical governance, a framework which helps all clinicians to practice safely, deliver effective care, and improve quality of clinical services (RCN 2003). The NHS is committed to management of risk and has operational systems in place to identify, analyse, and control risks, resulting in changes within practice. A risk management consideration is avoiding hyponatraemia in acutely ill hospitalised children, which may occur during inappropriate rehydration or with maintenance fluids. Although the majority of healthcare trusts have structures in place for addressing clinical risk, reducing litigation is an ongoing problem for management as clinical negligence claims appear to cost the NHS millions of pounds each year (Wai Hung Yau et al. 2020). For up-to-date guidance on how to identify and quantify risks of all types, clinical and non-clinical, and assesses priorities for action, visit NHS England » An operational risk management strategy for trusts.

EXAMPLES OF RISK

- Prevention of fire/noise in the hospital
- Security of children on the ward
- The play environment (Stower 2000)
- Pharmacological side-effects
- Breach in nurse's 'duty to care'

A study by Verdu (2003) investigated whether a decision tree can aid pressure ulcer management. It hypothesised that nurses who use a decision tree in pressure ulcer care assess wound grade more accurately and select more appropriate dressings. Sixty-six nurses were randomly assigned to two groups. Each nurse reviewed written information and pictures of three cases of pressure ulceration, and then graded and selected a dressing for the lesions. The absence or presence of a decision tree was used as an independent variable and the results found baseline characteristics were comparable for both groups. There was no statistically significant difference between the grades selected by the two groups. But significantly more of the decision tree users selected an appropriate dressing ($p < 0.02$). The study concluded that decision trees could help nurses to make complex clinical decisions and that further studies undertaken in a clinical setting are needed.

FOLLOWING AN INCIDENT

Upon reflection (Johns 1995), should an incident occur, it is important that professional discussion following the incident takes place, to enable the individuals involved to learn for themselves what happened, why it happened, what needs to be improved, and the lessons learnt. According to Vincent (2001) 'when a patient safety incident occurs, the issue is not who is to blame, but how and why did it occur', because it would appear that when blame comes into the room truth may leave it. Indeed, handling the truth takes courage: sharing it and learning from it takes leadership.

Furthermore, decisions cannot always wait for senior staff, for example when dealing with verbal complaints from parents. Children's nurses need to become empowered and confident leaders in order to make decisions on a daily basis.

SUMMARY

Within this chapter risk assessment and management have been explored, highlighting the need to prevent or minimise risks within the nursing process of providing care. However, clear communication pathways and interdisciplinary working are essential if risks are to be minimised. Everyday incidents in clinical practice occur; therefore, children's nurses should not become complacent, instead assertive with clinical judgement, encouraging discussion about their concerns.

REFERENCES

Ali, P., Santy-Tomlinson, J. & Watson, R. (2014) *Assessment and Diagnosis of Acute Limb Compartment Syndrome: A Literature Review*. London: RCN/BOA.

Anthony, D., Willock, J., & Baharestani, M. (2010) A comparison of Braden Q, Garvin and Glamorgan risk assessment scales in paediatrics. *Journal of Tissue Viability*, 19(3), 98–105. doi: 10.1016/j.jtv.2010.03.001.

Bowden, D. (1996). Calculate the risk. *Nursing Management*, 3(4), 10–11.

Braden, B. & Bergstrom, N. (1987). A conceptual schema for the study of the etiology of pressure sores. *Rehabilitation Nursing*, 12(1), 8–12.

Brunton, K. (2005). The evidence on how nurses approach risk assessment. *Nursing Times*, 101(28), 38.

Chadwick, R. & Tadd, W. (1992) *Ethics and Nursing Practice*. London: Macmillan Education.

Coyne, I.T. (1998). Researching children: Some methodological and ethical considerations. *Journal of Clinical Nursing*, 7(5), 409–416.

Doyle, M. & Dolan, M. (2002) Violence risk assessment: Combining actuarial and clinical information to structure clinical judgements for the formulation and management of risk. *Journal of Psychiatric and Mental Health Nursing*, 9(6), 649–657.

Griffiths, P. & Jull, A. (2010) How good is the evidence for using risk assessment to prevent pressure ulcers? *Nursing Times*, 106, 14.

Johns, C. (1995) Framing learning through reflection within Carper's fundamental ways of knowing in nursing. *Journal of Advanced Nursing*, 22(2), 226–234.

Liversedge, H. (2019) Preventing medical device-related skin damage. *Nursing Standard*. doi: 10.7748/ns.2019.e11375.

Lomas, C. (2009) Top nurse warns risk assessment tools are not backed by evidence. www.nursingtimes.net/whats-new-in-nursing/acute-care/top-nurse-warns-risk-assessment-tools-are-not-backed-by-evidence/5009295.article [Accessed 14 June 2010].

Luker, K.A. & Kendrick, M. (1992). An exploratory study of the sources of influence on the clinical decisions of community nurses. *Journal of Advanced Nursing*, 17(1), 108–112.

Miller, V.G. (1993). Measurement of self perception of intuitiveness. *Western Journal of Nursing Research*, 15(5), 595–606.

Monkey-Poole, S. (1998). Calculating risk community mental health nursing: The decision analysis approach. *Mental Health Care*, 21(92), 56–59.

NICE (2015) Pressure ulcers: Prevention and management. *Clinical Guideline [CG179]*. London: NICE.

Norton, D., Exon-Smith, A.N., & McLaren, R. (1962) *An Investigation of Geriatric Nursing Problems in Hospital*. Edinburgh: Churchill Livingstone.

Royal College of Nursing (2003) *Clinical Governance: An RCN Resource Guide*. London: RCN.

Royal College of Nursing (2022) *Peripheral Neurovascular Observations for Acute Limb Compartment Syndrome RCN Consensus Guidance.* London: RCN.

Shields, C. & Clarke, S. (2010) Using neurovascular assessment tool within children's A & E. *International Journal of Orthopaedic and Trauma Nursing.* doi: 10.1016/j.ijotn.2010.04.002.

Stower, S. (2000). Keeping the hospital environment safe for children. *Paediatric Nursing,* 12(6), 37–42.

Verdu, J. (2003) Can a decision tree help nurses to grade and treat pressure ulcers? *Journal of Wound Care,* 12(2), 45–50.

Vincent, C. (2001) *Clinical Risk Management, Enhancing Patient Safety,* 2nd edn. London: BMJ Publishing Group.

Wai Hung Yau, C., Leigh, B., Liberati, E., Punch, D., Dixon-Woods, M., & Draycott, T. (2020) Clinical negligence costs: taking action to safeguard NHS sustainability. BMJ, 368. doi: 10.1136/bmj.m552.

Waterlow, J.A. (1997). Pressure sore risk assessment in children. *Paediatric Nursing,* 9(6), 21–24.

Willock, J., Baharestani, M., & Anthony, A. (2007). A risk assessment scale for pressure ulcers in children. *Nursing Times,* 103(14), 32–33.

CHAPTER 3
Safeguarding to Protect Children, Young People, and Their Families

Julie Brown and Sonya Clarke

LEARNING OUTCOMES

- Understand the main concepts of safeguarding and child protection, defining key terms
- Be familiar with the legislation and policy underpinning safeguarding practice in the United Kingdom
- Describe and discuss safeguarding assessment, recognizing the risk factors for, and the indicators of child maltreatment
- Understand the process of appropriate escalation and referral of safeguarding concerns
- Understand the professional responsibility in recognizing and appropriately responding to safeguarding concerns

INTRODUCTION

The term child protection was predominately concerned with protection from abuse and neglect, whereas the term 'safeguarding' is a much broader term. Working together to safeguard children (2018) defines safeguarding as protecting children from maltreatment, preventing impairment of health or development, ensuring that children grow up in circumstances consistent with the provision of safe and effective care, and taking action to enable all children to have the best outcomes. Child protection is therefore part of safeguarding and refers to action taken to protect children who are suffering or likely to suffer significant harm.

Article 19 in the United Nations Convention of the Rights of the Child (UNCRC 1989), ratified by the UK in 1991, states that all children have a right to be protected from *all forms of physical or mental violence, injury or abuse, neglect or negligent treatment, maltreatment or exploitation including sexual abuse*.

Martin et al. (2020, p. 379) acknowledges safeguarding children as, *the action taken to protect children from harm, [and] is an important aspect of paediatric care*. We must accept our mutual responsibility as citizens and professionals to be aware of the danger signs and to act on concerns by prompt referral to the appropriate agency. Nurses are well placed to recognise and intervene when safeguarding issues arise and the Nursing and Midwifery Council (NMC) clearly identify the nurse's responsibility to 'raise concerns immediately if [they] believe a person is vulnerable or at risk' (NMC 2018: Section.17). The Royal College of Nursing (RCN 2021) reiterates that it is the responsibility of all nurses, not only on safeguarding specialists to safeguard and promote the welfare of children and young people and state that all organisations must play their full part and work together with a clear, child centered approach to deliver effective safeguarding services.

MALTREATMENT, ABUSE, AND NEGLECT

The terminology of safeguarding can be confusing with terms being used interchangeably in the literature. This chapter will primarily use the term 'maltreatment', as defined by The World Health Organisation (WHO) (2020) as.

'the abuse and neglect that occurs to children under 18 years of age. It includes all types of physical and/or emotional ill-treatment, sexual abuse, neglect, negligence and commercial or other exploitation, which results in actual or potential harm to the child's health, survival, development, or dignity in the context of a relationship of responsibility, trust or power'

Care Planning in Children and Young People's Nursing, Second Edition. Edited by Sonya Clarke and Doris Corkin.
© 2024 John Wiley & Sons Ltd. Published 2024 by John Wiley & Sons Ltd.

Responsibility and professional accountability of the Registered Children's Nurse in safeguarding children and young people.

As a Registered Children's Nurse, you are legally responsible for safeguarding the children and young people in your care. You will do this in line with local policies and procedures and in line with local and national legislation and guidance.

Professionally you are accountable to the Nursing and Midwifery Council to 'Raise concerns immediately if you believe a person is vulnerable or at risk and needs extra support and protection' Section 17 NMC Code of Conduct (NMC 2018).

To achieve this, you must:

- Take all reasonable steps to protect people who are vulnerable or at risk from harm, neglect, or abuse.
- Share information if you believe someone may be at risk of harm, in line with the laws relating to the disclosure of information.
- Have knowledge of, and keep to the relevant laws and policies about protecting and caring for vulnerable people (NMC 2018).

In order to protect children and young people from harm, and help improve their wellbeing, all healthcare staff must have the competencies to recognise child maltreatment, opportunities to improve childhood wellbeing, and to take effective action as appropriate to their role (RCN 2019). The Royal Colleges and other integral professional bodies have jointly published a framework which identifies the core competencies required for healthcare staff, even those primarily working with adults, to fulfil their role in safeguarding children. It outlines five levels of safeguarding competency, which relate to the role of the practitioner. It is recommended that all clinical staff working with children, young people and their families reach a minimum of Level 3 competence. Refer to Box Activity 3.1.

ACTIVITY 3.1

- Access the intercollegiate framework Safeguarding Children and Young People: Roles and Competencies for Healthcare Staff
- Reflect on the need for such a framework and how its development has evolved
- Identify the level of training you require to fulfil your role in safeguarding children and young people and reflect on your competencies in this area of practice

ADVERSE CHILDHOOD EXPERIENCE AND RISK FACTORS FOR MALTREATMENT

Children carry childhood trauma into adulthood, and this can impact their physical and mental health in later life. Adverse Childhood Experiences (ACE's) are situations which lead to an elevated risk of children and young people experiencing damaging impacts on health across the lifespan (Department of Health (DoH) 2015); these include abuse, neglect, domestic violence, having a parent with a mental illness, or alcohol dependency. Experiencing multiple ACE's can lead to death or injury in childhood and negatively affect mental and physical health in adulthood and lead to premature death. The responsibility therefore of the healthcare professional is to have the knowledge and skills to identify those children and young people experiencing, or at risk of experiencing ACE's and intervene to reduce their impact. It also places a responsibility to acknowledge the past experience and trauma experienced by children and young people and to understand the impact this has in later life (Gilliver 2018). For more information about ACE's and their implications for health and wellbeing, please visit the Safeguarding Board for Northern Ireland (SBNI) website.

All children are classed as vulnerable; however, some children are more vulnerable to maltreatment than others (Table 3.1). Adverse childhood experiences and other risk factors interplay to put children and young people at risk of maltreatment. Whilst there is no one definitive indicator for maltreatment, the more risk factors are present, the greater the likelihood of harm to the child.

Table 3.1 Risk Factors for Abuse (Permission granted by Elsevier).

Child Factors	Parent/Family Factors
<1 year of age – heightened risk of child maltreatment due to increased vulnerabilities as a non-mobile, non-verbal child. Statistically the greatest number of child deaths attributed to child maltreatment occur in the <1-year age group.	Domestic abuse – impacts emotionally and physically upon the child and is the key risk factor for abuse.
Disability or complex health needs – increases vulnerability due to potential immobility, speech and language needs, communication difficulties, learning needs.	Substance misuse – impacts upon parental capacity and child safety.
Adolescence – a time when needs may be overlooked or attributed to being a difficult teenager.	Mental health needs – parental capacity may be impaired and pose additional risk for the child.
Child is a young carer – looking after a parent can mean a child's needs are overlooked and unmet.	Poor attachment between parent and child can lead to internalising and externalising problems.
Mental health needs – increased risk if parental capacity is limited to support the child.	Extreme poverty/debt – impacts upon parental capacity and child safety.
Looked after children – A child may be in care due to abuse or neglect, and/or may be exposed to abuse or neglect whilst in the care system.	Very young parents – emotionally unprepared for parenthood, may be socially isolated and out of work.
Delayed physical/emotional/social development – environmental factors and parental capacity to meet the child's needs and provide appropriate stimulation through positive interaction with the child.	Parents who have a history of abuse/neglect or have been in care may not have learned how to be a parent themselves, or have very poor role models.
Preterm/low birthweight child – increased vulnerability due to additional needs and impact upon parental capacity.	Family instability, dysfunction, or chaos – e.g. multiple partners, homelessness, criminality, and prison.
Home-schooled children – may not have been seen outside of the home.	Social isolation and lack of support, for example extended family and friends, may include travelling families, being new to an area.
Friends with links to gangs – risk of child sexual exploitation.	Significant stress, for example divorce, bereavement, military families with deployment, injury, frequent moves.
Asylum seekers and refugees – linkages for both parents and children with prostitution, child sexual exploitation, drug smuggling, human trafficking, modern slavery, self-harm, unmet health needs, and mental health issues.	

RECOGNITION OF CHILD MALTREATMENT	All health professionals need to be aware of the signs of child maltreatment act accordingly. Children's Nurses must have the skills to undertake a comprehensive, holistic nursing assessment, which includes consideration of safeguarding, for every child and young person in their care. There is no one definitive 'red flag' to identify the maltreatment of a child and a series of seemingly minor, unrelated incidents can be just as concerning as any one incident in isolation. Health professionals must place the interests of children at the core of their practice and share their concerns appropriately with other health professionals. The National Institute for Health and Care Excellence (NICE 2017) clinical guideline Child maltreatment: when to suspect maltreatment in under 18's. identifies the signs of possible child maltreatment in children and young people and is a key tool for healthcare professionals in identifying cases of concern.
CATEGORIES OF MALTREATMENT	Child maltreatment can be classified into four main categories (DoH 2017); physical abuse, sexual abuse, neglect, and emotional abuse. It is important to consider that the harm suffered by children and young people from maltreatment is not always straightforward to identify, may present differently between individuals and may change due to context or family circumstances and over time. We must also be aware that a child or young person may experience multiple forms of maltreatment.
PHYSICAL ABUSE	Physical abuse may involve hitting, pinching, shaking, throwing, poisoning, biting, burning or scalding, drowning, suffocating, or otherwise causing physical harm to a child. Physical harm may also be caused when a parent or carer feigns the symptoms of or deliberately causes ill health to a child whom they are looking after (fabricated induced illness (FII)) (RCN 2021; Royal College of

Paediatrics and Child Health 2021). Infants who are not yet mobile, who present with physical injury should always be regarded with a high level of suspicion.

Indicators of physical abuse may include:

- Bruising
- Burns and scalds (thermal injuries) particularly if they are in an unexpected place, or in the shape of an implement (e.g. Cigarette, iron)
- Human bites
- Intracranial injury
- Lesions and cuts, including knife wounds
- Fractures (new and old), particular suspicion afforded for multiple fractures in the absence of a medical condition predisposing to fragile bones or if the fracture is occult (identified on X-Ray but not clinically evident)
- Female genital mutilation (FGM)

Other indicators of physical abuse may include:

- Delay in seeking medical attention
- Physical chastisement
- No explanation/inadequate/changing explanation of injuries
- Recurrent injuries – particularly if forming a pattern
- Inadequate parental concern

SEXUAL ABUSE AND EXPLOITATION

Sexual abuse is any sexual activity with a child. The term comprises acts of physical contact (both penetrative and non-penetrative), and non-contact activities, such as encouraging children to behave in sexually inappropriate ways. The sexual abuse of children using online technologies is increasingly concerning. It is important to be aware that perpetrators of sexual abuse are not always adult males, they can be women or other children and that sexual abuse often takes place within families.

Physical indicators of sexual abuse may include:

- Genital, anal, or perianal injury
- Recurrent anal or genital symptoms (bleeding, discomfort, or discharge)
- The presence of foreign bodies in anal or vaginal cavities
- The presence of sexually transmitted infections or underage pregnancy

Other indicators of sexual abuse may include:

- Knowledge or interest in sexual acts inappropriate to a child's age
- Using sexual language or having sexual knowledge that you would not expect the child/young person to have
- Asking others to behave sexually or play sexual games
- Unexplained behavioural or emotional changes

(RCN 2019)

Child sexual exploitation (CSE) is a type of child sexual abuse. It occurs where an individual or group takes advantage of an imbalance of power to coerce, manipulate or deceive a child or young person under the age of 18 into sexual activity (Department for Education 2017). For more information on Child Sexual Exploitation, visit the NSPCC Learning Portal 'Protecting children from sexual exploitation'.

| EMOTIONAL ABUSE AND CHILD EXPLOITATION | Emotional abuse is the persistent emotional ill-treatment of a child such as causing severe and continuing adverse effects on the child's emotional development. It may involve conveying to children that they are worthless or unloved, inadequate or valued only insofar as they meet the needs of another person (RCN 2021). Furthermore, emotional abuse may involve inappropriate age or developmental expectations being imposed on children. |

Indicators of emotional abuse may include:

- Parents/carers who humiliate, intimidate, persistently chastise, or are overly critical of the child. It may include not allowing the child to express their views, or 'making fun' of what they say or how they communicate.
- Children who are reluctant to go home
- Parents/carers who withdraw from the child or blame them for their problems
- Children who are withdrawn or anxious, display negative emotions around adults. May check in with the parents before answering questions or giving opinions. Fearful of doing something wrong.
- Children with extreme behaviours and self harm

These signs can present singly or in clusters of behaviours, depending on each child's environment and specific situation. It is crucial for the health professional to recognise the behaviours exhibited in the child according to their age and stage of development and in the context of mental health issues or learning disability. It is also important to acknowledge that emotional abuse can be perpetrated by other children in the form of bullying and harassment online and in person. Refer to Box Activity 3.2.

ACTIVITY 3.2

Write 250 words on the effects of emotional abuse on a pre-school child.

Child exploitation is often classified independently as category of abuse and can take the form of forced marriage, modern slavery, radicalisation to terrorist groups, involvement in drug trafficking, and sexual exploitation. It has been included here under the category of emotional abuse because by definition, child exploitation is the coercion, abuse of power, deceit, control, and manipulation over a child or young person for person gain.

| NEGLECT | Neglect is the persistent failure to meet a child's basic physical and/or psychological needs, likely to result in the serious impairment of the child's health or development (RCN 2021). Neglect can be deliberate or triggered by the care giver's lack of capacity to meet the child's needs. Refer to Box Activity 3.3. Neglect can start during pregnancy. |

This area can be sub-divided into the following:

- Health neglect
- Physical neglect
- Educational neglect
- Emotional neglect/Stimulation neglect
- Nutritional neglect

Indicators of neglect may include:

- Children that are hungry and/or dirty

- Children that do not have adequate clothing appropriate for the climate
- Children not receiving basic healthcare may miss healthcare appointments
- Failure to thrive, failure to gain weight, or obesity in childhood
- Poor attendance at school
- Children may present with extreme behaviours and/self-harm (RCN 2021)

ACTIVITY 3.3

A three-year-old child is admitted to the ward with a failure to gain weight.
- What concerns would you have?
- What questions would you ask to gain a comprehensive picture?
- Who might you discuss your concerns with?

Bools (2020) highlights the challenges in both identifying and managing the fabrication or induction of illness (FII) in a child by their parent or carer – although relatively rare, the situation can lead to serious physical and/or emotional harm to the child. To assist in the management of suspected FII, statutory guidance titled Safeguarding Children in Whom Illness is Fabricated or Induced (HM Government 2008) was published. This is supported by more recent guidance from the RCPCH (2021). Refer Box Activity 3.4.

FABRICATED INDUCED ILLNESS

ACTIVITY 3.4

Access the National Institute for Health and Care Excellence (NICE (2017)) clinical guideline on child maltreatment. Child maltreatment: when to suspect maltreatment in under-18s. Reflect on your clinical practice in identifying signs of child maltreatment and discuss this guideline with your colleagues.

This inquiry, which was reported in the Laming Report (2003), described the systematic maltreatment of Victoria at the hands of her great aunt Marie Therese Kouao and her partner Carl Manning. This seminal inquiry was at the time, the most extensive investigation into the failings of the child protection system in the United Kingdom. It was the first inquiry to triangulate the role of social services, NHS and police in the protection of children using their respective legislative frameworks. During the period from 1998 to 2000, the inquiry concluded that there were twelve key occasions when opportunities to intervene to protect Victoria were overlooked. These missed opportunities in the system were described by Lord Laming as 'lamentable' and 'a gross failure of the system' and he stated that it must never happen again.

INQUIRY INTO VICTORIA CLIMBIÉ

The inquiry made a total of 108 recommendations, clearly set out for all the agencies involved. Refer to Box Activity 3.5.

ACTIVITY 3.5

Access www.victoria-climbie-inquiry.org.uk and read the introduction, which gives an overview on Lord Laming's report.

Refer to the sections on recommendations and identify the key agencies who failed in their duty to protect.

Select the healthcare recommendations and having reviewed them identify the key themes.

Discuss these with your colleagues.

The inquiry acknowledged that there were significant omissions and failures in the healthcare system, particularly with regards to documentation and reporting mechanisms. It highlighted the 'failure of nursing staff' to document their observations and concerns contemporaneously. The consequent discrepancy between the levels of concern expressed by the nurses in question in their oral evidence at the trial and that reflected in the nursing documentation from the time, was a matter which arose with 'depressing regularity' (Laming 2003). The consideration of safeguarding was not evident in the nursing documentation, despite this being of high suspicion in Victoria's admission to hospital. Collectively this indicates that essential principles of assessment, record-keeping, care planning and communication had not been adhered to.

Following the death of Victoria Climbié in 2000 and the subsequent report by Lord Laming in 2003, the Government produced the green paper 'Every Child Matters' and the first national guidance for child protection Working together to Safeguard Children (updated 2018). The Laming Inquiry also led to the revised Children Act (2003), which allowed for the introduction of co-ordinated multi-agency Children's Trusts and the creation of a national child database to log all contact of children under 16 with health, police, and social services. These measures, amongst others initiated as a result of the case, changed the landscape of child protection in the United Kingdom (UK).

ESCALATION OF CONCERN – REFERRAL PROCESSES

A referral, in the context of child protection, occurs when a person contacts Children's Services due to concerns about the safety and well-being of a child or young person. Children's Services have a legal duty to investigate circumstances where a concern has been raised about the safety and well-being of a child or young person. Even though the investigation is the responsibility of 'social workers' within Children's Services, they do work closely with the Police, healthcare workers, and other professionals who are connected to the child, young person, and/or family. Any person can make a referral including a parent, wider family member, friend, doctor, teacher, nurse, or health visitor. Variations may exist within the UK; as each country's governing body guides the referral and assessment process. For example, within Northern Ireland, a referral should be made to the Single Point Entry (SPOE, Referral Gateway) or ring the regional emergency social work service – out of hours. Northern Ireland has a Children and Young People (safeguardingni.org). Safeguarding Board which ensures organisations work together to keep children and young people safe.

To support staff, conduct high quality assessments that clearly identify children's needs and lead to these needs being met, an inter-agency assessment model was developed in Northern Ireland. This framework is called UNOCINI (DHSSPS 2007:8), which stands for Understanding the Needs of Children in Northern Ireland. The UNOCINI Assessment Framework has been developed to:

- improve the quality of assessment within stakeholder agencies.
- assist in communicating the needs of children across agencies.
- avoid the escalation of children's needs through early identification of need and effective intervention.

UNOCINI has three assessment areas which are each divided into four domains:

- the needs of the child or young person.
- the capacity of their parents or carers to meet these needs.
- wider family and environmental factors that impact on parental capacity and children's needs.

Click on the link to view the unocini-forms.doc (live.com)

The UNOCINI form is embedded within NI's Heath and Social care – it is used by children's nurses who provide care to CYP in all care settings.

POLICIES AND PROCEDURES

There is no nationally agreed guidance for safeguarding children in the UK. England, Scotland, Wales, and Northern Ireland each have their own laws and systems in place to protect children and young people and keep them safe. Whilst these systems and practices may vary, they are based on the same key principles. Table 3.2 presents the key legislation and policy relating to each of the four nations in the United Kingdom.

The key legislation that you might be aware of are listed in chronological order:

The Children Act 1989 (as amended).

The United Nations Convention on the Rights of the Child 1989.

The Human Rights Act (1998).

The Education Act (2002).

The Female Genital Mutilation Act (2003).

Prohibition of Female Genital Mutilation (Scotland) Act (2005).

The Equality Act (2010).

The Children and Families Act (2014).

Modern Slavery Act (2015).

Counter Terrorism and Security Act (2015).

The Children and Social Work Act (2017).

Working Together to Safeguard Children (2018).

Keeping Children Safe in Education (2019).

For further information on the listed key legislation, visit Safeguarding Children Legislation | Virtual College (virtual-college.co.uk)

Local Safeguarding Children Boards (LSCBs) in England and Wales, and the Safeguarding Board Northern Ireland (SBNI) replace the Area Child Protection Committees. These are local inter-agency forums that bring together the local authorities, police, and health professionals to work more effectively in safeguarding children.

Safeguarding is concerned with child protection, multidisciplinary working and creating a broader understanding of child protection to include prevention and family support. The scope of the LSCBs and SBNI aims to protect all children from maltreatment, to target specific groups in a proactive manner, to safeguard and promote the welfare of children potentially more vulnerable, and to protect children who are suffering from significant harm.

Table 3.2 Key legislation and policy relating to safeguarding children and young people in the UK.

Nation	Responsible Body	Legislation	Policy
Northern Ireland	Northern Ireland Executive through Department of Health (DoH)	Children (Northern Ireland) Order (1995)	DHSSPS (2007) Co-operating to safeguard children and young people in Northern Ireland
England	Department for Education (DfE)	Children Act 1989	Working together to safeguard children: A guide to inter-agency working to safeguard and promote the welfare of children (2018)
Scotland	Scottish Government	Children (Scotland) Act 1995	National Guidance for child protection in Scotland (2014)
Wales	Welsh Government	Social Services and Well Being Act 2014	Working together to Safeguard People (2018)

The National Society for Prevention of Cruelty to Children (NSPCC) is an independent organisation working to place pressure on government to improve child protection systems and legislation across the UK. They provide a wealth of guidance, information and support around child protection and safeguarding issues for anyone working with children. For further information, visit Keeping children safe | NSPCC. The NSPCC has also generated a National Case review repository detailing cases from across the UK, you can access the repository here.

Table 3.1 includes a number of strategic documents published to inform nursing and midwifery services across the UK in order to secure the continued development of effective services which safeguard children, young people, and their families.

These legislative and policy frameworks provide guidance and clear direction, including specific details of the roles and responsibilities of all those involved in the care and delivery of services to children.

ACTIVITY 3.6

List the range of policies and procedures in your region that you must be aware of.

All healthcare professionals are responsible for ensuring timely and appropriate responses to safeguard children regardless of the setting or specialty. Safeguarding children is everyone's business; therefore, all health professionals must be competent and knowledgeable in order to safeguard and promote the welfare of children.

Getting_the_right_start_National_Service_Framework_for_Children_Standard_for_Hospital_Services.pdf (publishing.service.gov.uk), this seminal 2003 guidance document clearly states that all staff should understand their roles and responsibilities in safeguarding children and also promote the welfare of children and young people. In order to do this all staff will need training, updating, and support to function effectively. This was echoed in the Laming Inquiry (2003, p11), which states that *all staff appointed to any of the services where they will be working with children and families must have adequate training for the positions they will fill.*

More recent guidance – Safeguarding Children and Young People: Roles and Competencies for Healthcare Staff (2019) is an intercollegiate document which provides a clear framework and identifies the competencies required for all healthcare staff. Levels 1–3 relate to different occupational groups, while level 4 and 5 are related to specific roles.

Likewise, where a child who is the subject of concern has a parent with a learning disability, the health professionals in this situation are well placed to identify and respond to the increased vulnerability and potential risk of abuse to children with special needs. The health professionals involved must act in the best interests of the child and discuss such concerns with other agencies.

All professionals must be mindful that the protection of the child is of paramount importance and where there are concerns, they should follow agreed procedures. These concerns or referrals must be shared and discussed with the line manager, named doctor, or safeguarding nurse. Refer to Activity 3.7.

ACTIVITY 3.7

Find out who is the named doctor and/or safeguarding nurse in your area.

Discuss what you should do when you have a concern.

Discuss the key stages of the referral process.

Safeguarding children is a complex aspect of practice; therefore, nurses will require support through effective supervision, and this should be available to nurses at a level that reflects their involvement with children and families. Indeed, a quality supervision process should result in a more efficient and confident nursing workforce.

Safeguarding children is a complex aspect of practice; therefore, nurses will require support through effective supervision, and this should be available to nurses at a level that reflects their involvement with children and families. Indeed, a quality supervision process should result in a more efficient and confident nursing workforce.

RECORD-KEEPING

Record-keeping is an integral part of nursing and a key responsibility of the registered nurse. The NMC requirement to 'Keep clear and accurate records relevant to your practice' (Section 10 NMC 2018) applies across all care settings and to both written and electronic records. The NMC accepts that, until there is national agreement between all healthcare professionals on standards and format, records may differ depending on the needs of the child. All records must however be a clear, objective, and concise record of events, contemporaneous, dated and signed, and stored securely in line with local and national policy. The records should also be recorded in such a manner that the text cannot be erased or deleted without a record of such a change. Any justifiable alterations or additions should be dated, timed, and signed or clearly attributed to a named person so that the original entry can still be read.

Laming (2003) stated: 'I regard the keeping of proper notes and the accurate recording of concerns felt about a child as being a fundamental aspect of basic professional competence.'

The subject of a record does have the right in law to request access to their record at any stage. Therefore, it is important that all information regarding a child should be collated in one set of notes, as recommended by Laming (2003). They should also be in chronological order and demonstrate the collaboration between professionals where decisions were made, and actions taken.

Health professionals have a key part to play in safeguarding and promoting the welfare of children and must be clear about their own roles and responsibilities and be aware of the roles and responsibilities of other professionals. They must also be confident about their own standards, respectful of others, and be mindful of the attitudes required for effective collaboration and negotiation. Good communication skills are also essential in order to contribute to the assessment and investigations of concerns about a child. They must also demonstrate skills in engaging children, parents, and other professionals and actively seek knowledge to deliver improved services to children and young people, and comply with statutory requirements regarding training and working together.

SUMMARY

The overarching aim of this chapter is to introduce the reader to the main concepts of safeguarding and child protection. This included the defining of key terms and identification of UK legislation and policy. It also describes and discusses safeguarding assessment, whilst recognizing the risk factors and indicators of child maltreatment. It is also hoping the reader will gain a greater understanding of the escalation process and referral of safeguarding concerns alongside the professional responsibility in recognizing and appropriately responding to safeguarding concerns.

In summing up, the second edition has been updated to reflect the current thinking and challenges around safeguarding and child protection in today's society. This chapter is mindful of the negative impact COVID-19 pandemic continues to have on children's nursing and on the children and young people who endured school closures, lock down, and reduced access to health and social care services (Fallon et al. 2020). It also champions all UK pre-registration children's nurses to complete a national level safeguarding training as part of their programme, prior to registration with the NMC. Finally, in context and of pertinent concern, the authors draw the reader's attention to a press report in July 2022 – Baby P's mother Tracey Connelly released from prison – BBC News.

REFERENCES

Bools, C. (2020) Safeguarding children when fabricated or induced illness is suspected or proven: Reviewing the experiences of local safeguarding children boards in England. *Child Abuse Review*, **29**, 559–573. doi: 10.1002/car.2653.

Children and Families Act (2014) Children and families act 2014 (legislation.gov.uk) [Accessed 1 August 2022].

Children and Social Work Act (2017) Children and Social Work Act 2017. (legislation.gov.uk) [Accessed 1 August 2022].

Counter Terrorism and Security Act (2015) Counter-terrorism and security act 2015. (legislation.gov.uk) [Accessed 1 August 2022].

Department for Education (2017) Child sexual exploitation: Definition and a guide for practitioners, local leaders and decision makers working to protect children from child sexual exploitation. *Crown Copyright*. Available online at https://assets.publishing.service.gov.uk/government/uploads/system/uploads/attachment_data/file/591903/CSE_Guidance_Core_Document_13.02.2017.pdf [Accessed 19th July 2022].

Department of Health (2015) The impact of adverse experiences in the home on the health of children and young people. UCL Institute of Health Equity. Crown Copyright. Available online at https://www.instituteofhealthequity.org/resources-reports/the-impact-of-adverse-experiences-in-the-home-on-children-and-young-people/impact-of-adverse-experiences-in-the-home.pdf [Accessed 7th July 2022].

Department of Health and Social Services and Public Services in Northern Ireland (DHSSPS) (2007) *Understanding the Needs of Children in Northern Ireland (UNOCINI)*. Belfast: DHSSPSNI.

Education Act (2002) Education Act 2002. (legislation.gov.uk) [Accessed 1 August 2022].

Equality Act (2010) Equality Act 2010. (legislation.gov.uk) [Accessed 1 August 2022].

Fallon, D., McGhee, K., Davies, J., MacLeod, F., Clarke, S. & Sinclair, W. (2020) Capturing the Impact of the COVID-19 Pandemic on Children's Nursing. *Comprehensive Child and Adolescent Nursing*, Sep **43**(3), 166–170. doi: 10.1080/24694193.2020.1788346. Epub 2020 Jul 13.

Female Genital Mutilation Act 2003 (England, Wales, Northern Ireland) Female Genital Mutilation Act 2003 (legislation.gov.uk) [Accessed 1 August 2022].

Gilliver, C. (2018) Trauma-informed care in response to adverse childhood experiences. *Nursing Times*, **114**(7), 46–49. Available online at https://www.nursingtimes.net/roles/nurse-educators/trauma-informed-care-in-response-to-adverse-childhood-experiences-08-06-2018 [Accessed 7 July 2022].

HM Government (2008) *Safeguarding Children in Whom Illness Is Fabricated or Induced: Supplementary Guidance to Working Together to Safeguard Children*. London: HMSO.

HMSO (1995a) *Children (Northern Ireland) Order*. Belfast: HMSO.

HMSO (1995b) *Children (Scotland) Act*. Scotland: HMSO.

Human Rights Act (1998) Human Rights Act 1998 (legislation.gov.uk) [Accessed 1 August 2022].

Keeping Children Safe in Education (2019) Keeping children safe in education - GOV.UK (www.gov.uk) [Accessed 1 August 2022].

Laming Report (2003) *The Victoria Climbié Inquiry: Report of an Inquiry by Lord Laming*. Norwich: The Stationery Office (TSO).

Martin, E., Kraft, J., Wilder, R. & Bryant, H. (2020) Safeguarding children in trauma and orthopaedics. *Orthopaedics and Trauma*, **34**(6), 379–389.

Modern Slavery Act (2015) Modern Slavery Act 2015 (legislation.gov.uk) [Accessed 1 August 2022].

National Institute for Health and Care Excellent (NICE) (2017) Child maltreatment: when to suspect maltreatment in under 18's: Clinical guideline. Available online at https://www.nice.org.uk/guidance/cg89/resources/child-maltreatment-when-to-suspect-maltreatment-in-under-18s-pdf-975697287109 [Accessed 19th July 2022].

National Guidance for child protection in Scotland (2014) https://www.pkc.gov.uk/media/39931/National-Guidance-for-Disabled-Children/pdf/National_Guidance_for_Disabled_Children [Accessed 10th March 2023].

Nursing and Midwifery Council (2018) The Code: Professional standards of practice and behaviour for nurses, midwives and nursing associates. Available online at https://www.nmc.org.uk/globalassets/sitedocuments/nmc-publications/nmc-code.pdf [Accessed 30th June 2022].

Prohibition of Female Genital Mutilation (Scotland) Act (2005) *Prohibition of Female Genital Mutilation (Scotland) Act 2005* https://www.legislation.gov.uk/asp/2005/8/contents [Accessed 10th March 2023].

Royal College of Nursing (2019) Safeguarding children and young people: roles and competencies for healthcare staff. Available online at https://www.rcn.org.uk/professional-development/publications/pub-007366 [Accessed 10th March 2023].

Royal College of Nursing (2021) *Safeguarding Children and Young People: Every Nurse's Responsibility*. London: RCN. Available online at https://www.rcn.org.uk/Professional-Development/publications/safeguarding-children-and-young-people-every-nurses-responsibility-uk-pub-009-507 [Accessed 30th June 2022].

Royal College of Paediatrics and Child Health (RCPCH) (2021). Perplexing Presentations (PP)/Fabricated Induced Illness (FII) in children – guidance. London: RCPCH. Available online at: https://childprotection.rcpch.ac.uk/resources/perplexing-presentations-and-fii [Accessed 19th July 2022].

The United Nations Convention for the Rights of the Child (1989) *Ratified by the United Kingdom Government in 1991*. Geneva: United Nations.

Working Together to Safeguard Children (2018) Working together to safeguard children - GOV.UK (www.gov.uk) [Accessed 1th August 2022].

World Health Organisation (2020) Child maltreatment factsheet. Geneva: WHO. Available online at https://www.who.int/news-room/fact-sheets/detail/child-maltreatment [Accessed 30th June 2022].

Ethical, Legal, and Professional Implications When Planning Care for Infants, Children, and Young People (ICYP)

CHAPTER 4

Orla McAlinden and Sonya Clarke

INTRODUCTION

Infants, children, and young people's nurses (ICYP), also known as children's, paediatric, or CYP nurses, are required to understand their role as an advocate for children, young people, and their families, and work in partnership with them. They must deliver child and family-centred care; empower children and young people to express their views and preferences, and maintain/recognise their rights and best interests. This is alongside each child and young person's individuality, including their stage of development, ability to understand, culture, learning or communication difficulties, and health status. They will be able to communicate effectively with them, their parents, and carers. This is in addition to underpinning knowledge, clinical and decision-making skills, and also in addition to the standards for competence that apply to all fields of nursing in the UK (NMC 2018; RCN 2015, 2017). Today's nursing curricula and nursing practice consequently requires all nurses to gain mandatory knowledge and training on the concepts equality, diversity, and inclusion (EDI) (Stonehouse 2021).

When assessing, planning, delivering, and evaluating care ICYP nurses must practice in an anti-discriminatory way, remaining alert to the legal, moral, and ethical implications of their practice. This chapter will enable the ICYP nurse (and others) to recognise and meet the professional/ethical/legal imperatives expected from any registered nurse (RN) working with infants, children, young people, and their families.

Where exactly in a nursing curriculum ethics and law should be introduced is arguably a matter for those who are involved in the consultation, design, and delivery, and evaluation of a higher education programme. However, the curriculum design must include the views and needs of those who may be in receipt of care, that is to say the voices of parents, children, and young people as a co-production enterprise (Bruce et al. 2021; Lundy 2007, 2019).

The central issue is that all nurses seeking to register with the UK's regulating body, Nursing Midwifery Council (NMC) as a Registered Nurse (RN Child) must demonstrate they have achieved all the proficiencies required by the NMC in order to do so. Their programme will have met the initial and ongoing scrutiny of the NMC if completed in the UK and the individual academic institutions and, thereafter, the respective auditing teams such as internal audits by Northern Ireland Practice Education Committee (NIPEC) or similar statutory bodies throughout the UK.

The clear intention is that those exiting from a higher educational nursing programme will:

- *in all four fields of nursing, demonstrate competencies across the four domains and seven platforms*:
- *professional values, communication, and interpersonal skills;*
- *nursing practice, decision-making, and leadership;*
- *management and team working.*

A nursing student (and the RN subsequently) needs to demonstrate that academically and clinically they can meet the requirements of NMC Future Nurse Future Midwife (2018). The addition of a 'declaration of good character' is another requirement, which clearly indicates that there is a need to use fundamental skills and knowledge in a way that is morally acceptable.

It is therefore, not sufficient to just 'know' and 'do or not do'. The ICYP nurse must be able to demonstrate that the knowledge underpinning action or omission is based on the best available contemporary evidence and mindful of the imperatives of current legislation and ethical behaviours (Aveyard & Sharp 2017). It follows from this that the ICYP nurse needs to be aware of what role ethical action and legislation has upon all domains and platforms of practice – and the nurse should then be seen to practice consistently in a way that shows internalisation and commitment to those principles (Cornock 2020; Cornock & McAlinden 2018; Dimond 2019; RCN 2015, 2017). Refer to activity box 4.1– 4.8.

ACTIVITY 4.1

List below some of the reasons why an ICYP nurse would need to be informed about the law and ethical actions.

Why law?
Why ethical actions?
Ethics and morality
Principles or virtues?

Quite commonly, in practice ICYP nurses are in a position of uncertainty. Arguably, ethical thinking and moral reasoning have the effect of making those involved more empowered to take an effective course of action, more able to articulate what their concerns are, and why they deserve consideration or action. Unease or uncertainty about a certain action or situation prompts one to reflect upon what the correct response should be in any given situation. This reflection is a moral reflection because it is about the notion that something is important and it is therefore worth worrying about the 'rightness' or 'wrongness' of a particular course of action (Avery 2026; Beauchamp & Childress 2012, Dowie 2017; Standing 2020). This is the case in both academic endeavour and clinical practice (Standing 2020).

DECISION-MAKING

There are different models for ethical decision-making described in the literature (Dowie 2017) and choosing is usually a matter of personal preference or ease of understanding. All of them begin with identifying an issue and end with taking a decision of some sort. What happens between the beginning and end steps will influence the end decision.

ACTIVITY 4.2

Read these NHS articles then reflect on an aspect of your clinical practice, which highlights these approaches.

https://www.england.nhs.uk/shared-decision-making
https://www.england.nhs.uk/blog/alf-collins-3

The principles referred to in the NHS model above are:

- Beneficence (doing good or correct things)
- Non-maleficence (not doing bad or wrong things)
- Respect/autonomy (recognise that individuals should be able to make their own decisions)
- Justice (treat all cases alike unless they differ in some relevant respect)

The 'users' of health and social care hold their own perceptions and expectations of these services and the public servants (for we are public servants) who manage and deliver that care. This public accountability is one compelling reason why we, as healthcare professionals in a multi- and interdisciplinary setting need to ensure that we can justify our actions and decisions on both ethical and clinical grounds. It should be noted that holding ethical views or being aware of ethical principles is not enough in itself – as nurses we need to demonstrate ability to apply this knowledge to our clinical practice. This means inclusion of legal and ethical policies, procedures, and standards as well as clarifying what goals and values we uphold as ICYP nurses (Cornock 2020a, 2020c; Dimond 2019; McAlinden 2018).

Some issues are more topical than others; some change and recede or magnify over time, but the fact remains that we need to constantly ensure that our practices can always be justified as moral as well as 'scientific' and within the law, including employment law. For a deeper understanding of ethical decision-making in practice see Standing (2020) and The Francis Inquiry Report (2013).

THE LAW

This emphasises that the accountable practitioner is one who recognises that law underpins practice and is therefore fundamental to the theory and practice of nursing (Cornock 2020; Dimond 2019; McAlinden 2018).

The NMC Code (2018) uses the 'principles' based approach to the care of patients and clients and also indicates how law intertwines and informs healthcare practices.

The NMC Code (2018) is a combination of rules; some are positive rules (legally binding) and some normative rules (what a person 'should' do rather than what legislation imposes). This is because it reflects the reality of what happens in life and in health and social care.

A simple way to view this is perhaps:

- The law 'spells out' the minimum acceptable standard of care expected.
- The NMC code sets out the best possible standard of care expected.

So together: The law + the Code = professional standard of care

DUTY OF CARE, DUTY OF CANDOUR, ACCOUNTABILITY, NEGLIGENCE

As an RN, you are accountable for your actions and omissions to society in general and your individual patient/family in particular as well as to your employer. You have a 'duty to care' for patients, which can be challenged by those in your care or your employers if they believe that you as an RN have not fulfilled that duty. If a patient/family/employer considers that this is the case then they may claim negligence, which is where harm occurs as a result of a nurse's carelessness. You also have a 'duty of candour'. The duty of candour expectation emerged after the findings of the Mid Staffordshire case – Francis Report in 2013 and the Gosport War Memorial Hospital scandal (2018). The Francis Report (2013) found major issues of concern about treatment of patients and other matters including professional disengagement, lack of patient voice and advocacy, inadequate risk assessment, and poor standards and performance with the wrong priorities being upheld.

The Gosport inquiry (2018) believed that of 833 deaths Dr Barton certified between 1988 and 2000, 456 died and possibly 200 more had their lives shortened because of the prescription practices used by Gosport hospital. The dangers of unsupervised death certification had previously been considered by the Shipman Inquiry (2003–2005) and if the recommendations of that enquiry had already been in place these tragic events would not be permitted today. This prompted a new version of the Code (2018) as well as the NMC Professional Duty of Candour guidance (2019) as part of the Health and Social Care Act 2008 (Regulated Activities) Regulations 2014: Regulation 20. Most recently the Muckamore Abbey Inquiry into abuse at this hospital (Feb 2023) raises further concerns about how care is managed and delivered to vulnerable people.

Healthcare professionals must:

- tell the patient (or, where appropriate, the patient's advocate, carer, or family) when something has gone wrong.
- apologise to the patient (or, where appropriate, the patient's advocate, carer, or family).

- offer an appropriate remedy or support to put matters right (if possible).
- explain fully to the patient (or, where appropriate, the patient's advocate, carer, or family) the short and long-term effects of what has happened.
- be open and honest with their colleagues, employers, and relevant organisations, and take part in reviews and investigations when requested.
- be open and honest with their regulators, raising concerns where appropriate.
- support and encourage each other to be open and honest, and not stop someone from raising concerns.

This is a statutory duty for care organisations across all four UK nations. https://www.nmc.org.uk/standards/guidance/the-professional-duty-of-candour/read-the-professional-duty-of-candour

Negligence

If those in your care or your employers believe that you as an RN have not fulfilled your duty of care you may be challenged in law under the tort of negligence.

Three elements of negligence are:

- There was a duty of care owed.
- That this duty of care was breached, and
- As a result of the breach the patient suffered harm (physical or psychological).

Note: all three elements must be proven in law and following from this the nurse is liable to be sued for compensation for the consequential harm. At this point, it is also important to realise that the requirements of 'The Code' (NMC 2018) will have been infringed and so the RN will come under the scrutiny of the NMC and their employer. This is a very clear example of where the Code not only meets but also extends beyond the standards expected in law (Cornock 2020).

Advocacy

Save the Children UK | Global Children's Charity define advocacy as:

'a set of organised activities designed to influence the policies and actions of others to achieve positive changes for children's lives based on the experience and knowledge of working directly with children, their families and communities'.

ICYP nurses can advocate for their client group in many ways, by speaking up for them, by facilitating their voice being heard, by representing their viewpoint when they cannot be present or heard. It can be a formal or informal process; it may involve the family – or just the child or young person.

ACTIVITY 4.3

Think of a time when you did not respond on someone else's poor attitude towards a child or young person:

Why did you not speak up?
What might have been the consequences of you speaking up? (patient, staff member, yourself)?
What courses of action did you feel were available to you?
(Tip: this could be about CYP reaction to painful experience, or fear, or emotional dysregulation due to a prior traumatic experience. You might have your own examples from practice.)

ACTIVITY 4.4

Watch the video https://www.youtube.com/watch?v=urAyr3tqKZo Reflect on the various ways you could be an advocate for others.

ACTIVITY 4.5

Reflect and discuss the following statements with others in a group:

- Nurses find it difficult to challenge the decisions made by others (give example).

- Factors hindering nurses in their advocacy role include age, gender, attitude to power, personality, role conflict, or social situations (give example).

- Professional hierarchies make it more difficult for nurses to raise concerns about patient care (give example).

- There are things nurses can do to improve their confidence in being an advocate here are things nurses can do to improve their confidence in being an advocate.

The antecedents of advocacy for children stems from the nineteenth and early twentieth century. A timeline can be used to demonstrate development of what was essentially a paternalistic concern for children in the earlier years.

ACTIVITY 4.6

For all relevant reports and legislation specific to your country visit the appropriate governmental websites and make a note of pertinent material.

England: https://www.gov.uk
Northern Ireland: www.dhsspsni.gov.uk
Scotland: www.scotland.gov.uk
Wales: https://www.legislation.gov.uk/browse/wales
Republic of Ireland: https://www.gov.ie/en
Irish Health Reports: https://www.gov.ie/en/organisation/department-of-health

From 1970 onwards concerns took the shape of a more inclusive view of the health and social welfare of children and young people. This development recognised importantly that this group of individuals need to have a voice of their own and their rights extended beyond the purely paternalistic concerns of previous years. Legislation and governmental reports such as Platt (Committee of the Central Health Services Council 1959), Court (Committee on Child Health Services 1976), up to Kennedy (DH 2001) urged advocacy and listening to and learning from the voice and developmental needs of children and families. The advent of pressure groups such as the National Association for the Welfare of Children in Hospital (NAWCH) slowly pushed back the boundaries of care for this group and influenced the development of advocacy in the wider social context. By the early 1990s, NAWCH changed its name to Action for Sick Children (ASC). This change of name highlighted the need for a more encompassing focus for children and young people who were ill but were not necessarily hospitalised which better reflected the contemporary needs of children and young people. Sadly, ASC are now defunct, a casualty of austerity measures and an economic downturn.

The growth of advocacy for children and young people has been slow and has a tendency to remain adult-led rather than focused on the needs of the child or young person. England and Wales were ahead of Scotland and Northern Ireland in the landmark establishment of independent advocacy positions for children, with the appointment in 1987 of the first UK Children's Rights Officer and the development of the first national advocacy service to cover England and Wales in 1992.

A Children's Commissioner was appointed in Wales in 2001, in Northern Ireland in 2003 and in Scotland in 2004. England appointed their Children's Commissioner in 2005 under the provisions of the Children Act (HMSO 2004). Unlike the other countries mentioned, the English Commissioner must consult with the Secretary of State before it is possible to hold an independent inquiry.

Although undoubtedly welcome, there is still a large discrepancy between the dates in the timeline and the actual appointment of the UK Children's Commissioners. Advocacy exists but there are differing levels, definition models and also a recognised limitation to the advocacy role that some nurses and healthcare professionals can uphold in certain situations (www.childrenscommissioner.gov.uk/report/advocacy-for-children).

UNITED NATIONS CONVENTION ON THE RIGHTS OF THE CHILD: INFANTS, CHILDREN, AND YOUNG PEOPLE

The concept of child rights emerged in the 1920s, with one of the earliest pioneers Janusz Korczak (holocaustresearchproject.org) and then with the Declaration of Geneva in 1924. The Declaration on the Rights of the Child followed in 1959, although it should be noted that this declaration was not legally binding. The 1970s saw a further development in the interest of children's rights.

The United Nations (UN) Convention on the Rights of the Child (adopted by the UN General Assembly in 1989 was ratified by the UK in 1991 and came into legal force in 1992 in the UK) and the first legally binding legislation in relation to the rights of children and young people. This convention was also to be the most universally ratified of all the UN instruments, showing 'intent' at least of member states to recognise and uphold the rights of children and young persons. In 2021, Scotland joined the list of signatory countries.

Children and young persons have differing needs and perspectives at various stages of their social, cultural, and developmental continuum (Bee and Boyd 2013). Dependence upon others is normal at the beginning of the lifespan and this tends to decrease with developmental progress and move towards a more independent lifestyle. At all early stages, children require nurture, care, and protection and are 'socialised' throughout their early childhood by the dominant culture of their community/society and the specific manner of their parenting. Others, often parents or the law bring influence to bear which is claimed to be in the 'best interests' of the child. Whilst this is considered acceptable in the early years of childhood, it is increasingly less acceptable as children and young people become seen as social entities in their own right (Lundy 2007).

Some categories of children and young people will require particular or increased attention. These include: transitional care, children going into or leaving the care system, those who are fostered or adopted, entering or leaving the prison or young offender's system, refugees and asylum seekers from political, conflict, and sexual exploitation situations (The Children Act 1989 guidance and regulations. Vol 3, 2015).

Lundy (2007, 2019), 'The Lundy Model' strategy is primarily aimed at children and young people under the age of 18, but also embraces the voice of young people in the transition to adulthood up to the age of 24. It is influenced by the United Nations Convention on the Rights of the Child (UNCRC) and the EU Charter of Fundamental Rights. Based on four key concepts – *Space, Voice, Audience and Influence*, it espouses rights based participatory engagement with children. Lundy (2007) notes that those involved in developing children's services may need reminded that the UNCRC (1989) is a universal legal imperative and not a just a 'nicety'.

The same should be true for health and social care policy, education, research, and practice. This is and will continue to be a central consideration expected in law, of all nurse practitioners in demonstrating that the best interests of the child or young person are taken into consideration. The voice of the child and young person must be heard and consideration given to the implications of all our actions (Article 12, UNCRC 1989; Clarke 2021).

ASSENT, CONSENT, AND REFUSAL OF CONSENT

Assent

Assent helps to develop a **child's** autonomy, plays the role of educational tool, and supports communication between the researcher and the **child.** Oulton et al. (2016) contend appropriate assent is a valuable process that has important consequences for children's/young people's participation in research. It should focus on practical ways of supporting researchers to work in partnership with children, thus ensuring a more informed, voluntary, and robust and longer lasting commitment to research. In a study by Clarke in 2021, informed assent was sought from children to seek their view of an overnight stay in hospital – informed consent was also sought from the child's parent/guardian. Child assent and parental consent were required for the child to participate. During recruitment, one child gave assent but their parent refused to give consent with another parent wanting to give their consent and their child refusing to give their assent. Both children did not participate in the study.

Assent has important consequences for children's participation in research, including the likelihood of reducing the risks of coercion, promoting open discussion, and establishing trust.

Consent

The NHS states that persons aged 16 years or over are entitled to Consent to treatment – Children and young people – NHS (www.nhs.uk) if they have sufficient capacity to decide on their own medical treatment, unless there is significant evidence to suggest otherwise.

Competence of children in giving consent is another notable advance, which supports the value of listening to what children say and experience. Gillick vs. West Norfolk & Wisbech Area Health Authority (1985) enabled minors under 16 to consent if the doctor is satisfied with the criteria as follows:

- Capacity of child to consent
- Voluntariness of child to consent
- Understanding of risks and benefits (informed consent)

Importantly in the eyes of the law, this 'Gillick competence' can be applied to other medical/surgical/dental treatment if in the opinion of the treating doctor the child can be said to have sufficient understanding and intelligence and is capable of making a 'reasonable' assessment of the advantages and disadvantages of proposed treatment, with sufficient discretion to make a choice in his or her own interest. Furthermore, it is important to remember that informed consent is a process and not a one-off event and that doctors and healthcare professionals sometimes influence parent/child consent either way (Taylor 2018) https://www.healthline.com/health/informed-consent#other-uses last accessed 5 April 2021.

ACTIVITY 4.7

View the legal body that oversees the operation of the Mental Capacity Act (2005).

The Courts can overrule a child's refusal to consent in cases which are life threatening, but all cases should be considered on their own merits in accordance with the principle of justice (treating each case the same unless there is a significant difference). It is very important that all health professionals act at all times in such a way as to help build a child's capacity to understand what they are involved in, and not to exert undue influence upon their decision-making (UNCRC 1989 and http://capacityltd.org.uk https://www.unicef.org/adolescence).

ACTIVITY 4.8

View this online tutorial from UNCRC:
https://www.youtube.com/watch?v=TFMqTDIYI2U

CHALLENGES TO HEALTHCARE DECISIONS AND ACTIONS

There continues to be many challenges under the Human Rights Act (1998) and UNCRC (1989). This is due to a number of factors, including more awareness by the public of their perceived 'rights' and retribution, but also because of the competing complexity of meeting healthcare needs which may indeed infringe some aspects of human rights.

As the care of children and young people involves other practitioners and therapists, not only nurses, there is a clear implication here in relation to how multidisciplinary teams (MDT) and interdisciplinary teams should work. There should be a shared understanding of the complexities of ethical, legal, and professional imperatives and guidelines, and legislation should be observed to the letter. All multidisciplinary working practices, particularly the assessment and referral processes are an essential element of the communication process when dealing with the care of children and young persons. This is particularly important where the care management and delivery crosses the interfaces.

EVIDENCE-BASED PRACTICE

In the quest for underpinning evidence it would seem to be easy to fall foul of the belief that evidence is the 'be all and end all' of care interventions. Aveyard and Sharp (2017, Bruce et al. 2021; Cornock 2020a, 2020b, 2020c) remind us that just as there are different 'hierarchies' of evidence so, too, different clinical issues may be best served by differing 'kinds' of evidence, and explores the notion that in some cases clinical judgement and expertise is more important, as external evidence can inform practice but never totally replace individual clinical expertise. This is an important distinction because it recognises the value of individual professional judgement in the decision-making process.

In general, it is accepted that the safe and competent RN/practitioner should always seek out an action, which is in the best interests of the child and family and is also the best from the available current evidence. It should go without saying that in order to meet the requirements of the law, as well as ethical practice, the nurse must keep their knowledge, skills, and competence up to date and relevant to their field of practice throughout their working life (http://www.nmc-uk.org).

DOCUMENTATION WITHIN CARE PLANNING

Good record keeping, whether at an individual, team, or organisational level, has many important functions. These include a range of clinical, administrative, and educational uses (Douglas & Ruddle 2009; McGeehan 2007; NMC 2010; Oliver 2010; Scovell 2010; Woodward 2007) such as:

- Showing how decisions related to patient care were made and why variations may occur.
- Supporting the delivery of services.
- Supporting effective clinical judgements and decisions.
- Supporting patient care and communications.
- Making continuity of care easier.
- Providing documentary evidence of services delivered.
- Promoting better communication and sharing of information between members of the multi-professional healthcare team.
- Helping to identify risks and enabling early detection of complications.
- Supporting clinical audit, research, allocation of resources, and performance planning.
- Helping to address complaints or legal processes.

Essential to the provision of good care, record-keeping is a very high-risk activity. Different contexts of care and different systems for record-keeping are used from country to country and in different organisations. Challenges include the move from written paper-based reports to electronic systems and issues around confidentiality and disclosure. Hinchcliff and Rogers (2008) note that the burden to respect the confidentiality of our patients is considerable and point out that in community settings the issue of confidentiality of record – keeping may require more rigor in protection than is automatically available in an acute care setting. The NHS Confidentiality Code of Practice (DH 2001) provides further guidance on record-keeping and confidentiality to that issued by the NMC. NHS employees will be expected to understand and follow the NHS code.

The NMC Code (2018) states that records should show effective communication within the MDT; they must be an accurate record of care planning, treatment, and delivery for the individual. Records should be consecutive and completed as soon as possible after the event. They should also show clear evidence of decisions taken and that the information is shared appropriately. Recording and documenting for assessment, intervention, and referral processes should follow best practice guidelines to ensure transparency of all interventions and consultations and the informed consent of those involved as clients.

Despite this clear directive there are many instances year on year, of incomplete care plans, poor or absent documentation or records which have a disproportionate lean towards physical care and medical problems rather than the holistic needs of a patient care plan. Documentation should, according to the Patient Health Service Ombudsman (2005) include the items of information and education provided to patients in the clinical setting to assure effective communication between healthcare professionals. These authors assert that this should also include any developmentally appropriate comfort and communication methods used in family-centred care delivery within the context of the rights of the child.

Social networking sites have widespread usage today. Technology facilitates the spread of information in an instant and with a global reach. The implication for nurses is significant; remember that anything written, uploaded, transmitted, or otherwise broadcast is in the public domain. What one individual might see as venting their emotions after a stressful day can be seen by others as offensive, libellous, or as whistle-blowing. Material or media considered explicit or inappropriate will result in a nurse putting their registration at risk. The NMC Code states that you are accountable for your actions at all times and for upholding the Code in your personal life as well as your professional activities (RCN 2009).

Therefore, exercise caution before you 'hit that post/send button' on your PC or mobile device and be certain that you understand and uphold the principles in NMC (2019) Social Media Guidance. Think through content of your post, act professionally to ensure public protection at all times.

The need to exercise great conscience (accountability) in nursing and social care practice, with particular relevance to the care of children and young people is identified in this chapter. Acting ethically or doing the right thing can be fraught with difficulties. It will be necessary to seek guidance and clarity in all deliberations and actions. Advocacy is an ethical stance, which should be enshrined in all health and social care enquiry and action. Each individual children's nurse should be aware of the contents and meaning of the most current NMC Code, both in their personal and professional life.

SUMMARY

The nurse should be aware that the standard expected in professional practice is at least that expected in law and indeed often exceeds the legal expectation. All nurses should be able to demonstrate that they are practising with due regard for the benefit of, and in the best interests of their clients. Record keeping and care delivery are very high-risk activities in which all healthcare professionals must follow the standards set by professional bodies. Accountability of the practitioner is essential and a secure knowledge and skills base must be constantly updated according to need and within the guidance of current NMC Code (2018), the employment contract and that country's legislation. A child-rights based approach is a legal imperative, not an optional extra in the planning, delivery and evaluation of all education practice and research involving children, young people and their families. Capacity building should be an informed approach embedded in all aspects of our practice and communication as children's nurses.

REFERENCES AND ADDITIONAL RESOURCES

Avery, G. (2026) *Law and Ethics in Nursing and Healthcare: An Introduction Second Edition: An Introduction*, 2nd edn. London: Sage Publications.

Aveyard, H. & Sharp, P. (2017) *A Beginner's Guide to Evidence-Based Practice in Health and Social Care*. London: Open University Press.

Beauchamp, T.L. & Childress, J.F. (2012) *Principles of Biomedical Ethics*. New York: Oxford University Press.

Bee, H. & Boyd, D. (2013) *The Developing Child*, 13th edn. United States of America: Pearson New International Edition.

Bruce, E. & Williss, J.G. (2021) *The Great Ormond Street Hospital Manual of Children and Young People's Nursing Practices*. London: Wiley Blackwell.

Clarke, S. (2021) An exploration of the child's experience of staying in hospital from the perspectives of children and children's nurses using child-centered methodology. *Comprehensive Child and Adolescent Nursing* 1 April 2021 online. https://www.tandfonline.com/doi/full/10.1080/24694193.2021.1876786?scroll=top&needAccess=true [Accessed 5 April 2021].

Committee of the Central Health Services Council (1959) *The Welfare of Children in Hospital (Platt Report)*. London: HMSO.

Committee on Child Health Services (1976) *Fit for the Future (Court Report)*. London: HMSO.

Cornock, M. (2020) Clinical negligence. *Orthopaedic & Trauma Times*, **32**, 10–13.

Cornock, M. (2020a) A summary of law and ethics for the new health care practitioner. *Orthopaedic & Trauma Times*, **36**, 30–37.

Cornock, M. (2020b) To indemnify or not: Professional indemnity arrangements. *Orthopaedic & Trauma Times*, **38**, 6–11.

Cornock, M. (2020c) Revisiting informed consent. *Orthopaedic & Trauma Times*, **38**, 6–11.

Cornock, M. & McAlinden, O. (2018) Chapter 8 Law and policy for children and young people's nursing in Price, J. & McAlinden, O. (2018) *Essentials of Children and Young Peoples Nursing*, 2nd edn due 2023). London: Sage Publications.

Department of Health (2001) The Kennedy report: Learning from Bristol. The Report of the Public Inquiry into Children's Heart Surgery at the Bristol Royal Infirmary 1984–1995. Cm 5207 (1).

Dimond, B. (2019) *Dimond's Legal Aspects of Nursing: A Definitive Guide to Law for Nurses*. London: Pearson.

Douglas, E. & Ruddle, G. (2009) Implementation of the NHS knowledge and skills framework. *Nursing Standard*, **24**(1), 42–48.

Dowie, I. (2017) Legal, ethical and professional aspects of duty of care for nurses. *Nursing Standard*, 13 December 2017 **32**, 16–19.

Francis Inquiry Report (2013) Independent report of the mid Staffordshire NHS foundation trust public inquiry. [Accessed 5 April 2021].

Gillick vs. Wisbech & West Norfolk AHA (1985) *House of Lords*. London: All ER 402.423.

Gosport Independent Panel Report (2018) https://www.gov.uk/government/publications/gosport-independent-panel-report-government-responseandwww.enablelaw.com/news/expert-opinion/gosport-war-memorial-hospital-deaths-what-happened.

Health and Social Care Act 2008 (Regulated Activities) regulations 2014: Regulation 20 https://www.cqc.org.uk/guidance-providers/regulations-enforcement/regulation-20-duty-candour [Accessed 5 April 2021].

Hinchcliff S. & Rogers, R. (2008) *Competencies for Advanced Nursing Practice*. London: Edward Arnold.

HMSO (2004) *The Children Act*. London: HMSO.

Human Rights Act (1998) *Chapter 42. Elizabeth II*. London: Stationery Office.

Is anyone listening? https://www.youtube.com/watch?v=urAyr3tqKZo [last Accessed 5 April 2021].

Lundy, L. (2007) Voice is not enough: Conceptualising Article 12 of the United Nations Convention on the rights of the child. *British Educational Research Journal*, **33**(6), 927–942.

Lundy, L. (2019) National strategy on children and young People's participation in decision-making. *Department of Children, Equality, Disability, Integration and Youth*. Eire.

McAlinden, O. (2018) Chapter 11 Infant Wellbeing and Health or 'How to Grow a Healthy Adult' in Price, J. and McAlinden, O. (2018) Essentials of children and young peoples nursing Sage London 1st edition.

McGeehan, R. (2007) Best practice in recordkeeping. *Nursing Standard*, **21**(17), 51–55. Muckamore Abbey Hospital Inquiry. Health-ni.gov.uk [last Accessed 6 May 2023].

NMC (2018) *Standards for Competence that Apply to Specific Fields of Nursing: Children's*. London: NMC. https://www.nmc.org.uk/globalassets/sitedocuments/registration/toc-14/toc-14-blueprint---childrens-nursing.pdf [Accessed 11th March 2023].

NMC (2019) Social media guidance www.nmc.org.uk/standards/guidance/social-media-guidance [last Accessed 5 April 2021].

NMC Professional Duty of Candour guidance (2019) https://www.nmc.org.uk/standards/guidance/the-professional-duty-of-candour/read-the-professional-duty-of-candour [last Accessed 5 April 2021].

Nursing and Midwifery Council (2010) *Record-keeping: Guidance for Nurses and Midwives*. London: NMC.

Nursing and Midwifery Council (2018) *The Code: Professional Standards of Practice and Behaviour for*

Nurses, Midwives and Nursing Associates. London: NMC. https://www.nmc.org.uk/standards/code [last Accessed 13 August 2021].

Oliver, A. (2010) Observations and monitoring: Routine practices on the ward. *Paediatric Nursing*, **22**(4), 28–32.

Oulton, K., Gibson, F., Sell, D., Williams, A., Pratt, L. & Wray, J. (2016) Assent for children's participation in research: Why it matters and making it meaningful. *Child Care Health Development*, **42**(4), 588–597. https://pubmed.ncbi.nlm.nih.gov/27133591 [Accessed 11th March 2023].

Patient Health Service Ombudsman (2005) Making an Impact. Annual Report 2009–10. https://www.ombudsman.org.uk [Accessed 11th March 2023].

Royal College of Nursing (2009) *Legal Advice for RCN Members Using the Internet.* London: RCN.

RCN (2015) Recordkeeping. The Facts London RCN Publications. Code 005 343.

RCN (2017) *Standards for Assessing, Measuring and Monitoring Vital Signs in Infants, Children and Young People.* London: RCN Publications. Code 005 942.

Scovell, S. (2010) Role of the nurse-to-nurse handover in patient care. *Nursing Standard*, **24**(20), 35–39.

Shipman Inquiry (July 2003–2005) Reports 1–6. Chairman Dame Janet Smith DBE https://www.gov.uk/government/organisations/shipman-inquiry [last Accessed 5 April 2021].

Standing, M. (2020) *Clinical Judgement and Decision Making in Nursing (Transforming Nursing Practice Series).* London: Learning Matters.

Stonehouse, D.P. (2021) Understanding nurses' responsibilities in promoting equality and diversity. *Nursing Standard*, Jun 2; **36**(6), 27-33. doi: 10.7748/ns.2021.e11531. Epub 2021 Apr 6. PMID: 33821596.

Taylor, H. (2018) Informed consent 1: Legal basis and implications for practice. *Nursing Times*, [online]; **114**(6), 25–28 https://www.nursingtimes.net/roles/nurse-educators/informed-consent-1-legal-basis-and-implications-for-practice-21-05-2018 [last Accessed 5 April 2021].

The Children Act 1989 guidance and regulations. Volume 3: Planning transition to adulthood for care leavers. October 2010 revised January 2015.

United Nations Convention on the Rights of the Child (UNCRC) (1989) UNCRC.

Woodward, S. (2007) Learning and sharing safety lessons to improve patient care. *Nursing Standard*, **20**(18), 49–53.

CHAPTER 5

Young People and Truth Telling

Catherine Monaghan

INTRODUCTION

Having open, honest, and clear communication channels with a patient is a key component for patient-centred care, which can in turn facilitate the delivery of high quality nursing care (Newell & Jordan 2015). Providing young people with the correct information about their condition can help maximise the person's autonomy; however, there are times where it is less straightforward when the young adult is uncertain about involving their parents. Ethical issues arise on a daily basis which challenge nurses to think critically about the ethics of their day-to-day practice (Butts & Rich 2020).

Ethical issues will be analysed from traditional perspectives: deontology and utilitarianism, and in addition to this a virtue-based approach will be explored. It could be argued that the process of telling the individual about their diagnosis should not be based on ethical principles/theories alone. Carman et al. (2022) assert that virtues such as honesty and compassion need to be considered.

It is not the intention of this chapter to address in detail whether it is right or wrong to disclose the truth about the individual's diagnosis. The aim is to explore what good practice is and how the children's nurse can enhance best practice by examining key points which should be considered when caring for a young person with a terminal illness.

A framework is useful in assessing the nature of a dilemma, for example the DECIDE model (for further reading see Thompson et al. 2000). In this chapter the framework will reflect the steps in the nursing process: assess, plan, implement, and evaluate. A scenario and guidance notes are used to illustrate and explore crucial ethical points. This chapter will be useful for educational purposes when used as a framework for discussion in student nurse education. Case study 5.1 presents an example of truth telling.

CASE STUDY 5.1

Sara was 16 years old and she had sailed with her father for many years. Even though the boat was small it still needed a crew of two to sail comfortably. A year ago the boat had been a place of fun and sport where both of them enjoyed the thrill of sailing. Today, however, it had become a place of quiet reflection for Tom, her father. So much had changed within the last ten months.

Sara had been diagnosed with myelodysplastic syndrome, a defect in stem cells leading to bone marrow failure, involving red and white cells plus platelets (Kumar & Clark 2005). Both Tom and his wife were fraught with anxiety about what lay ahead for their daughter. Tom approached the children's nurse who had been involved in Sara's care and asked how best to disclose this news with his daughter (see guidance note 1, Assess).

Their initial reaction was to protect their daughter from pain arising from being told that her condition had become worse (see guidance note 2, Plan). On the other hand, they knew that their daughter would want to know and have the right to know. Both parents considered who would share this information with Sara. The team of healthcare professionals who were caring for Sara were asked to tell Sara about her situation (see guidance note 3, Implement). The children's nurse involved in Sara's care planning reflected on the situation (see guidance note 4, Evaluate).

Care Planning in Children and Young People's Nursing, Second Edition. Edited by Sonya Clarke and Doris Corkin.
© 2024 John Wiley & Sons Ltd. Published 2024 by John Wiley & Sons Ltd.

ASSESS

Throughout the assessment phase, consider the following questions which the children's nurse might want to address in Sara's case:

- What different ethical approaches might be employed?
- What are the ethical principles that need to be explored?
- Can a virtue ethics approach offer guidance in Sara's situation?

Guidance note 1

The children's nurse will begin by assessing the situation, the context and the individuals involved. By reflecting on the situation and approaching it from a deontological perspective, the nurse will ascertain that they have a professional duty and obligation to tell the truth to Sara. The nurse is less concerned with the consequences and it is more their belief that it is their duty to adhere to the principle of veracity at all times. The nurse believes that it is morally indefensible to engage in any act of lying or deceit. Furthermore, the nurse feels bound by the *Code of Professional Conduct* (NMC 2018), which reminds us that all actions are performed in the patient's best interest. The nurse believes that as an individual Sara has the right to be told the truth regardless of the consequences of telling her. Such an approach reflects Kant's duty-based moral theory, which demands an absolute adherence to rules and duties and respect for autonomy (Kendrick 1994). The children's nurse is concerned that Sara will not be able to exercise autonomy if she is not informed of her diagnosis.

In contrast, if the nurse believes that Sara should be told the truth but at the same time takes a utilitarian approach, they will be concerned that the consequences of the truth may cause more harm rather than 'good'. This is where a conflict of principles can arise. The nurse is motivated to do 'good' (principle of beneficence) and avoid harm which is the principle of non-maleficence. For further reading see Beauchamp And Childress Four Principles Framework (NursingAnswers.net 2018).

Utilitarians appraise the moral worth of an act by considering the consequences or end result; the act should bring about the greatest benefit for the greatest number (Vearrier & Henderson 2021). Thus, Sisk et al. (2016) encourage practitioners to consider how best to provide the greatest benefit for patients while doing the least harm. The children's nurse will also know that Sara already has insight into her condition and suspects that something has changed. Feelings of fear and uncertainty may be expressed by the patient and according to Sisk et al. (2016) many children with a terminal cancer illness will have some insight into their condition and know that something is wrong even when they are not informed. Asikli and Er (2021) reported on how 18 children, during their stay in pediatric oncology and haematology clinics, viewed the nurse and physician's care. The virtue most emphasised by the children was honesty. Of particular significance the children conveyed the importance of communication from the nurse and physician and the need to be honest about their cancer condition. The children also valued their parents' honesty towards them as a child and that they were kept informed.

Traditional objective moral theories such as deontology and utilitarianism may not be appropriate alone, and virtue ethics, which includes virtues such as honesty, compassion and integrity, should be considered. For further reading and discussion of virtue ethics, refer to Oakley (2015). See Table 5.1.

PLAN

Throughout the planning phase, consider the following questions which the children's nurse might want to address in Sara's case:

- What options does the children's nurse have when planning to share the information about her condition with Sara?
- What consequences are likely to occur?

Table 5.1 A summary of the ethical principles, ethical approaches, and virtues relevant to Sara's situation.

Ethical principles	Ethical approaches	Virtues
Veracity	Deontology/duty – obligation	Compassion
Beneficence	Utilitarianism	Honesty
Non-maleficence	Virtue-based approach	Integrity
Justice		Kindness
Confidentiality		Understanding
Autonomy		

Guidance note 2

In order for the children's nurse to make effective planning, issues such as when this information will be shared with Sara, who will disclose such information, and where the best venue is for this to take place need to be decided. The children's nurse needs to consider first of all who will be best placed to give this information. In general, a member from the healthcare profession tends to adopt the role of informing the patient about their diagnosis. According to Ekberg et al. (2021), considerable advancement has been achieved in developing high-quality evidence to inform conversations with patients about their condition and end of life concerns. However, when it comes to communicating a cancer diagnosis with a young person it is not without great difficulty. Sometimes a family member may feel they are best placed to impart such information, but this can prove to be an immense emotional challenge for the parent/guardian and there should always be support for the individual and patient. Henry et al. (2021) point out that clinicians need to be cognizant of the individual's and family needs, decision-making preferences and cultural norms when sharing a diagnosis. For further reading and discussion refer to Wiener et al. (2013) and Henry et al. (2021).

It is acknowledged that factors such as age and maturity play a key role in the detail and extent of cancer-related information that is shared with a child (Asikli and Er 2021). They further assert that parents should be included thus considering how much information the child wants to obtain and in a way that the child will understand.

Initially, Sara's parents did not want Sara to be told about the change in her condition. The issue of paternalism versus autonomy arose here. Her father felt that if Sara heard such information she would not be able to cope and that the truth could possibly destroy any hope that his daughter had. If the children's nurse agreed with Sara's parents and they had decided to withhold such information, then both the nurse and parents would have been exercising paternalism. Bartholdson et al. (2015) point out that it can present a challenge for the healthcare professional when there is a decision to withhold the information from the patient and to consider a decision based on 'the professional knows best' or respect for the patient's autonomy.

On the other hand, let us consider at how non-disclosure of the truth/information might affect the patient. Limited information sharing can lead to the patient not possessing important information which can affect the ability to make sound decisions about their care and future treatment plans. Sisk et al. (2016) point out that by keeping the younger person informed you are treating them with the utmost respect. However, they similarly argue that the child should not be forced into disclosure discussions or feel they have been lied to. Rost and Mihailov (2021) offer an informed debate around disclosure. Whilst they argue disclosure can strengthen the child–parent, child–physician and parent–physician relationship, they equally point out the need to consider the child's wishes. In order for the young person to be able to make informed decisions, the truth needs to be disclosed and answers to questions asked need to be given in a meaningful and sensitive manner. It is necessary that the correct amount of information must be shared with young people at the right level for their current understanding. Raz et al. (2016) point out that sensitivity and careful judgement in how this information is shared must be considered. Thus Sisk et al. (2016) argue that effective communication that reflects the child's needs is paramount. Therefore, each situation must be carefully assessed and planned on an individual basis and the interests of the young person must remain the focus and central in the decision-making process.

Table 5.2 Possible outcomes if the truth is shared with the young person or if information is withheld.

Positive aspects: telling truth	Negative aspects: not telling truth
Patient autonomy	Paternalism
Compliance	Patient non-compliance
Trust	Issue of deceit
Informed choices	Decreased sense of security
Hope	Despair
Open communication	Secrecy
Engagement	Exclusion
Family-centred approach	Isolation
Decision-making	Vulnerability

If the information is shared with Sara, then she can make informed choices in partnership with the healthcare professional and her parents. According to Bartholdson et al. (2015), autonomy is a key prevailing ethical principle. All parties can then engage with Sara in decision-making about the right care for her. This reflects a more family-centred approach. See Table 5.2.

IMPLEMENT

Consider the following questions which the children's nurse might want to address once an action plan has been established as to who will share Sara's information with her.

- How will this information be shared with Sara?
- In addition to the virtues highlighted below what other virtues might the children's nurse possess?
- What important aspects of communication must be considered?

Guidance note 3

Careful thought must be given to how information is imparted. A virtue ethics approach is appropriate here and in Sara's situation the nurse must be able to demonstrate compassion, a friendly and caring approach, sensitivity, and respect. When any aspect of care is being implemented, the young person needs to feel valued, and meaningful communication must take place. This can be facilitated in a venue where the individual is able to discuss their concerns. Hence, the child should be encouraged to ask questions about their condition and to express their anxieties and fears (Asikli & Er 2021). The children's nurse needs to take into consideration what has already been communicated to Sara, what she has already heard or not heard and indeed misunderstood. Thought must be given to the choice of words and terminology used when communicating with Sara about her situation. Explanations should not be misleading and time needs to be afforded so that Sara is able to express her feelings.

In order for the nurse and Sara's parents to be able to communicate effectively with Sara there needs to be trust and this trust will only develop and be therapeutic whenever the children's nurse/patient relationship embraces truth telling. If the professional is striving to achieve being honest with the individual, then truth is the vehicle that surely facilitates us reaching that goal (Asikli & Er 2021). Whenever the individual knows the truth about their illness this can help with the psychological and emotional adjustment (Raz et al. 2016). However, Gillam et al. (2022) cautions how truth telling may affect the child's overall best interests, either negatively or positively. Therefore, each child's situation must be viewed as unique to that child and their family. Knowing what Sara's wishes are can facilitate proper support services to be implemented into Sara's treatment plan.

At this point let us consider possible reasons why the truth may not be communicated (see Box 5.1).

> **BOX 5.1**
>
> Possible reasons why the truth may not be communicated with the young person.
>
> The young person clearly states that she does not wish to receive this information at present.
>
> This situation, however, must be continually assessed as this may change.
>
> Medical staff may not always be in a position to know the truth about the individual's condition.
>
> Consideration must be given to the development level of the child/young person as well as cultural background.

EVALUATE

Consider the following questions which the children's nurse might want to address in the process of evaluation:

- What needs to be evaluated in relation to Sara, her parents, the nurse, and practice?
- What important aspects of evaluation need to be considered?

Guidance note 4

In Sara's situation there are four areas that need to be evaluated throughout the disclosure process. Evaluation is an ongoing process; therefore, the children's nurse will continually need to assess what the impact of revealing the truth has on Sara. The nurse must continuously assess for any signs of distress that Sara may experience and monitor how she copes with this. The diagnosis and deterioration in her condition is Sara's information and needs to be shared with her as opposed to Sara being told. This, however, must be communicated in a sensitive and caring approach.

Sara's parents have engaged in a family-centred approach rather than adopting a paternalistic view. If a partnership approach is adopted and implemented it helps facilitate a more open channel for Sara's parents to approach the children's nurse and, where appropriate, seek support services which they may require, such as advice and counselling. Appropriate and timely information throughout all aspects of Sara's care is paramount for both Sara and her parents. As a result, they will feel empowered to be able to make informed choices and be able to take an active role and fully engage in decisions being made about Sara's situation and treatment plan. This must be continuously monitored and ways to enhance this partnership must be explored.

The children's nurse must equally evaluate their own involvement in the process of truth telling. Being involved in facilitating the truth being shared with a young person can be viewed as extremely difficult and cognisance must be taken of the impact it can have on the children's nurse. Reflection on how the children's nurse can manage and cope in such delicate and emotional situations must be encouraged and promoted. The children's nurse needs to be knowledgeable and well equipped to deal with situations such as these. Robaee et al. (2018) further support the need to provide a supportive environment in hospitals and to consider strategies for diminishing feelings of ethical and moral distress; where the nurse is faced with ethical challenges and uncertainty how to manage the situation. Best practice in this area, which can be an ethical minefield, requires proper training and support. Good education and mentoring of staff is, therefore, essential in achieving a positive outcome for patient, family, and professional. Griffiths et al. (2015) stressed that nurses working within palliative care require training to be specific to their practice Thus, training needs should address and include the nurse becoming skilled in developing effective and meaningful communication skills and in developing a reflective approach. See Table 5.3.

Table 5.3 Four areas which need to be evaluated throughout the disclosure process and possible issues arising in each.

Young person	Parent/guardian	Nurse	Practice
Coping	Partnership	Reflection	Guidelines
Central to decision-making process	Support and advice	Critical thinking	Research focused
Approach		Training needs	Cultural needs

SUMMARY

As Butts and Rich (2020) point out, the nurse must think critically about the ethics of day-to-day practice. Consideration should be given to informing the child with the support from the family (Asikli & Er 2021). Open discussion should be encouraged whilst appreciating the need for sensitivity, cultural differences and respect for the child. In addition, all documentation throughout the process must be accurately recorded. In Sara's situation, it would appear to be morally indefensible to withhold the information from the patient (Bartholdson et al. 2015). Furthermore, they assert that each situation is fluid; the children's nurse must take into consideration what is happening with the young person, what the parent/guardian is experiencing, and what different views and ethical principles each professional holds. Asikli and Er (2021) argue that it is necessary for the nurse to be honest in order for the patient to trust them. Consideration must also be afforded to different cultural backgrounds and beliefs (Weiner et al. 2013).

REFERENCES

Asikli, E. & Er, R.A. (2021) Paediatric oncology patients' definitions of a good physician and good nurse. *Nursing Ethics*, **28**(5), 656–669.

Bartholdson, C., Lutzen, K., Blomgren, K. & Pergert, P. (2015) Experiences of ethical issues when caring for children with cancer. *Cancer Nursing*, **38**(2), 125–132. doi: 10.1097/ncc.0000000000000130.

Butts, J.B. & Rich, K.L. (2020) *Nursing Ethics. Across the Curriculum and into Practice*, 5th edn. London: Jones and Bartlett Publishers.

Carman, C.S., Peter, E., Ramos, F.R.S. & Brito, M.J.M. (2022) The process of moral distress development: A virtue ethics perspective. *Nursing Ethics*, **29**(2), 402–412.

Ekberg, S., Parry, R., Land, V., Ekberg, K., Pino, M., Antaki, C., Jenkins, L. & Whittaker, B. (2021) Communicating with patients and families about illness progression and end of life: A review of students using direct observation of clinical practice. *BMC Palliative Care*, **20**(186), 1–12.

Gillam, L., Spriggs, M., McCarthy, M. & Delany, C. (2022) Telling the truth to seriously ill children: Considering children's interests when parents veto telling the truth. *Bioethics*, **36**(7), 765–773.

Griffiths, J., Ewing, G., Wilson, C., Connolly, M. & Grande, G. (2015) Breaking bad news about transitions to dying: A qualitative exploration of the role of the district nurse. *Palliative Medicine*, **29**(2), 138–146.

Henry, M., Nichols, S., Hwang, J.M., Nichols, S.D., Odiyo, P., Watson, M., Ali, A., Parker, P., Kissane, D., Asuzu, C. & Lounsbury, D.W. (2021) Barriers to communicating a cancer diagnosis to patients in a low-to-middle-income context. *Journal of Psychosocial Oncology Research and Practice*, **3**(2), 1–6.

Kendrick, K. (1994) Tools which aid the decision-making process: Addressing moral dilemmas in nursing practice. *Professional Nurse*, **9**, 739–742.

Kumar, P. & Clark, M. (2005) *Clinical Medicine*, 6th edn. Edinburgh: Elsevier Saunders.

Newell, S. & Jordan, Z. (2015) The patient experience of patient-centred communication with nurses in the hospital setting: A qualitative systematic review protocol. *JBI Database System Rev Implement Rep*, **13**(1), 76–87. doi: 10.11124/jbisrir-2015-1072. PMID: 26447009.

Nursing and Midwifery Council (2018) *The Code. Professional Standards of Practice and Behaviour for Nurses, Midwives and Nursing Associates*. London: NMC.

NursingAnswers.net (2018 November) Beauchamp And Childress Four Principles Framework. [online]. Available from: https://pubmed.ncbi.nlm.nih.gov/34876096/ [Accessed 28th February 2023].

Oakley, J. (2015) A virtue ethics perspective on bioethics. *BIOETHICS Update*, **1**, 41–53.

Raz, H., Tabak, N., & Kreitler, S. (2016) Psychological outcomes of sharing a diagnosis of cancer with a pediatric patient. *Frontiers in Pediatrics*, **4**(70), 1–10. doi: 10.3389/fped.2016.00070.

Robaee, N., Atashzadeh-Shoorideh, F., Ashktorab, T., Baghestani, A. & Barkhordari-Sharifabad, M. (2018) Perceived organizational support and moral distress among nurses. *BMC Nursing*, **17**(1), 1–7.

Rost, M. & Mihailov, E. (2021) In the name of the family? Against parents' refusal to disclose prognostic information to children. *Mental Health Care and Philosophy*, **24**(2), 1–12. doi: 10.1007/s11019-021-10017-4.

Sisk, B.A., Bluebond-Langner, M., Wiener, L., Mack, J. & Wolfe, J. (2016) Prognostic disclosures to children: A historical perspective. *Pediatrics*, **138**(3), 1–10. e20161278.

Thompson, I.E., Melia, K.M. & Boyd, K.M. (2000) *Nursing Ethics*. Edinburgh: Churchill Livingstone.

Vearrier, L. & Henderson, C.M. (2021) Utilitarian principlism as a framework for crisis healthcare ethics. *HSC Forum*, **33**(1–2), 45–60. doi: 10.1007/s10730-020-09431-7.

Wiener, L., McConnell, D.G., Latella, L. & Ludi, E. (2013) Cultural and religious considerations in pediatric palliative care. *Palliat Support Care*, **11**(1), 47–67.

Sexual Health

CHAPTER 6

Jim Richardson

INTRODUCTION

When addressing nursing considerations, the issues identified through considering the box case study 6.1 and the questions posed will help to identify those aspects of the situation which will require further nursing assessment, planning, and, ultimately, the nursing interventions which will help Kylie to address her sexual health needs (see case study below).

CASE STUDY 6.1

Kylie is a 16-year-old girl who lives with her parents and younger sister. She attends school enthusiastically and plans to study to become a primary schoolteacher.

Kylie has a 24-year-old boyfriend of two months and although she is sexually active, she has not sought advice about contraception.

She now wants to speak to a nurse as she thinks she may be pregnant.

Questions

1. What constitutes good sexual health?
2. What do young people need to promote their own sexual health?
3. What problems might young people experience in maintaining their sexual health and wellbeing?

ANSWERS TO QUESTIONS

Question 1. What constitutes good sexual health?

Good sexual health can be defined by concrete factors such as the absence of sexually transmissible disease. However, there are more abstract perspectives too, such as freedom of expression of the sexual self.

It is worth considering the definition of sexual health to ensure that all dimensions are identified. The World Health Organisation (WHO 2002) defined sexual health as:

A state of physical, emotional, mental and social wellbeing related to sexuality. It is not merely the absence of disease, dysfunction or infirmity. Sexual health requires a positive and respectful approach to sexuality and sexual relationships, as well as the possibility of having pleasurable and safe sexual experiences, free of coercion, discrimination and violence. For sexual health to be attained and maintained, the sexual rights of all persons must be respected, protected and fulfilled.

This rather long statement serves to highlight the complexity of sexual health. Some of the key ideas from a nursing perspective include:

- Sometimes we think of sexual health rather narrowly in terms of sexually transmissible infection and unintended pregnancy. While these factors are important, they are not the whole story.
- People may need help to achieve the sexual life they want, free of social pressures (such as the peer group for young people), coercion (such as being pushed into engaging in sexual activity against their better judgement or before they feel ready to do so).

Care Planning in Children and Young People's Nursing, Second Edition. Edited by Sonya Clarke and Doris Corkin.
© 2024 John Wiley & Sons Ltd. Published 2024 by John Wiley & Sons Ltd.

- Sexual bullying and violence are too common and young people need to be equipped with the skills to protect themselves.
- Sexual health is not merely a matter of physiological or mechanical issues. It is important that young people learn how to conduct their sexual lives in a way that is emotionally and psychologically rewarding and satisfying.
- Sexually transmissible infections are prevalent among young people and there is evidence that they are rather taken for granted by this age group. However, the long-term consequences of some of these can be severe, for example chlamydia. Misinformation about these infections remains widespread among young people.
- Some young people actively opt for early parenthood. However, the UK has among the highest rates of teenage pregnancy in the Western world and this is even more marked in areas of relative deprivation. Many of these pregnancies will be unintended and have the potential to limit the life opportunities of these young parents.

In the light of these factors, it is important for nurses working with children and young people to consider what young people need to be able to protect and improve their own sexual health and wellbeing. Equally significant will be a consideration of factors which serve as barriers to young people being able to act in their own best interests in this central facet of their health. Exploration of these issues will allow the children and young people's (CYP) nurse to identify their learning needs so that they are equipped with the knowledge and skills necessary to help young people meet their health needs.

SOME FACTS

In Scotland, in 2019, 17,336 diagnoses of chlamydia were made. This represents a 6% increase compared to 2018. (Health Protection Scotland 2021).

In Wales, between 2005 and 2008, 44 per 1000 young women between the ages of 15 and 17 became pregnant. However, this rate was 25.4 per 1000 in 2019. (Teenage Pregnancy.net 2021; Welsh Assembly Government 2010).

In England, between 2019 and 2020 there was a 46% reduction in the number of those diagnosed as having genital warts. This may relate to the pandemic lockdown but remains high compared to similar countries. (UK Government 2021).

In Northern Ireland in 2019, 60% of victims of sexual crimes were girls below the age of 18. (The Strategic Investment Board 2020).

All of these indicators are significantly more negative than those found among our Western European neighbours (UNICEF 2004). These facts indicate rather starkly the need for improvement in sexual health promotion among our young people.

QUESTION 2. WHAT DO YOUNG PEOPLE NEED TO PROMOTE THEIR OWN SEXUAL HEALTH?

The first and most obvious need is for accurate and constructive information in relation to sex. Young people readily identify this need but often have difficulty accessing this information:

- While many young people get their sex-related information at home, many parents find it difficult to discuss sex with their children, often because they feel ill-equipped themselves to discuss this matter. This attitude can also lead to young people feeling unable to bring their sexual concerns to their parents (Rhondda Cynon Taff Fframwaith 2009).
- The school can play an important role in ensuring the sex education of young people. However, this provision is patchy and variable in quality. Sometimes sex-related information offered is excellent and versatile, tailored to the needs of the young people and covering all aspects of sexuality. On the other hand, some young people receive information relating to the biology of sex with little reference to relationship aspects of a healthy sexual life. Excluded and hard-to-reach young people suffer a further disadvantage in this respect.

- For many young people, the principal source of sex-related information is the peer group. This may be unhelpful and inaccurate and lead to negative feelings about sex and sexuality and risky behaviour.
- Young people who are gay, lesbian, bisexual, or transgendered can be particularly disadvantaged in this key element of their lives. Their particular needs must be identified and respected, although currently that generally is not the case for most.
- This is an area which is sensitive, complex, and rapidly evolving requiring the provision of specialist services. CYP nurses offering a service to these young people must rigorously maintain, among others, two key principles: respect for the young person and their identity and prevention of any harm, physical, psychological, social, etc.
- The media offer distorted images of sexuality in our sexualised society. Young people can be led to believe that this is reliable and dependable information and may base their expectations on this.
- Expectations of sexuality and sexual health can vary between ethnic, religious, and cultural groups. Sex-related information will have to be couched in formats which are sensitive to these expectations.

Young people need access to services which exist to promote their sexual health:

- Contraceptive and sexual health (CASH) services need to be orientated towards the needs of young people and specifically address the needs of this age group.
- Sexual health services which offer diagnosis and treatment of sex-related disorders need to be readily available and accessible as well as youth-friendly.
- Counselling in relation to sexual wellbeing needs to be available. This is particularly important for those who have experienced sexual coercion or exploitation (Scottish Government 2010).
- Dedicated facilities for the support of victims of sexual violence are particularly crucial.

CYP nurses and other professionals who work with young people are in a position to help this group with their informational needs. There are a number of approaches to this (NIHCE 2014) and might still include approaches such as:

- Drop-in services offered by specifically prepared professionals. Young people particularly value the services of groups such as school nurses and youth workers.
- Educational programmes delivered by specially prepared peer educators can be effective.
- Mass health education campaigns can be effective, especially when channelled through media and platforms used by young people.
- Projects designed to improve access to contraception services can be very useful (Health Development Agency 2004).

On occasion, the most important role of the CYP nurse is, having assessed sexual health-related needs, being aware of appropriate local services, and being able to refer to these effectively.

QUESTION 3. WHAT PROBLEMS MIGHT YOUNG PEOPLE EXPERIENCE IN MAINTAINING THEIR SEXUAL HEALTH AND WELLBEING?

- Being unaware of what good sexual health is and how this can be achieved is the first and most obvious need and can be answered by good educational provision.
- Young people sometimes meet professionals and others who have negative, judgemental, flawed, and damaging attitudes and assumptions. This, in place of a proper and comprehensive assessment of need, constitutes a real barrier.
- Young people have a real concern for confidentiality in relation to their sexual health needs and can be impeded from accessing services. This can naturally be particularly marked in rural and

remote settings. There is some evidence that young people perceive health professionals as being sensitive to confidentiality needs.

- Assertiveness and negotiation skills within relationships is something many young people find difficult to achieve.
- If an atmosphere conducive to open discussion and questioning is not created, embarrassment can be a real hurdle to communication.
- A lack of awareness that substance and alcohol use can lead to errors of judgement and risky behaviour.
- Victimisation, exploitation, and abusive relationships are sources of substantial damage to sexual health in every respect.

From consideration of this range of factors, it begins to become evident how care in relation to sexual health for Kylie might be approached. The first step to care will always be to assess need. Refer to Box Activity 6.1

ACTIVITY 6.1

Draft an assessment approach to establishing Kylie's sexual health needs. You may find Mitchell and Wellings (1998) helpful in doing this. Once you have done this, it will be straightforward to draft a plan of care which will address Kylie's sexual health needs. Bear in mind that the plan will be drafted in negotiation with Kylie and will fully take into account Kylie's perceptions of her needs in this respect.

SUMMARY

The sexual health of young people in the UK could be improved in every dimension. Sexual wellbeing is an important part of people's lives and is a significant determinant of perceptions of quality of life. Children's and young people's nurses can contribute to this aspect of their patients' care needs but need the appropriate knowledge and skills to be able to do this effectively and in an appropriate manner.

REFERENCES

Health Development Agency (2004) *Teenage Pregancy and Sexual Health Interventions.* London: Health Development Agency.

Health Protection Scotland (2021) www.hps.scot.nhs.uk/publications/hps-weekly-report/volume-54/issue-21 [Accessed 19th September 2021].

Mitchell, K. & Wellings, K. (1998) *Talking about Sexual Health.* London: Health Education Authority.

National Institute for Health and Clinical Excellence (2014) Contraceptive Services for the under 25s. https://www.nice.org.uk/guidance/ph51 [Accessed 28th February 2023].

Rhondda Cynon Taff Fframwaith (2009) *Developing a Strategy for Preventing Teenage Pregnancy, Supporting Teenage Parents and Meeting Sexual Health Needs.* Pontypridd: Rhondda Cynon Taff Fframwaith.

Scottish Government (2010) *Draft National Guidance: Under-age Sexual Activity–Meeting the Needs of Children and Young People and Identifying Child Protection Concerns.* Edinburgh: Scottish Government.

Strategic Investment Board (2020) Sexual Health Strategy Northern Ireland, Interim *Report.* www.sibni.org. [Accessed 19th September 2021].

Teenagepregnancy.net. [Accessed 19th September 2021].

UK Government (2021) STI rates remain a concern despite fall in 2020. https://www.gov.uk/government/news/sti-rates-remain-a-concern-despite-fall-in-2020 [Accessed 19th September 2021].

UNICEF (2004) *A League Table of Teenage Births in Rich Nations.* Florence: UNICEF.

Welsh Assembly Government (2010) *Sexual Health and Wellbeing Action Plan for Wales, 2010–2015.* Cardiff: Welsh Assembly Government.

World Health Organisation (2002) *Definition of Sexual Health.* https://www.who.int/health-topics/sexual-health#tab=tab_2 [Accessed 15th November 2010].

CHAPTER 7

Integrated Care Pathways

Pauline Cardwell and Lucy Simms

In Chapter 1 a review of the development of the nursing process and several models of nursing were outlined in relation to children's nursing. In more recent times, healthcare delivery has focused on developing services which are inclusive of patient and health professionals' views and flexible to ensure evidence-based practice is supported within the finite resources of service provision. Thus, the goals of planning and delivering effective patient-focused care and services which meet the needs of patients has been developed and supported using integrated care pathways. Health delivery systems globally are under increasing pressure to provide effective services to meet the increasing needs of society, whilst working with finite resources in aiming to do so (National Council for the Professional Development of Nursing and Midwifery (NCNM) 2006). Whilst family-centred care has developed within the field of children's nursing and is utilised alongside the nursing process to organise and aid care delivery, there is an increasing acknowledgement and development of integrated care pathways (ICP). Such developments are purported to support inter-professional working and improve the effectiveness of care delivery and seamless service delivery with organisation and communication across agencies and professionals (NICE 2018). These pathways are increasingly used in care planning and delivering patient care relevant to various conditions and settings, whilst also aiding practitioners in making timely decisions, alongside other health professionals, which are appropriate to the needs of the child and family.

Within this chapter, the origin and elements of ICPs will be discussed and consideration will be given to the development of ICPs for specific patient groups within a clinical environment. The chapter will draw on information from national and international examples when considering their contribution to care delivery. In addition, how these pathways can support the implementation of best practice guidelines and standardised care planning and delivery to children and their families will be included. To illustrate and appreciate the structure and support ICPs offer in delivering care to children and their families, an ICP for the management of bronchiolitis will be utilised in this chapter to outline how these documents can support care planning and delivery.

THE ORIGINS OF INTEGRATED CARE PATHWAYS

Integrated care pathways serve several purposes, including continuous quality improvement, reduction in variation of standards, minimising resource utilisation, and education of healthcare staff (Lee et al. 2021). Such reported activities have contributed to their development and utilisation in current healthcare practice. In attempting to identify the origins and use of these pathways, it is therefore necessary to consider the strengths of these innovations and their contribution to the delivery of healthcare in the twenty-first century. Wakefield (2004) identified the origins of ICPs as being utilised in the USA and Australia from the 1980s, with their introduction in the UK in the 1990s. In responding to the reforms and modernisation of health services in the UK, the need for an integrated approach to healthcare has been reinforced, whereby inter-professional, inter-organisational, and service user collaboration methods are seen as essential components of best practice (Yuliyanti et al. 2020). This translates into putting children and their families at the centre of service planning and delivery alongside multidisciplinary teams. According to Middleton and Roberts (2000) and Whittle and Hewison (2007) this represents the vision for the modern NHS and the means of enhancing high-quality service delivery have been sought through ICPs.

Several authors identify reasons from a governance perspective for the introduction and development of ICPs in the UK; these include demonstrating evidence-based care through the utilisation of best practice guidelines, such as national service framework standards, developing

Care Planning in Children and Young People's Nursing, Second Edition. Edited by Sonya Clarke and Doris Corkin.
© 2024 John Wiley & Sons Ltd. Published 2024 by John Wiley & Sons Ltd.

benchmarking standards, and thus addressing the clinical governance agenda (Allen et al. 2009; Campbell et al. 1998; Cunningham et al. 2008; MacLean et al. 2008; Wakefield 2004). Additional strengths of the ICP in care planning and delivery include reducing lengths of hospitalisation, facilitating decision making, and supporting clinical judgement skills. These skills standardise and define the patient's programme of care and assess the impact on patient outcomes in terms of education and self-management (Lee et al. 2021; MacLean et al. 2008; Whittle & Hewison 2007). Thus, ICPs have become part of contemporary healthcare practice in the UK and are developing globally.

WHAT ARE INTEGRATED CARE PATHWAYS?

Within this chapter the term ICP is utilised; however, it is important to appreciate that within the literature several terms are used to identify these initiatives, including integrated case management, care map, clinical pathways, critical pathways, and integrated care systems. The development and utilisation of these pathways are frequently individually unique to the unit or clinical environment in which they have been developed. They are created for specific purposes as creative solutions to issues in clinical practice and are developed for managing the care of particular patient groups or situations. De Luc (2001) and Yuliyanti et al. (2020) identify the inclusion of all professionals involved in 'hands on' care in developing the ICP relevant to the topic of interest, to develop and support the success of the initiative. Careful thought therefore needs to be given to their development and design if changes in practice are to be in the direction intended (Allen et al. 2009). Irrespective of their descriptive title it is important to consider what ICPs are.

Walsh (1998) identifies critical pathways as setting out plans of care to meet the needs of patients with the same medical problem, identifying goals to be achieved and defining outcomes against which progress can be measured, a view supported by Middleton and Roberts (2000). More contemporarily, ICPs are described as multidisciplinary care management tools which map chronologically, activities in healthcare systems which are to be achieved, whilst additionally having a quality improvement function (Allen et al. 2009). Subsequently, having identified agreed goals and outcomes of care provision with other health professions involved in providing care to the individual, it is necessary to create a tool for recording and documenting these aspects which can be used by all involved in the delivery of care for the infant and family. Integrated care pathways have been developed to provide a framework for clinical and treatment decisions regarding care provision which incorporate and support the use of best evidence, by streamlining and standardising care for specific patient groups (NCNM 2006). Baxter et al. (2018) succinctly suggests ICPs as being crucial in delivering care, which is safe, effective, patient-centred, timely, efficient, and equitable in the modern NHS. Indeed, the use of ICPs can be perceived to address the following aspects of professional practice:

- Patient-centred care
- High quality and safe-care delivery
- Evidence bases for care delivery utilised
- Timely delivery of care to meet needs of patient when required
- Efficiency through better management and use of services
- Equitable service for all patients.

The pathway aims to identify significant factors and progression points along the patient's journey in relation to a particular disease process or access point to services. Do refer to Box activity 7.1.

ACTIVITY 7.1

Think about what benefits using an ICP would have for you individually as a professional in your current clinical environment. Can you list what some of these might be?

WHAT ARE THE ELEMENTS OF AN INTEGRATED CARE PATHWAY?

The ICP will include several key aspects, which are initially based on the aim of tracing the expected journey of the infant through the illness. The patient's journey will have definitive start and end points and within the ICP will involve input from various health professionals who will contribute to care delivery and will aim to integrate evidence, clinical guideline information and recommendations (NICE 2015, 2021). In relation to ICP's it is also important to identify and appreciate boundaries for the ICP, to ensure its effective utilisation in clinical practice, for example an infant who is admitted with a secondary pneumonia to the primary diagnosis of bronchiolitis may require consideration of variances in the ICP which may impact on expected care trajectories.

A variance is any deviation from the proposed standard of care listed in the pathway. It is the difference between the care stated within the time and the actual event (Du et al. 2020). A variance from expected outcomes is important to detect deviations early and should be addressed and documented to include scrutiny of reasons as to why the deviation has occurred. According to Du et al. (2020), variations from the pathway identify patients who are not progressing as expected and obviously allows for early and appropriate interventions to be instigated. Recording of variances assists professionals utilising personal autonomy to individualise care for the patient and their family as well as aiding communication of these differences. In addition, variances provide valuable information which may be collated and analysed alongside other assessment tools such as Paediatric Early Warning Systems (Hall 2006), and as a result improvements for future practice may be identified.

The ICP, which outlines the programme of care that has been developed for infants with bronchiolitis, will include areas to guide holistic medical and nursing assessments of the patient in the initial stages of the journey (NHS 2021). From a nursing perspective and in conjunction with the nursing process, these activities facilitate designing plans which meet the infant and family's individual needs, through the delivery of timely care and effective interventions. Additionally, areas of care particular to the individual infant's condition, investigations, communications, teaching, and discharge plans are usually included in the document (see Appendix 2).

The ICP is aimed at providing a multi-professional tool to detail and log the infant's journey through the illness or disease process, assisting professionals to create comprehensive documents which are developed by those involved in care delivery. The plan may also include criteria to help identify parameters of recovery or deterioration to assist the health professional in making timely decisions regarding management of the infant's condition. Timelines may be used within the pathway to monitor the patient's journey through the healthcare systems, with a multi-professional focus. The inclusion of such information assists the professional practitioner to make timely clinical assessments and decisions based on the current condition of the infant and identify required interventions aimed at meeting the needs of the patient. As with many of the documents used in clinical practice these may vary in design from facility to facility and thus it is useful to provide an illustration of some of the elements of an ICP, to explore their content. Refer to Box Activity 7.2.

ACTIVITY 7.2

Think about an infant presenting with a possible diagnosis of bronchiolitis. What do you think would be key symptoms and indicators of severity of the disease process to observe?

List some of the symptoms and describe the altered physiology relevant to the symptoms identified. Reflect on the information accessible in the NHS (2021) guidance.

CLINICAL SCENARIO

If you consider the earlier identified example of bronchiolitis in a two-month-old infant, using an ICP will provide the children's nurse with guidance on presenting symptoms which will help to identify the diagnosis and the immediate care needs of the infant and family (see Appendix 2). Bronchiolitis is a seasonal, acute, infectious lower airway infection, usually caused by a virus affecting the bronchioles, and can cause acute respiratory distress including difficulty breathing, cough, irritability, and even apnoea in young infants (NICE 2015, 2021; Scottish Intercollegiate Guidelines Network (SIGN) 2006). As the most common lower respiratory tract infection in infants, bronchiolitis has several key features, including coryzal symptoms, snuffles, cough, wheeze, feeding difficulties, increasing respiratory rate, respiratory distress, pyrexia, tachycardia, and fatigue (Pearce 2021; Stevens & Kelsall-Knight 2022). Nursing care management for infants with bronchiolitis is supportive, aimed at monitoring the infant's condition, relieving respiratory distress through use of prescribed therapies, and ensuring adequate hydration and nutrition, and delivering effective infection control. Nevertheless, the children's nurse must be able to accurately determine the critical status of the infant and identify their immediate needs at the initial point of contact. The value of having clear criteria on which to base these clinical decisions is beneficial to all professionals and supports the provision of services in a timely manner. Incorporating guidelines and evidence such as that produced by SIGN (2006) assists the health professional to provide a high-quality service which also meets the individual needs of the infant and family.

Signs of severe disease include:

- Respiratory rate > 70/minute
- Oxygen saturation ≤ 90%
- Nasal flaring/grunting
- Severe intercostal recession
- Cyanosis/history of apnoea
- Lethargy
- Poor feeding < 50% of feeding requirements

(NICE 2015, 2021)

The ICP may also give the children's nurse information regarding interventions and guidance in relation to supportive care to the infant and family.

Subsequently, an example of a care pathway has been developed to illustrate some of the components of an ICP relating to the care of an infant with bronchiolitis.

HOW DO INTEGRATED CARE PATHWAYS CONTRIBUTE TO EVIDENCE-BASED PRACTICE?

In developing ICPs, an initial search of the literature which relates to the care pathway being created is undertaken. This will allow the development team to consider and integrate current clinical guidelines, information from recent studies and contemporary research in the area. The involvement of service users is also seen as key to ensuring the care pathway is responsive to patients' needs and focuses the development of the initiative by keeping the patient at the centre of care delivery. Access to sample ICPs from other organisations may assist in considering the challenges and modifications of the developing ICP required and may prevent 'reinventing the wheel' processes. Additionally, review of sample ICPs may also facilitate focusing those involved in the initiative on key variances and ensure that best practice evidence is integrated into the process.

The development of ICPs is also strongly advocated and supported by Government both nationally and regionally within the UK, as it clearly supports multi-professional working and partnerships which recognise the patient at the centre of service provision (Charles 2022; DH 2022). The impetus of these government guidelines is to utilise the expertise of clinicians in delivering on modernising the health service in the UK to deliver high quality, evidence-based care within an efficient, finitely resourced service. With the developing partnerships amongst professionals in delivering care through ICPs, these inter-professional workings can cross traditional boundaries between health and social care settings, ensuring that the patient's journey is supported throughout.

As identified earlier in the chapter, ICPs also assists in achieving the clinical governance agenda through the delivery of evidence-based care which encompasses best practice guidelines and is subject to regular clinical audit and review (Egbuta et al. 2021). Through this process of development, utilisation, and evaluation of ICPs cognisance of contemporary research, clinical guidelines, and current best practice, alongside review of clinical audit will be achieved. The ICP must be viewed as a dynamic and flexible tool which with regular review can incorporate changes occurring in clinical practice and which can adapt to meet the needs of patients for which the tool was designed.

SUMMARY

In this chapter we have considered what an ICP is and how it contributes to the delivery of healthcare in the twenty-first century. ICPs have enjoyed the support of clinicians, academics, and governmental policy in their development and growth in healthcare service delivery systems. The origins and use of ICPs have been explored, considering what they are and are not and what elements contribute to their structure and functionality. In developing such innovations an examination of how they require input from all professionals involved in the delivery of care is crucial to the success of such initiatives. This chapter has outlined major aspects of ICPs. However, it is by no means exhaustive and further independent study may assist in developing your appreciation of ICPs in contemporary healthcare services.

ACKNOWLEDGEMENTS

I would like to thank Dr Mike Smith, Consultant Paediatrician, for his generosity of time, support, and feedback on the first edition of this chapter.

REFERENCES

Allen, D., Gillen, E. & Rixson, L. (2009) Systematic review of the effectiveness of integrated care pathways: What works, for whom, in which circumstances? *International Journal of Evidence Based Healthcare*, **7**, 61–74.

Baxter, S., Johnson, M., Chambers, D., Sutton, A., Goyder, E. & Booth, A. (2018) The effects of integrated care: A systematic review of UK and international evidence. *BMC Health Serv Res*, **18**(350), 2018.

Campbell, H., Hotchkiss, R., Bradshaw, N. & Porteous, M. (1998) Integrated care pathways. *British Medical Journal*, **316**, 133–137.

Charles, A. (2022) *Integrated Care Systems Explained: Making Sense of Systems, Places, and Neighbourhoods*. The King's Fund. https://www.kingsfund.org.uk/publications/integrated-care-systems-explained

Cunningham, S., Logan, C., Lockerbie, L., Dunn, M.J.G., McMurray, A. & Prescott, R.J. (2008) Effect of an integrated care pathway on acute asthma/wheeze in children attending hospital: Cluster randomised trial. *The Journal of Pediatrics*, **152**, 315–320.

De Luc, K. (2001) *Developing Care Pathways: The Tool Kit*. Oxford: Radcliffe Medical Press.

Department of Health and Social Care (2022) *Guidance on the Preparation of Integrated Care Strategies*. London: DH.

Du, G., Huang, L. & Zhou, M. (2020) Variance analysis and handling of clinical pathway: An overview of the state of knowledge. *IEEE Access*, **8**, 158208–158223.

Egbuta, U., Howley, C., Selvarajoo, A., Iqbal, M. & Meskauskait, D. (2021) An audit of Individual Care Plan (ICP) in Dublin North City and County (DNCC) child and adolescent mental health service (CAMHS). *BJPsych Open*, **7**(S1), S77–S78.

Hall, J. (2006) Quality improvement. Chapter 2. In: *Integrated Care Pathways in Mental Health*. London: Churchill Livingstone. Elsevier.Howard, D.

Lee, K.S., Yordanov, S., Stubbs, D., Edlmann, E., Joannides, A. & Davies, B. (2021) Integrated care pathways in neurosurgery: A systematic review. *PLoS One*, **16**(8), e0255628.

MacLean, A., Fuller, R.M., Jaffrey, E.G., Hay, A.J. & Ho-Yen, D.O. (2008) Integrated care pathway for *Clostridium difficile* helps patient management. *British Journal of Infection Control*, **9**(6), 15–17.

Middleton, S. & Roberts, A. (2000) *Integrated Care Pathways: A Practical Approach to Implementation*. Oxford: Butterworth Heinemann.

National Council for the Professional Development of Nursing and Midwifery (2006) *Improving the Patient Journey: Understanding Integrated Care Pathways*. Dublin: NCNM.

National Institute for Health and Care Excellence (2015, updated 2021) Bronchiolitis in children: Diagnosis and management, NICE guideline [NG9].

National Institute for Health and Care Excellence (NICE) (2018) Chapter 38: Integrated care: Emergency and Acute Medical Cover in Over 16's service delivery and organisation, NICE guideline 94.

NHS (2021) *Bronchiolitis Pathway: Guideline for the Management of Bronchiolitis*. Southampton: Oxford Retrieval Team.

Pearce, L. (2021) Bronchiolitis: How to recognise and flag symptoms requiring emergency care, Nursing. *Children and Young People*, **33**(6), 14.

Scottish Intercollegiate Guidelines Network (SIGN) (2006) *Bronchiolitis in Children–a National Clinical Guideline*, **91**. Edinburgh: SIGN.

Stevens, R., & Kelsall-Knight, L. (2022) Clinical assessment and management of children with Bronchiolitis. *Nursing Children and Young People*, **34**(2), 13–21.

Wakefield, L. (2004) An integrated care pathway for diabetic ketoacidosis. *Paediatric Nursing*, **16**(10), 27–30.

Walsh, M. (1998) *Models and Critical Pathways in Clinical Nursing–Conceptual Frameworks for Care Planning*. London: Baillière Tindall.

Whittle, C. & Hewison, A. (2007) Integrated care pathways: Pathways to change in health care? *Journal of Health Organisation and Management*, **21**(3), 297–306.

Yuliyanti, S., Utarini, A. & Trisnantoro, L. (2020) A protocol study of participatory action research: Integrated care pathway for pregnant women with heart disease in Indonesia. *BMC Health Services Research*, **20**(1), 932.

CHAPTER 8
Interprofessional Assessment and Care Planning in Critical Care

Carolyn Green and Doris Corkin

INTRODUCTION

Caring for a critically ill child can be very complex and challenging. Critical illness can be defined as a clinical state which may result in respiratory, cardiac, neurological, gastrointestinal, metabolic, renal, and haematological complications (Nadel & Kroll 2007).

Managing the care of a critically ill child requires rapid and systematic clinical assessment to detect physiological instability so that timely, prompt, and effective resuscitation and stabilisation may occur before the onset of organ failure. The cornerstones of paediatric intensive care management are the optimisation of a patient's physiology, the provision of advanced organ support, and the identification and treatment of underlying pathological processes. This is best achieved through a multidisciplinary team approach, with shared responsibility and decision making (Jackson & Cairns 2021).

This chapter will outline the approach required by the interprofessional team when involved in the assessment and subsequent care planning for a child with a critical illness. The case study relating to a child with meningococcal sepsis will illustrate each stage of the process within an ABCDE framework (Resuscitation Council UK 2021).

CASE STUDY

Martha, a two-year-old girl, has been admitted to hospital following emergency referral by her GP with a history of being unwell for the past 24 hours with high temperature, vomiting, and refusing to feed. The GP reported that she had an increased heart rate and respiratory rate, some non-blanching petechiae, and felt that she might be presenting with symptoms of meningococcal disease and/or sepsis. The GP administered parenteral benzyl penicillin and secured intravenous access before Martha was transported to hospital by ambulance. Martha was accompanied by her mother who was extremely anxious about her daughter's condition. She was concerned that her child's hands and feet were very cold and remarked on her pale, mottled skin. Although Martha was constantly crying she was, according to her mother, becoming drowsy.

The history given by Martha's mother and the GP's initial diagnosis of meningococcal disease and/or sepsis and subsequent administration of parenteral benzyl penicillin suggests that this child's condition is critical.

Note two major clinical forms of meningococcal disease are **meningitis** and **septicaemia** but most will have a mixed presentation. Meningitis can be bacterial or viral with the bacterial causes of infection including *Neisseria meningitidis*, *Meningococcus*, *Streptococcus pneumoniae*, *Escherichia coli*, *Staphylococcus aureus*, and *Haemophilus influenzae* type B (Alamarat & Hasbun 2020). Meningococcal disease is not only associated with increased risk of mortality but also long-term morbidity. Despite the successful introduction of the serogroup meningococcal vaccines since 1999, meningococcal disease still remains one of the leading causes of death from infection in early childhood globally (Wright et al. 2021).

The disease has an early non-specific stage, with signs such as fever, lethargy, irritability, nausea, and poor feeding. Cold extremities and abnormal skin colour are associated with developing invasive meningococcal disease (Thompson et al. 2006), which progresses rapidly to clinical meningitis and/or septicaemia. Clinical meningitis is characterised by fever, lethargy, vomiting, headache, photophobia, neck stiffness, and positive Kernig's sign and Brudzinski's sign. Petechiae or purpura may also be present. Meningococcal septicaemia is characterised by fever, petechiae, purpura, and shock.

Care Planning in Children and Young People's Nursing, Second Edition. Edited by Sonya Clarke and Doris Corkin.
© 2024 John Wiley & Sons Ltd. Published 2024 by John Wiley & Sons Ltd.

Sepsis is a leading cause of morbidity and mortality in children worldwide and is defined as life-threatening organ dysfunction caused by a dysregulated host response to infection (Singer et al. 2016). Sepsis with shock is a life-threatening condition, and in 2020 the Surviving Sepsis Campaign proposed a definition for septic shock in children: 'severe infection leading to cardiovascular dysfunction (including hypotension, need for treatment with a vasoactive medication, or impaired perfusion)'. Early identification and appropriate resuscitation and management are therefore critical to optimising outcomes for children with sepsis (Surviving Sepsis Campaign 2020).

Over the past decade there has been a significant improvement in survival from sepsis in the developed world. This has been attributed to the fact that the basic principles of sepsis have become widely accepted, in part by global initiatives such as the Surviving Sepsis Campaign (2020) and the formulation of national guidelines such as NICE NG51 (2016).

The main principles of progressive sepsis care are:

- early recognition of sepsis
- appropriate balanced resuscitation
- rapid identification of the source of infection
- timely source control
- early and effective antimicrobial therapy
- haemodynamic support, consideration of adjunctive therapies and high-quality supportive care.

(Jackson & Cairns 2021)

Martha's symptoms would suggest that she has progressed from the non-specific early stage of meningococcal disease and is rapidly developing disease patterns associated with meningococcal septicaemia.

Achieving the best possible outcomes for Martha as previously stated requires rapid and systematic clinical assessment to detect physiological instability so that timely, prompt, and aggressive resuscitation and stabilisation will occur before the onset of organ failure. However, improving health outcomes for this child lies outside the scope of any single practitioner (Headrick et al. 1998). This assumption remains very evident in emergency care situations when the number of professionals involved and the importance of their ability to work collaboratively increases with the complexity of the child's condition. The delivery of high-quality care with optimal patient safety in these situations is dependent on effective interprofessional team management. This highlights the need for developing interprofessional working models (DH 2005), whereby expertise in assessment, planning, and treatment interventions are timely and promote stabilisation of the critically ill child. Interprofessional team-based models of care bring a range of professionals together to share different knowledge and experiences and aim to bridge gaps and negotiate overlaps in roles and minimise risk (Schot et al. 2020).

INTERPROFESSIONAL WORKING

A powerful incentive for greater teamwork among professionals is created when there is respect and understanding of the role of each of the team members and recognition of the unique contribution of each individual in a critical care situation. In a well-practised team, each member knows in advance their role and regards the leader as the person who co-ordinates, directs the assessment, and consults with other members regarding problem identification and subsequent care or management planning. Therefore interprofessional working models require that the level of equality of esteem and power in formal decision-making is balanced within the professional roles of doctor and nurse (Stocker et al. 2016). Indeed effective multidisciplinary team working is at the heart of providing high quality and safe care (DHSSPS 2007).

The role of education in encouraging interprofessional working is crucial in promoting collaboration, team working, and establishing roles and responsibilities (WHO 2010), particularly in a critical care situation. Education and competency-based training of interprofessional teams should include recognition of the acutely ill child, clinical assessment, appropriate interventions, and recognition of deterioration whereby senior assistance becomes necessary. Simulation as an educational strategy involves not only technological and computerised facilities, but includes important human interactions. High fidelity simulation using Simbaby provides opportunities for users at all levels, from novice to expert, to practice and develop skills with the knowledge that mistakes carry no penalties or fear of harm to patients or learners (Bradley 2006; Corkin & Morrow 2011).

Using simulations within an interprofessional educational programme seeks to provide participants with a meaningful learning experience and has become increasingly recognised as having great potential in delivering elements of healthcare education (Bradley 2006; McNaughten et al. 2020). It integrates the cognitive, psychomotor, and affective domains in a non-threatening and safe environment (Underberg 2003). Irrespective of a healthcare practitioner's chosen speciality, cognitive and psychomotor skills pertinent to assessing a patient's respiratory function, cardiovascular status, and level of pain must be acquired (Rogers et al. 2001). Human patient simulators enable the replication of rarely witnessed critical events, ensuring all healthcare practitioners are exposed to the same standard of training. In addition, complex skills such as communication, critical thinking and decision-making, and team working thus receive attention.

Interprofessional development of protocols for the assessment and management of the sick child include physiological warning systems, whereby clinical parameters outside the normal ranges (see Table 8.1) indicating deterioration are subsequently detected and medical interventions can be implemented at an early stage.

The Glasgow Meningococcal Septicaemia Prognostic Scoring Tool is a scoring system which may determine the severity of the child's illness and subsequent deterioration (see Table 8.2).

Note the UK Sepsis 6 Trust Screening Tool (Nutbeam & Daniels 2022) can be used to support the implementation of the National Institute for Health and Clinical Excellence guidelines (2019), for management of sepsis and identification of early warning signs (see Table 8.3).

Agreed assessment methods must consider the unpredictability of the timeframe, the multiple parameters that require observation and the swift spiral effect of deterioration in the sick child (Teasdale 2009). Prioritisation and effective action requires identification of one's own limitations and promptly identifying the most appropriate person within the multidisciplinary team to carry out an appropriate assessment and ensure that immediate action is taken (DHSSPS 2007).

This requires the utilisation of an effective communication tool such as SBAR. This is a situational briefing model which uses a clear structure ensuring the provision of all relevant information organized in a logical fashion (Lee et al. 2016). It helps ensure that important information is transmitted in a predictable structure, when summoning senior nursing and medical staff when support for the management of a child's deteriorating condition is vital. The SBAR tool is regarded as a communication technique that increases patient safety and is current 'best practice' to deliver information in critical situations (Muller et al. 2018).

Table 8.1 Normal ranges (Meningitis Research Foundation 2010).

Age	Respiratory rate	Heart rate	Systolic BP
< 1	30–40	110–160	70–90
1–2	25–35	110–150	80–95
2–5	25–30	95–140	80–100
5–12	20–25	80–120	90–110
> 12	15–20	60–100	100–120

Table 8.2 Glasgow meningococcal septicaemia prognostic scoring tool (Scottish Intercollegiate Guidelines Network 2008).

Clinical signs	Points
BP < 75 mmHg systolic, age < 4 y < 85 mmHg systolic, age > 4 y	3
Skin/rectal temperature difference > 3°C	3
Modified coma scale score < 8 or Deterioration of > or =3 points in 1 hour	3
Deterioration in hour before scoring	2
Absence of meningism	2
Extending purpuric rash or widespread ecchymoses	1
Base deficit (capillary or arterial) >8.0	1
Maximum score	15

Add scores to give result Score > or = to 8, or an escalating score is indicative of serious and rapidly progressing disease.

Table 8.3 UK Sepsis Trust Screening Tool for under 5s (https://sepsistrust.org).

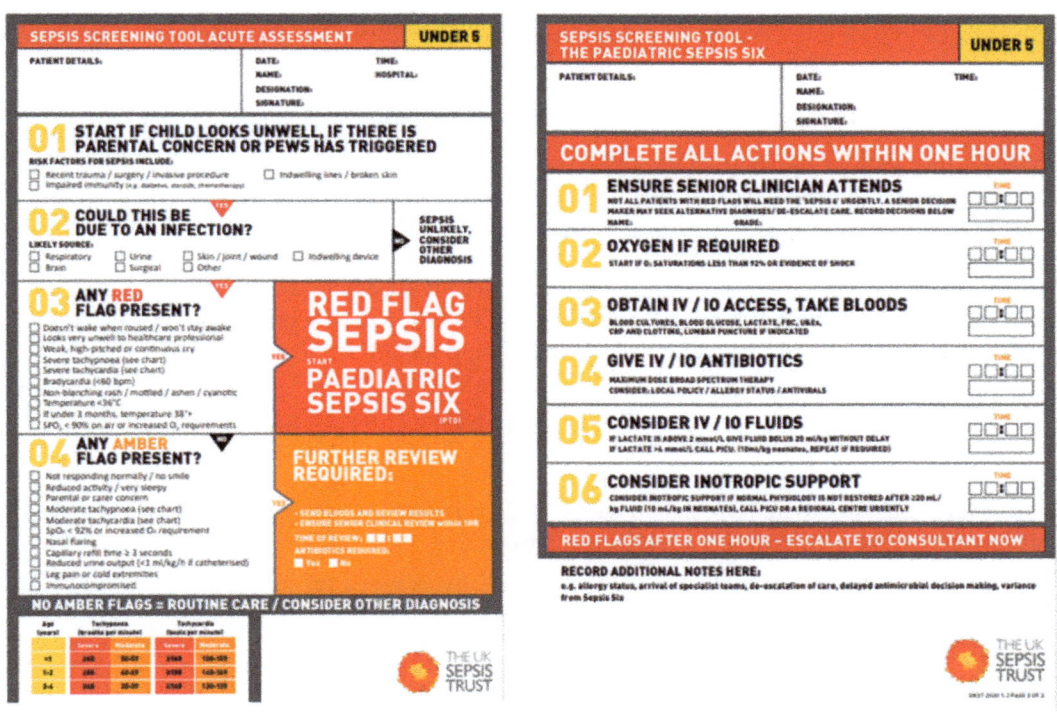

SBAR stands for the following (Leonard et al. 2004);

- S = Situation (a concise statement of the problem)
- B = Background (circumstances leading up to situation or clinical background)
- A = Assessment (analysis and consideration of options – what you found/think)
- R = Recommendation (action requested/recommended – what you want)

IMMEDIATE ASSESSMENT OF THE CRITICALLY ILL CHILD

The hospital ward or emergency department will have been informed of Martha's anticipated arrival and this provides an opportunity for the nursing and medical team to prepare for immediate assessment and management of her clinical state in a systematic and organised way. Do refer to activity 8.1 and 8.2.

ACTIVITY 8.1

With reference to the SBAR model, write down what you consider necessary to report regarding Martha's condition when communicating with the doctor.

ACTIVITY 8.2

Based on the formula, work out Martha's estimated weight and WETFLAG values.

The hospital environment where the child is admitted to will have:

- Facilities to ensure adherence to infection control procedures.
- Oxygen and suction with correct size of masks/catheters.
- Emergency equipment available and an appropriately stocked resuscitation trolley with the necessary drugs and fluids.

Fluid volumes, drug dosages, and correct equipment size will depend on the weight of the child. Martha's mother may know what her weight is; if not then it may be worked out quickly to avoid delay in treatment interventions. A formula for estimating weight in kilograms is:

$$\text{Weight}(kg) = (\text{age} + 4) \times 2$$

A WETFLAG mnemonic can be prepared with the specific calculations relating to the child prior to their arrival. This is a clinical aid memoire used to reduce risk in emergency calculations (Sherif et al. 2021).

- **W** – Weight (kg)
- **E** – Energy (4 Joules/kg)
- **T** – Endotracheal Tube Size (Age/4 + 4)
- **F** – Fluids (10 ml/kg or 20 ml/kg)
- **L** – Lorazepam (0.1 mg/kg)
- **A** – Adrenaline (0.1 ml/kg of 1:10,000)
- **G** – Glucose (2 ml/kg 10% Dextrose)

Assessment of the child will be rapid and sequential, with simultaneous management of life-threatening problems as they arise. Evaluation and systematic reassessment after each treatment intervention is essential. A combination of clinical features, laboratory results, ongoing monitoring, and repeated assessment over time provide a foundation for predicting progress and informing care planning and treatment (SIGN 2008).

Martha's mother must be supported and encouraged to remain with her daughter and provided with information about her condition. Her concerns must be seriously considered and investigated.

The use of the structured ABCDE approach promoted by the Resuscitation Council UK (2021) is a framework that helps when assessing and monitoring, to ensure that potentially life-threatening problems are identified and dealt with in order of priority.

ABCDE ASSESSMENT FRAMEWORK

ASSESSMENT OF AIRWAY

The aim is to assess if the airway is patent or if there are signs of obstruction as indicated by difficulty in breathing, increased respiratory effort, and noisy breathing, for example stridor, wheeze, coughing, or grunting. Silence may be a sign of complete obstruction. Do refer to Box 8.1 to 8.4.

Assessment is based on the following observations:

- Detect airway obstruction – look at the child's chest/abdomen for signs of respiratory movement.
- Listen to breathing sounds and feel for air movement at the child's face and mouth.
- Assess child's responsiveness and ability to talk, cry, or cough.
- Unless contraindicated, assess for possible cause of airway obstruction by looking in the mouth for gastric contents or mucous.

    Martha is crying at the time of initial assessment which indicates patency of airway.

ASSESSMENT OF BREATHING AND VENTILATION

The aim in assessing breathing and ventilation is to determine whether there is adequate gas exchange to provide sufficient oxygen for Martha's tissue requirements and prevent her from developing respiratory acidosis.
    Assessment is based on observation of:

- The work of breathing, as it may be compromised due to pulmonary oedema resulting from capillary leakage.
- Body position and visual movements of chest and abdomen and breathing pattern.
- Use of accessory muscles.
- Evidence of minimal movement of chest wall.
- Sternal supraclavicular substernal or intercostal recession.

BOX 8.1 PROBLEM IDENTIFICATION

Potential problem for obstruction due to intense muscle contraction associated with the release of tumour necrosis factor and other inflammatory mediators. Secretions such as vomitus may further impede the airway.
    A progressive developing hypoxic state will result in apnoea.

Goal: to maintain patency of the airway to ensure adequate respiratory ventilation to prevent hypoxia, vital organ failure, and cardiorespiratory arrest.

Care interventions with rationale

- Observe Martha for signs of airway obstruction – if obstruction is evident place child in supine position.
- Open the airway by performing a jaw thrust or chin lift manoeuvre and head tilt – check for possible airway obstruction.
- Clear excessive secretions, vomitus or other secretions using appropriate size and type of suction catheter, maintaining suction pressure as low as possible and taking care to prevent adverse effects such as hypoxia.
- If Martha's airway becomes compromised insert correctly sized airway adjunct, for example Guedel airway (oropharyngeal airway) to open a channel between the base of the tongue and posterior pharyngeal wall (Resuscitation Council 2021).
- If airway patency cannot be maintained tracheal intubation will be required to be carried out in a controlled and safe environment.

BOX 8.2 PROBLEM IDENTIFICATION

Martha is presenting with signs of increasing hypoxia as indicated by increased respiratory rate and effort.

She has the potential to become fatigued if hypoxia state persists, with progression to respiratory failure and bradypnoea.

Goal: to immediately ensure effective delivery of oxygen through a patent airway to maintain O_2 saturations above 95% and prevent metabolic acidosis, cellular damage, and cell death from hypoxia.

Care interventions with rationale

- Apply high flow oxygen 10–15 litres through a non-rebreather oxygen facemask to ensure Martha receives adequate oxygenation to allow normal metabolism of cells.
- Attach pulse oximetry to assess oxygen saturations which aim to be maintained above 92–95%.
- A reading below 92% for Martha with 100% mask oxygen could be an indication that she requires assisted ventilation.
- Respiratory rate, heart rate, and oxygen saturations should be monitored relative to the child's condition and accurately documented.
- Reference to early warning scoring system to ascertain clinical deterioration.
- Support respiratory effort by nursing Martha, who is distressed, in upright position unless her clinical state contraindicates this position.
- Keep communicating with the multidisciplinary team informing them of Martha's condition.
- If breathing is absent or if Martha is hypoventilating, that is, with slow respiratory rate or weak respiratory effort, she should be supported with oxygen by valve mask device and an airway adjunct needs to be inserted. Effective bag-mask ventilation remains the cornerstone of providing effective emergency ventilation (Nadkarni & Berg 2009).
- If Martha is exhausted and needs ongoing respiratory support or cardiorespiratory arrest is imminent tracheal intubation will be necessary.

BOX 8.3 PROBLEM IDENTIFICATION

Martha is presenting with signs of compensated shock as indicated by tachycardia and tachypnoea. Her cold hands and feet and skin colour represent changes in peripheral circulation and are the early symptoms of sepsis (Thompson et al. 2006).

Potential problem of progressing to decompensated shock which will be evident if Martha presents with bradycardia and lowered blood pressure and increased capillary refill time.

Goal: to immediately enhance circulatory function to provide adequate delivery of O_2 and nutrients to meet the metabolic demands of tissues.

Care interventions with rationale

- Monitor the heart rate, pulse quality, and skin temperature, oxygen saturations and blood pressure. Compare findings on Paediatric Early Warning Score Chart or Glasgow Meningococcal Septicaemia Prognostic Scoring Tool, see Table 8.2 and report to medical team.
- Assist in obtaining additional vascular access and blood samples if possible.
- Monitor capillary refill, which is normally less than two seconds. If >2 seconds then assist in administering immediate fluid resuscitation of **10–20** ml fluid/kg of a balanced isotonic crystalloid, for example, Plasmolyte or alternatively 0.9% Normal saline, administered usually as a bolus infusion to restore circulating volume, blood pressure, and tissue perfusion. **Reassess following administration of fluid bolus.**
- Continue to monitor heart rate, blood pressure, peripheral perfusion, and oxygen saturations throughout fluid resuscitation and report.
- Maintain accurate record of fluid input and output.
- Follow prescription for required fluid maintenance – see Table 8.4. However, it may be necessary to restrict fluids so recheck prescription and discuss with the doctor if concerned.
- Check blood glucose as increased cellular activity increases the metabolic demands for glucose. Hypoglycaemia may cause seizures.
- After each treatment intervention reassessment of Martha's status is necessary to ascertain response or identify further deterioration.
- Call senior medical staff and additional nursing support if concerned.
- If the pulse rate falls below 60 and there are no or minimal signs of life commence cardiopulmonary resuscitation.

Intraosseous access may be necessary to deliver fluids and emergency drugs such as inotropic support, which may be administered to increase contractility of the heart and cardiac output. The child would need to be **transferred to paediatric intensive care** for further management (NICE 2018).

Table 8.4 IV Fluid Therapy in children and young people within hospital (NICE 2015).

Body weight	Daily fluid requirement ml/kg	Hourly fluid requirement ml/kg
First 10 kg	100	4
Second 10 kg	50	2
Subsequent kg	20	1

BOX 8.4 PROBLEM IDENTIFICATION

Martha is presenting with signs of early neurological impairment as she is irritable but becoming drowsy and is vomiting.

Goal: to recognise early signs of neurological disturbance, that is, raised intracranial pressure, so that treatment interventions aimed at preventing complications of hypoxia and hypoperfusion may be commenced.

Care interventions with rationale

- Maintain oxygenation to ensure adequate oxygen perfusion to Martha's brain.

- Monitor blood glucose levels to ensure they are maintained within normal limits to prevent seizure activity.

- Monitor temperature and administer antipyretic drugs as prescribed to prevent seizure activity (NICE 2019).

- Assess neurological status using the APVU scoring system and Glasgow Coma Scale to detect signs of raised intracranial pressure.

- Immediately summon medical assistance if there are signs of raised intracranial pressure – if Martha becomes drowsy, pupils are abnormal, pulse rate decreases, or presents with seizures.

- Assist in preparation and checking of drugs for administration. Initial antibiotic treatment will commence before definitive microbiological diagnosis. This is crucial for optimising the outcome of bacterial meningitis (Holub et al. 2007).

- Prepare child and family for lumbar puncture if considered necessary by the doctor to obtain sample of cerebral spinal fluid for diagnostic purposes to determine causative organisms and sensitivities to antibiotic treatments.

- Presence of nasal flaring.
- Respiratory rate fast, slow, or normal – see Table 8.1 for normal respiratory rate values according to age. Tachypnoea is the first indication of respiratory insufficiency.
- Evidence of central cyanosis indicates severe hypoxia and is a pre-terminal state.
- Air movement if audible on auscultation.
- Arterial oxygen saturation, although this may be unreliable when a child has poor peripheral circulation. A saturation of <90% in room air or <95% in supplemental oxygen indicates respiratory failure.

ASSESSMENT OF CIRCULATION

The aim is to assess adequate cardiovascular function to maintain oxygenation and tissue perfusion.

Assessment is based on observation of the following:

- Hypovolaemia, due to increased vascular permeability causing water and plasma proteins to leak out of capillaries as indicated by:
- Skin colour for pallor or mottling.
- Cold hands and feet due to vasoconstriction, which reduces blood flow to the skin, which in turn increases capillary refill time.
- Respiratory function, as previously indicated for increased respiratory rate.
- Pulse rate for indication of tachycardia or bradycardia.

- Pulse quality reflects the adequacy of peripheral perfusion. A weak central pulse may indicate decompensated shock and a peripheral pulse that is difficult to find, weak or irregular suggests poor peripheral perfusion and maybe a sign of shock.
- Blood pressure – see Table 8.1 for ranges across the age span. Low recording is an indication of decompensated shock.

HYPONATRAEMIA

Children and young people are sensitive to dehydration/volume depletion and have different fluid requirements compared to adults. As children's total body water composition may be up to 75–80% of their body weight, they are more prone to water and electrolyte imbalance than young adults, particularly during periods of acute illness (Stewart et al. 2018). Intravenous (IV) fluids can be harmful in these patients and it is important that healthcare professionals understand the principles of paediatric fluid prescription and administration. Whether IV fluid therapy is needed for fluid resuscitation, routine maintenance, replacement, or redistribution, it is vital that the correct composition, volume, and timing of IV fluid therapy is used (NICE 2015).

Hyponatraemia is one of the most common electrolyte abnormalities in children and is defined as a sodium level of less than 135 mmol/l. Regarding important blood values for infants, children, and young people, please check with local hospital laboratory as ranges can vary between age groups (RCPCH 2016). The normal range for Sodium levels in serum is 135–146 mmol/l. It represents an excess of water in relation to sodium in extracellular fluid and is described as severe or significant if below 130 mmol/l. Hyponatraemia can result in cerebral oedema causing neurological symptoms and significant morbidity and mortality. Warning signs may be non-specific and include confusion, irritation, reduced consciousness, and headache. As symptoms are generalized it is important to take on board parents' views of changes in their child (DoH 2019). All children are potentially at risk of hyponatraemia therefore any child or young person receiving IV fluid therapy requires precise measurement of fluid and electrolyte status to ensure they are prescribed the appropriate fluid (NICE 2015).

ASSESSMENT OF DISABILITY

Review care planning (see Chapter 16), for reference to detailed disability assessment to identify Martha's neurological status, which may be deranged as a result of respiratory failure, cardiovascular failure, and her neurological condition, meningitis. Meningitis causes severe inflammation of the meninges and capillary leak, which gives rise to fluid and electrolyte imbalance. This causes fluid shift and predisposes the child to developing cerebral oedema, thus raising intracranial pressure. Inadequate oxygen perfusion of the brain as a result of shock causes altered levels of consciousness. Hypoglycaemia and high body temperature may cause seizure activity.

Assessment is rapid and is determined by:

- The APVU score (Resuscitation Council 2021)
  - **A** alert
  - **P** response to painful stimuli
  - **V** response to voice
  - **U** unresponsive
- Ongoing monitoring using the Glasgow Coma Scale
- Appropriate pain assessment tools
- Kernig's and Brudzinski's signs as indicated previously are positive in a child with meningococcal meningitis
- Neck stiffness and photophobia may be evident

Glasgow Meningococcal Septicaemic Prognostic Scoring Tool (see Table 8.2) will determine the severity of Martha's condition.

EXPOSURE

To carry out an assessment of the body for signs of bruising, rashes or other skin abnormalities the child will need to be exposed for a brief period of time. Rashes will require further assessment to determine if it is non-blanching as this may be an indication of septicaemia. A rash may develop in minutes or initially present as a blanching, maculopapular rash. A generalised petechial rash, or a purpuric rash in any location, in an ill child is strongly suggestive of meningococcal septicaemia (Theilen et al. 2008).

Those who have been exposed to prolonged contact in a household setting with a child with meningococcal disease during the seven days before the onset of illness should be offered chemoprophylaxis. Chemoprophylaxis should be offered to healthcare workers who have been directly exposed to droplet or respiratory secretions during the acute illness phase, prior to completion of 24 hours of antibiotic (SIGN 2008).

DEBRIEFING

Debriefing after Martha's clinical status has been stabilised is an important reflective process for individuals involved and for the team. The process of debriefing allows interprofessional teams to reflect on their experience, support each other, share perspectives, identify learning opportunities, and agree on improvement needs (Diaz-Navarro et al. 2021). This creates opportunities for shared learning across disciplines as well as identifying the need for improvement in practices, which ultimately contributes to promoting safe effective care for the critically ill child.

POSSIBLE CHALLENGES OF CARING

The children's nurse has a professional duty to be open and honest and communicate challenging information (Crawford et al. 2020). However, it may be difficult to navigate the legal, ethical, and emotional issues of caring for a critically ill child, especially when there are disputes with parents over medical treatment and/or withdrawal in the best interests of the child, is being considered (Huxtable 2018):

- Appreciate decisions are not taken lightly – most cases will not need to go to court.
- Trust, clear communication skills and shared decision-making important to avoid conflict.
- Nurse must ensure documentation is in order, as Coroner may request a written report.
- Emotional intelligence will be key, remember link with professional body.
- Important that healthcare staff involved in cases reflect and learn from challenging situations.

SUMMARY

Enhancing patient safety requires timely, effective team working and collaboration, whereby formal decision-making and care interventions are informed by the knowledge and skills within each of the professional roles.

Achieving the best possible outcomes for a critically ill child requires rapid and systematic clinical assessment to detect physiological instability, so that prompt and aggressive resuscitation and stabilisation will occur before the onset of organ failure. In emergency care situations there is a need for interprofessional working models, whereby expertise in assessment, planning, and treatment interventions are timely and promote stabilisation of the critically ill child. The use of the structured ABCDE approach (Resuscitation Council 2021) as a framework will help ensure that potentially life-threatening problems are identified and dealt with in order of priority. Debriefing after a critical care event will enable professionals to reflect on their practice and identify strategies which may improve future care management of the critically ill child.

REFERENCES

Alamarat, Z. & Hasbun, R. (2020) Management of acute bacterial meningitis in children. *Infection and Drug Resistance*, Nov 11(13), 4077–4089.

Bradley, P. (2006) The history of simulation in medical education and possible future directions. *Medical Education*, **40**, 254–262.

Corkin, D. & Morrow, P. (2011) Interprofessional education: sustaining simulation in practice. *Education Through Simulation News*, (14), 1–3. www.laerdal.co.uk.

Crawford, D., Corkin, D. & McKenzie, G. (2020) Equipping children's nurses to de-escalate conflict and communicate challenging information. *Nursing Children and Young Children* doi: 10.7748.

Department of Health (2005) *Creating a Patient-Led NHS*. Department of Health. London: Stationery Office.

Department of Health (NI) Regional Paediatric Fluid Management Group (2019) Regional Policy for the Administration of Intravenous Fluids to Children Aged from Birth (Term) until Their 16th Birthday: Reducing the Risk of Harm Due to Hyponatraemia. HSS(MD)2/2020. Belfast: Health and Social Care (HSC).

Department of Health and Social Services and Public Safety (DHSSPS) (2007) *Promotion of Safe, High Quality Health and Social Care in Undergraduate Curricula*. London: Stationery Office.

Diaz-Navarro, C., Leon-Castelao, E., Hadfield, A., Pierce, S. & Szyld, D. (2021) Clinical debriefing: TALK© to learn and improve together in healthcare environments. *Trends in Anaesthesia and Critical Care*, **40**, 4–8.

Headrick, L.A., Wilcock, P.M. & Batalden, P.B. (1998) Interprofessional working and continuing medical education. *British Medical Journal*, **316**(7133), 1–9.

Holub, M., Beran, O., Dzupova, O. et al. (2007) Cortisol levels in cerebrospinal fluid correlate with severity and bacterial origin of meningitis. *Critical Care*, **11**(2), 1–9. https://www.researchgate.net/publication/6421708_Cortisol_levels_in_cerebrospinal_fluid_correlate_with_severity_and_bacterial_origin_of_meningitis [Accessed 30 September 2022].

Huxtable, R. (2018) Clinic, courtroom or (specialist) committee: In the best interests of the critically ill child? *Journal of Medical Ethics*, **44**(7), 471–475.

Jackson, M. & Cairns, T. (2021) Care of the critically ill patient. *Surgery (Oxf)*, Jan **39**(1), 29–36.

Lee, S.Y., Dong, L. & Lim, Y.H. (2016) SBAR: towards a common interprofessional team based communication tool. *Medical Education*, **50**, 1167–1168.

Leonard, M., Graham, S. & Bonacum, D. (2004) The human factor: the critical importance of effective teamwork and communication in providing safe effective care. *Quality and Safety in Health Care*, **13**, 85–90.

McNaughten, B., Storey, L., Corkin, D., Cardwell, P., Thompson, A., Bourke, T. & O'Donoghue, D. (2020) Familiarity with the clinical environment, achieved by priming, improves time to antibiotic administration in a simulated paediatric sepsis scenario: a randomized control trial. *Archives of Disease in Childhood* Published Online First: 14th July 2020. doi:10.1136/archdischild-2020-318904

Meningitis Research Foundation (2010) Algorithm, 8thA edn. Management of Meningococcal Disease in Children and Young People. Meningitis Research Foundation. www.meningitis.org [Accessed 19th September 2022].

Müller, M., Jürgens, J., Redaèlli, M., Klingberg, K., Hautz, W. & Stock, S. (2018) Impact of the communication and patient hand-off tool SBAR on patient safety: a systematic review. *BMJ Open*, **8**(8), 1–10.

Nadel, S. & Kroll, J.S. (2007) Diagnosis and management of meningococcal disease: the need for centralised care. Federation of European Microbiological Societies. *Microbiological Review*, **31**, 71–83.

Nadkarni, V.M., Berg, R.A. (2009) Pediatric cardiopulmonary resuscitation. In: Wheeler et al. (ed). *Resuscitation and Stabilization of the Critically Ill Child*. London: Springer-Verlag.

National Institute Clinical Excellence (NICE) (2015) *IV Fluid Therapy in Children and Young People in Hospital NG29*. London: NICE.

National Institute Clinical Excellence (NICE) (2016) *Sepsis: Recognition, Diagnosis and Early Management NG51*. London: NICE.

National Institute Clinical Excellence (NICE) (2019) *Fever in under 5's: Assessment and Initial Management NG143*. London: NICE.

National Institute for Health and Care Excellence (NICE) (2018) *Bacterial Meningitis and Meningococcal Septicaemia in Children*. London: NICE.

New RCPCH reference ranges (2016) https://www.rcpch.ac.uk/sites/default/files/rcpch/HTWQ/Reference%20ranges%20Jan%2018.pdf.

Nutbeam, T. & Daniels, R. on behalf of the UK Sepsis trust. Available at sepsistrust.org/professional-resources/clinical [date last Accessed 30th September 2022].

Resuscitation Council (UK) (2021) *Paediatric Advanced Life Support Guidelines*. London: Resuscitation Council (UK).

Rogers, P.L., Jacob, H., Rashwan, A.S. & Pnsky, M.R. (2001) Quantifying learning in medical students during a critical care medicine elective: a comparison of three evaluation instruments. *Critical Care Medicine*, **29**(6), 1268–1273.

Schot, E., Tummers, L. & Noordegraaf, M. (2020) Working on working together. A systematic review on how healthcare professionals contribute to interprofessional collaboration. *Journal of Interprofessional Care*, **34**(3), 332–342.

Scottish Intercollegiate Guidelines Network (SIGN) (2008) *Management of Invasive Meningococcal Disease in Children and Young People. A National Clinical Guideline*. Scotland: NHS.

Sherif, A.G., Cobb, S., Huxstep, K. & Goyal, S. (2021) WETFLAG-HDU: How a simple QI project can have high impact. *Archives of Disease in Childhood*, **106**, 106–107.

Singer, M., Deutschman, C.S., Seymour, C.W., Shankar-Hari, M., Annane, D., Bauer, M., Bellomo, R., Bernard, G.R., Chiche, J., Coopersmith, C.M., Hotchkiss, R.S., Levy, M.M., Marshall, J.C., Martin, G.S., Opal, S.M., Rubenfeld, G.D., van der Poll, T., Vincent, J. & Angus, D.C. (2016) The third international consensus definitions for sepsis and septic shock (Sepsis-3). *JAMA*, **315**(8), 801–810.

Stewart, C.J., Silvestre, C. & Vyas, H. (2018) Maintenance fluid management in paediatrics. *Paediatrics and Child Health*, **28**(7), 344–347.

Stocker, M., Pilgrim, S.B., Burmester, M., Allen, M.L. & Gijselaers, W.H. (2016) Interprofessional team management in pediatric critical care: some challenges and possible solutions. *Journal of Multidisciplinary Healthcare*, Feb 24(9), 47–58.

Weiss SL, Peters MJ, Alhazzani W, Agus MSD, Flori HR, Inwald DP, Nadel S, Schlapbach LJ, Tasker RC, Argent AC, Brierley J, Carcillo J, Carrol ED, Carroll CL, Cheifetz IM, Choong K, Cies JJ, Cruz AT, De Luca D, Deep A, Faust SN, De Oliveira CF, Hall MW, Ishimine P, Javouhey E, Joosten KFM, Joshi P, Karam O, Kneyber MCJ, Lemson J, MacLaren G, Mehta NM, Møller MH, Newth CJL, Nguyen TC, Nishisaki A, Nunnally ME, Parker MM, Paul RM, Randolph AG, Ranjit S, Romer LH, Scott HF, Tume LN, Verger JT, Williams EA, Wolf J, Wong HR, Zimmerman JJ, Kissoon N, Tissieres P. (2020) Surviving sepsis campaign international guidelines for the management of septic shock and sepsis-associated organ dysfunction in children. *Pediatric Critical Care Medicine*, Feb **21**(2), e52–e106. doi: 10.1097/PCC.0000000000002198PMID: 32032273

Teasdale, D. (2009) Chapter 2. In: Dixon, M., Crawford, D., Teasdale, D. and Murphy, J. (eds). *Nursing the Highly Dependent Child or Infant*. London: Wiley-Blackwell.

Theilen, U., Wilson, L., Wilson, G., Beattie, J.O., Qureshi, S. & Simpson, D. (2008) Management of invasive meningococcal disease in children and young people: summary of SIGN guidelines. *British Medical Journal*, **336**, 1367–1370.

Thompson, M.J., Ninis, N., Perera, R., Mayon-White, R., Phillips, C., Bailey, L. & Harnden, A. (2006) Clinical recognition of meningococcal disease in children and adolescents. *Lancet*, **367**, 397–403.

Underberg, K.E. (2003) Experiential learning and simulation in health care education. *Surgical Services Management*, **9**(4), 31–36.

World Health Organisation (WHO) (2010) *Framework for Action on Interprofessional Education and Collaborative Practice*. Geneva: Department of Human Resources for Health, WHO.

Wright, C., Blake, N., Glennie, L., Smith, V., Bender, R., Kyu, H., Wunrow, H.Y., Liu, L., Yeung, D., Knoll, M.D., Wahl, B., Stuart, J.M. & Trotter, C. (2021) The global burden of meningitis in children: Challenges with interpreting global health estimates. *Microorganisms*, Feb 13 **9**(2), 377.

CHAPTER 9

Supporting the Planning of Care – Practice Assessor, Academic Assessor, Supervisor, and Student

Nuala Devlin

In 2018 the Nursing and Midwifery Council (NMC) published the Standards of Proficiency (NMC 2018a) and *Standards for Student Supervision and Assessment* (SSSA) (NMC 2018b) which superseded the Standards *to Support Learning and Assessment in Practice* (NMC 2006, 2008), which reflected the response to two earlier consultations on the standards themselves and on fitness to practice at the point of registration (NMC 2005; UKCC 1999). This new framework adopted by all universities in partnership with placement providers encompasses undergraduate, post-graduate, and associate nursing (England only) (NMC 2018).[1] It recognises the important and varied roles that registrants and other healthcare professionals contribute to the student's journey, offering flexibility and richness to the student's practice learning experience. A student will now be supported by practice supervisors (PS), practice assessors (PA), and academic assessors (AA). These roles will support the student in practice working collaboratively to support and guide the student's progression through theory and practice. Registrants who were previously mentors and sign off mentors as per the SLiAP standards (NMC 2006, 2008) will undertake training and transition to practice assessors and supervisors.

Registrants have a key role in supporting nursing students in practice (Aston & Hallam 2011). Elcock and Sookhoo (2007) suggest that the quality of support in pre-registration nursing education is highly variable and at times may be a cause for concern, particularly since registrants are the people assessing nursing students' fitness for practice at the point of registration, crucially separating the roles of supervision and assessment. Under this new framework, three new roles have been set up to support the student in practice. These roles are defined under the SSSA (NMC 2018) as practice supervisors (PS), practice assessors (PA), and academic assessors (AA). Working collaboratively these roles will support the student's progression in both theory and practice.

PRACTICE SUPERVISOR	• The practice supervisor can be any health and social care registrant who will understand the programme the student is undertaking. • The role is similar to the earlier mentor role as they will support and supervise the student, that said, they will not be assessing the student's competency. • They will supply feedback on the student's performance, acting as a role model within their own professional code. • Raise and respond to any concerns or issues relating to conduct and competence.

(NMC 2018a)

The ability and flexibility of working with practice supervisors will enrich the nursing students' practice learning environments. This unique perspective will offer the student nurse insight into the roles of other members of the multi-disciplinary team (MDT). Aiding the student in the practice environment, the PS will help the student show learning opportunities and link in with other practice supervisors where appropriate, to combine that knowledge. Crucially the PS will provide the student with feedback on your knowledge, skills, and professional attitude. They will provide feedback to the nursing students' practice assessor naming areas of achievement along with areas for future development.

Care Planning in Children and Young People's Nursing, Second Edition. Edited by Sonya Clarke and Doris Corkin.
© 2024 John Wiley & Sons Ltd. Published 2024 by John Wiley & Sons Ltd.

<ul><li>Will be a registered nurse</li><li>Have undertaken training in preparation of the role and be suitably prepared to assess nursing students in practice.</li><li>They will understand the student's programme including proficiencies, programme outcomes, and the assessment process.</li><li>The student will have a different practice assessor for each assessed part of the programme.</li></ul>	**PRACTICE ASSESSOR**

(NMC 2018b)

The practice assessor should be assigned to the student at the start of the placement, and they will handle the overall assessment in practice. They will provide the student with constructive feedback and their assessment of the student should be objective and evidence based, considering feedback from practice supervisors and other members of the team. They will oversee the placement opportunities working with the practice supervisor to ensure that the student can avail of all necessary opportunities. They will make an informed decision about the nursing students' progression, supplying detailed and constructive feedback to the nursing students in relation to their achievements and areas for further development. They will communicate with the academic assessor (AA) developing an action plan to help the student achieve the identified goals. A practice assessor needs to have some extremely specific skills to reflect what Nash and Scammell (2010) describe as essential in pre-registration supervision. These include knowledge of learning theory, including adult learning; practice-based teaching and assessment; integration of theory and practice; and a knowledge and insight of the curriculum, as well as developed communication and relationship skill (Nash & Scammell 2010).

Will be a registered nurse<ul><li>Understand your progression in practice.</li><li>Collate and confirm achievement of academic proficiencies.</li><li>Work in partnership with the PA to review and recommend (or not) the nursing students' progression to the next part of the programme.</li><li>The academic assessor will be one of the academic staff from the student's university.</li><li>The student cannot have the same academic assessor for two consecutive parts of the programme.</li></ul>	**ACADEMIC ASSESSOR**

(NMC 2018b)

The academic assessor will be familiar with the student's programme of study. Their role is to support the practice assessor and ensure that the student has received an objective assessment of their performance. The academic assessor should check that all feedback has been considered and that the practice assessor is an appropriately prepared registered nurse. The focus of the AA is one of collaboration and partnership, working with the practice setting and liaising with practice education facilitators, placing an emphasis on the support of practice assessors and practice supervisors in the assessing and supervising of nursing students in practice. These roles have a wide remit to enhance the quality of the practice learning experience and positively contribute to the development of a well-educated and practice-competent future nursing/midwifery workforce. It is important to recognise that practice assessors and practice supervisors support nursing students and help to ease learning by identifying goals, programmes of learning, and negotiating action plans. Assessment and the provision of prompt and proper feedback are vital to the role and any challenging issues are discussed and managed. It is hoped that the introduction of these roles will provide the student with a more balanced approach to supervision and assessment in practice.

OTHER ROLES THAT WILL SUPPORT THE STUDENT IN PRACTICE

PRACTICE EDUCATION FACILITATOR

The focus of the practice education facilitator role is one of collaboration and partnership, working within the practice setting and liaising with higher education institutions, placing an emphasis on the support of mentors in the assessing and supervising of nursing students in practice. These roles have a wide dispatch to enhance the quality of the practice learning experience and positively contribute to the development of a well-educated and practice-competent future nursing/midwifery workforce. More specifically the role entails:

- Practice assessor and practice supervision support.
- Support for learning in practice.
- Ensuring the quality of the practice learning environment.
- Communication links between the practice setting and higher education institution (HEI).
- Involvement in updating practice assessors and practice supervisors.
- Supporting practice assessors and nursing students where there are concerns about a student's performance in practice and aiding with the documentation of this, for example creating action plans.
- Auditing practice placements in liaison with the HEIs and clinical areas.
- Working with clinical placement managers to manage the local register of available mentors, ensuring that staff are updated, and the records are exact.
- Advising practice assessors where a student has shown a support need.
- Maintaining the local register of mentors and devising teaching materials.
- Contributing to the teaching of the practice assessor and practice supervisors' preparation programme in partnership with the HEIs.

It is important to recognise that practice assessors and practice supervisors support nursing students and help to ease their learning by identifying goals, planning programmes of learning, and negotiating action plans. Assessment and the provision of prompt and proper feedback are vital to the role and any challenging issues are discussed and managed.

PERSONAL TUTOR

Within the university the student is assigned a personal tutor. The role of the personal tutor is to provide pastoral, professional, and academic support ('Guide to the Personal Tutoring Policy'). They will normally be assigned to the student throughout your programme. They will be able to signpost the student to additional support services if needed. They provide a safe space for the nursing students to discuss their progression. The roles and responsibilities of the personal tutor will be outlined in the student's course handbook and may differ slightly in institutions.

LINK LECTURER

The role of the link lecturer is to provide constant support to both the student and practice staff. Universities may differ slightly with the approach or titles (they may be known as, e.g., clinical teachers, practice tutors). They will be designated members of the university who are assigned to specific placement areas and will work collaboratively with the student, practice education facilitator, practice assessor, and practice supervisors to ensure that the student can avail of the necessary learning opportunities which are needed for this stage of the programme.

To enter the NMC, registered nurses must achieve the standards of proficiency in the practice of their specific field of nursing – in this case children's nursing. One of these standards under platform 4 is to:

> *Work in partnership with people to encourage shared decision making in order to support individuals, their families and carers to manage their own care when appropriate ("Nursing associate (NMC 2018) / Institute for ...").*
>
> *(NMC 2018 pg. 16)*

To illustrate the need for collaborative working between practice assessor, supervisor of the practice education facilitator, link lecturer in supporting student nurses in the practice setting, the following case study will explore the key points relating to the development of skills in care planning. The case study is taken from the perspective of a student not performing to the required standard of practice.

CASE STUDY

Jane is a registered children's nurse working in a busy medical ward within the regional children's hospital. Jane is the practice assessor for an undergraduate Children's and Young People second-year nursing student, Kelly, and has been working closely with her on several care planning issues which had been identified as a core clinical skill and is concerned that she is failing the placement. Having undertaken the Future Nurse Future Midwife training,[2] Jane has become more self-aware and has found that the student appears to be lacking in motivation and her performance appears to be declining. Working collaboratively, Jane contacted the LL, PA, and AA to ensure that there was transparency so that together they could discuss and explore the issues of concern with Kelly's performance. Jane is aware of the need to reflect on the situation to learn from it as this is an ongoing process and a means of new learning and understanding (Gibbs 1988).

Initially Jane felt the student was failing the placement, as she appeared disinterested, lacked motivation, and rarely asked questions about the care of patients on the ward. Through discussion and critical reflection with the AA several key points were raised, and Jane reflected on one episode when the student was being supervised as she gave advice to an 11-year-old girl who had been recently diagnosed with Type 1 diabetes.[3] Jane reflected on what she had seen throughout was the student ignored the patient and spoke directly to her parents. As a result, the student was unable to perform care planning safely and effectively as clearly identified in the student's ongoing record of achievement (practice assessment document).[4] Specifically, the student was unable to:

- Set realistic goals in partnership with the child and family.
- Find the child's preference about care and respect choices within the limits of professional practice.
- Apply the philosophy of family-centred care.
- Demonstrate ability in formulating and documenting care interventions relevant to child's needs.
- Document in the care plan.

During this reflection with the AA, Jane acknowledged that it was possible that the student did not have any insight into diabetes, thus ignoring the patient and that this could affect the student's ability to plan care for the patient. The practice assessor was able to relate to the specific domains as outlined in the NMC standards to support supervision and assessment in practice (NMC 2018). For the student to progress, an action plan would need to be agreed between Jane and Kelly. Jane would have to discuss issues of poor care planning with the student, recognising that the discussion may be challenging but drawing on her experience, feedback from the PS, and support from the academic assessor.

The input from the AA gave Jane greater confidence in being able to give nursing students constructive feedback and Jane was also aware of the difference in learning styles and the importance of being flexible and responsive and of creating a good learning environment. Through considerable discussion with the student Jane learnt that the student had been reluctant to engage with the patient as her theory on the subject was limited and she was afraid of looking 'stupid in front of the child'. The student also stated that she was worried about her level of knowledge and understanding and was reluctant to ask questions not because she was disinterested, but because she felt she should know this. Subsequently, the student agreed to evaluate which areas she specifically needed to focus on within this placement. Furthermore, an action plan was constructed to help the student meet the specific issues raised and an action plan was devised:

- The PA agreed to have one-to-one teaching sessions with the student about the treatment of common conditions on the ward.
- The PA agreed to supervise and guide the student in relation to care planning.
- The student agreed to revise the common conditions on the ward as instructed by the mentor.

- The PA agreed to give the student constructive feedback in a prompt fashion.
- Both student and PA agreed to meet on a weekly basis to evaluate the ongoing needs of the student.

Through this mode of enabling, the needs of both the PA and student were acknowledged and therefore progress was achieved. The AA continued to watch the situation with Jane to ensure as a PA she felt supported.

DISCUSSION

Through critical reflection the practitioner can analyse events more clearly and recognise that it is an essential element of learning (Sharp & Maddison 2008). Although it may be a gradual process and is ongoing from earlier experiences it should not be seen as a checklist. The ability to plan care for individuals is a fundamental requisite of the role of the registered nurse. However, like many skills, it is something that must be taught, and it should not be assumed that the individual can carry out the task without focused instruction.

The ability to find underperforming nursing students and manage the situation properly requires skill and knowledge acquisition (Duffy 2003). Through the support of the academic assessor the practice assessor is supported and encouraged to develop a culture of learning where nursing staff act as role models and articulate their practice and decision-making while sharing knowledge (Benner et al. 1996). Indeed, prompt intervention can often mean that practice assessors are able to support 'failing' nursing students with sensitivity and confidence, which can lead to the student achieving a satisfactory outcome of learning objectives (Carlisle et al. 2009). The role of the practice assessor within the clinical setting is of vital importance for the experience of the student, where practice-based assessment is complex, and it is difficult to manage objectively (Carr 2004). It is imperative that the practice assessor is prepared and supported so that they have the necessary skills needed to support nursing students.

Critical analysis is often something that is feared as it invokes feelings of disapproval (Sharp & Maddison 2008). However, this crucial skill of self-awareness and critical thinking is embraced by the academic assessor, and it plays an integral role in the development of the practice assessor and how they can support nursing students in their area. In the above case study both practice assessor and student were able to resolve pertinent issues affecting the performance of the student by critically discussing the incident, gaining insight, and developing an action plan which met the needs of all parties.

SUMMARY

The author has attempted to inform future practice development. This balanced approach with the introduction of these new roles looks to support practice assessors and supervisors experiencing challenges managing a 'failing' student. Working collaboratively and cohesively with each other ensures nursing students are supported in a sensitive and professional manner. This is exemplified in the case study by Jane's sensitive and supportive management of Kelly, the nursing student.

NOTES

1. Nursing Associates - The Nursing and Midwifery Council (nmc.org.uk)
2. https://nipec.hscni.net/service/fnfm/proj-info-background
3. Type 1 diabetes is Type 1 diabetes that causes the level of glucose (sugar) in your blood to become too high. It happens when your body cannot produce enough of a hormone called insulin, which controls blood glucose. You need daily injections of insulin to keep your blood glucose levels under control.
4. A practice assessment document (PAD) is an integral part of the learning process. It provides clear evidence that the NMC Future Nurse: Standards of Proficiency for Registered Nurses (NMC 2018) have been achieved.

REFERENCES

Aston, L. & Hallam, P. (2011) *Successful Mentoring in Nursing*. Exeter: Learning Matters.

Benner, P. Tanner, C. & Chesla, C. (1996) *Expertise in Nursing Practice: Caring, Clinical Judgment and Ethics*. New York: Springer.

Carlisle, C., Calman, L. & Ibbotson, T. (2009) Practice-based learning: The role of practice education facilitators in supporting mentors. *Nurse Education Today*, Oct; **29**(7):715-21. doi: 10.1016/j.nedt.2009.02.018. Epub 2009 Apr 3.(Accessed 28 February 2023).

Carr, S.J. (2004) Assessing clinical competency in medical senior house officers: How and why should we do it? *Postgraduate Medical Journal*, **80**(940), 63–66.

Duffy, K. (2003). *Failing Nursing Students: A Qualitative Study of Factors that Influence the Decisions regarding Assessment of Nursing Students' Competence in Practice* https://www.researchgate.net/publication/251693467_Failing_Students_A_Qualitative_Study_of_Factors_that_Influence_the_Decisions_Regarding_Assessment_of_Students'_Competence_in_Practice [Accessed 28 February 2023].

Elcock, K. & Sookhoo, D. (2007) Evaluating a new role to support mentors in practice. *Nursing Times*, **103**(49), 30–31.

Gibbs, G. (1988) *Learning by Doing: A Guide to Teaching and Learning Methods*. ("Gibbs, G. (1988) Learning by doing A guide to teaching and ..."). London: FEU.

NMC (2018a): Future nurse: Standards of proficiency for registered nurses. Available: https://www.nmc.org.uk/standards/standards-for-nurses

NMC (2018b) Part2: Standards for student supervision and assessment. Available: https://www.nmc.org.uk/standards/standards-for-nurses

Nash, S., & Scammell, J. (2010) Skills to ensure success in mentoring and other workplace learning approaches. ("Skills to ensure success in mentoring and other workplace ...") Nursing Times.net www.nursingtimes.net/nursing-practice-clinical-research/nursingstudents/skills-to-ensure-success-in-mentoring-and-other-workplace-learning-approaches/5010479.article?referrer=RSS [Accessed 2 July 2010].

Nursing and Midwifery Council (2005). *Consultation on Fitness for Practice at the Point of Registration*. ("Research Online"). London: NMC.

Nursing and Midwifery Council (2006) Standards to Support Learning and Assessment in Practice: NMC Standards for Mentors, Practice Teachers and Teachers. ("Evaluating a New Role to Support Mentors in Practice ..."). London: NMC. https://www.nmc.org.uk/standards-for-education-and-training/standards-to-support-learning-and-assessment-in-practice [Accessed 28 February 2023].

Nursing and Midwifery Council (2008) Standards to Support Learning and Assessment in Practice: NMC Standards for Mentors, Practice Teachers and Teachers. *("New standards on the supervision and assessment of ...")* London: NMC. www.nmc-uk.org/Documents/Standards/nmcStandardstoSupportLearningAndAssessmentInPractice.pdf [Accessed 8 June 2010].

Sharp, P. & Maddison, C. (2008) An exploration of the student and mentor journey into reflective practice. Chapter 4. In: Bulman, C. & Schutz, S. (eds). *Reflective Practice in Nursing*, 4th edn. Oxford: Blackwell Publishing.

United Kingdom Central Council for Nursing, Midwifery and Health Visiting (UKCC) (1999). *Fitness for Practice, the UKCC Commission for Nursing and Midwifery Education*. London: UKCC.

CHAPTER 10

Holistic Care – Family Partnership in Practice

Erica Strudley-Brown

INTRODUCTION

Lifestyles are changing dramatically throughout the Western world (Knapp & Wurm 2019). In the past, attention has largely focused on the traditional model of a nuclear family and neglected diversity in family composition. Although family structures vary, many people would agree that the central purpose of the family is to create and nurture a common culture that encourages the wellbeing of the people concerned, providing physical and emotional support.

The prevalence of children with life-limiting and life-threatening conditions in the UK is increasing. There has also been an increase in the last few decades of services that provide palliative and end-of-life care for children. Notwithstanding, there remains little information about the quality of care for families using these services (Fraser et al. 2020).

One of the first dilemmas of having a child with a serious or life-limiting illness is the shattering experience of how to cope with something which was unexpected and how to accept, as a parent, what is unacceptable (Bally et al. 2020). Several authors write about the isolation, which parents face as they struggle to come to terms with their shock (Hinton & Kirk 2017; Smith et al. 2020). The task of coping is a process in which parents find themselves constantly adjusting to the new demands that their child's illness makes.

Each family is unique. The central purpose of the family is to create and nurture a secure and loving environment, looking after the well-being of the people concerned. Theorists describe how parents experience a distinct connection and closeness with their children, which is unparalleled in other relationships (Bohannon 1990; Bowlby 1980; Broberg 2000; Matthews & Marwit 2004). The diagnosis of a life-limiting or a life-threatening condition is likely to challenge parent ideas about nurturing and protecting their children. Consequently, parents may face intense feelings of guilt, impotence, and worthlessness (Langner & Langner 2021). Coyne et al. (2016) advocate that caring for a child with complex needs may also jeopardise family stability and their hopes for the future. Mitchell et al. (2019) argue how well families cope will be influenced by demands such as employment (or lack of it), family problems, the presence of other children, and the quality of support from partners and other family members.

Many parents can vividly recall the time when they were told their child's diagnosis (Brown 2020). They describe their initial reaction as one of extreme shock, a state that Goldman et al. (2012) liken to bereavement. Diagnosis is often a watershed between two different family lifestyles – the pre-diagnostic life with normal 'ups and downs' and post-diagnostic life, where parents feel that everything is at the mercy of their child's health. Understandably, the situation is likely to cause them anxiety (Stroebe 2021; Wolfelt 2021). Not only do families have to cope with the diagnosis, but they must acknowledge that the situation will end in their child's death. Several authors write about the isolation parents face as they struggle to come to terms with their shock (Jaaniste et al. 2017; Stroebe 2015).

FAMILY-CENTRED CARE

Family-centred care was implemented in major teaching hospitals from the late 1970s, and in 1988, Casey introduced a family-centred nursing model. Together with other models developed from the Casey (1988) principles, existing nursing models were revised and the family's need to be involved in the care of their child was considered. Built upon the principles of partnership and negotiation, these models encourage family members to participate in assessment, planning, and delivery of care.

Families often manage multiple providers of care. Given this complicated landscape, effective care-co-ordination across care providers is paramount in maintaining their child's optimal health by

Care Planning in Children and Young People's Nursing, Second Edition. Edited by Sonya Clarke and Doris Corkin.
© 2024 John Wiley & Sons Ltd. Published 2024 by John Wiley & Sons Ltd.

avoiding fragmented or duplicated services. Together for Short Lives (2018) emphasizes the importance of an individual needs assessment for each family by the care team that will play a central coordinating role in the child's care. The assessment will provide an important foundation for building trust, partnership, and support throughout the trajectory of the child's illness and after their death. Assessment of the family's needs involves ongoing in depth gathering, recording, and sharing of information, with the child and family at the heart of the process and provide the opportunity for the child and family's hopes, wishes, and concerns to be heard and for their holistic needs including faith or spiritual wishes to be explored (Brown et al. 2021). It should empower the family and ensure that they can take control of their lives and reframe the relationship between professionals and families from professionally led care to family-led care, where families are enabled to deliver the care their child needs to make the most of the opportunities and time they have together. Turnas (2020) emphasizes the important role that the palliative care workforce plays in the implementation and co-production of care and outlines how the care skills used by staff need to be inter-linked.

Many practitioners consider family-centred care to be a cornerstone of paediatric practice, yet there is no single definition of family-centred care (O'Connor 2019). One definition is, there *must be a willingness on behalf of the staff to collaborate positively and respectfully with parents and families* (Bevan & Bedells 2016, p25). Others interpret the concept as a list of elements of care. Thus, whilst family-centred care considers the wider needs of the child and family, in practice, this may be at a relatively superficial level, depending on the depth of the assessment and the interpretation and communication of the information received from individual families. Many families will experience multiple providers of care for their child including primary care, specialists, and education, and they may encounter barriers to accessing the support they need (Strudley-Brown 2021; Ufer et al. 2018).

Aoun et al. (2020, p. 76) emphasize the importance of collaborative partnership *between health professionals, patients and families when delivering and evaluating services*. Notwithstanding, the same authors report that a gap remains in clinical practice between the optimal approach and the reality. Smith et al. (2018) and Jones et al. (2014) endorse this viewpoint arguing that accessibility to services is problematic for many families.

Assessment will also depend on a definition of 'family' and whom the child considers as core members of their 'family'. For some children, their grandparents may be the main carers, for others their parent's partner may be a crucial support and influence, even though they are not related. The situation may be further complicated by former partner's relatives, stepsiblings, foster carers, home care teams, etc. (Tatterton 2019).

Family-centred care is grounded in the participation and involvement of the family but there is much evidence to suggest that this is not always a reality, and, in many cases, mere lip service is paid to the process. It is well recognized that experienced nursing staff are generally confident in enabling decision-making, but negotiation of care and the assessment of need may be affected by the expectations of both staff and parents, issues of control and the lack or quality of information. Family-centred care may also be less successful where resource issues such as staff shortages or poor facilities influence family involvement in care.

All families need to achieve a balance between stability and change, but roles and relationships may need to alter to accommodate developments in the physical, social, or emotional life of family members (Collins et al. 2020). This means that the assessment of care must be constantly revisited.

FAMILIES ADAPTING TO THEIR CHILD'S ILLNESS

Within each of the phases of illness experienced by the child, the family will have to develop strategies for adjusting and coping. These will differ throughout the trajectory of the illness, but they may include:

- Recognizing the symptoms, pain, and physical changes.
- Adjusting to medical intervention, treatment, and in some cases to palliative care.
- Developing strategies to manage stress.
- Communicating effectively with professional people and carers.

- Maintaining the family identity.
- Preserving relationships with partners and friends.
- Expressing emotions and fears (Brown 2020).

Several frameworks explore the adaptation process (Brown 2020); Hinton & Kirk 2017).

Families vary in the ways in which they deal with stress. Factors that influence family adjustment include:

- The demands of the illness, including onset, progression, severity of symptoms, and symptom visibility.
- The impact of the illness on everyday living.
- The personality of the child and family and their ways of communicating with each other.

Traditionally, there has existed a tension between the coping strategies adopted by parents and those preferred by professionals. Parents need to be encouraged and empowered to develop the coping strategies which are best for them. The challenge to professionals is in helping parents to develop those tactics, which will enable the strategies to work (Aoun et al. (2020)).

Professionals who work with parents after their child's diagnosis should not assume that because a family has been coping for some time they are no longer in need of constant support. The coping strategies which families learn and the skills they acquire need to be acknowledged. All parents will need:

- Continued support in adjusting to their emotional and psychological reactions
- Assistance in seeking professional support
- Support in recouping their physical strengths
- Assistance in ensuring resources to meet their needs
- Adequate information at each stage of the child's illness.

Discussions with the child and their family should enable various options for care in response to the needs of the child and their family as the status of the child's health changes, an approach called parallel planning Together for Short Lives (2018).

Models of care are different. Some children with life-limiting conditions are cared for in the community, some in children's hospices and some in hospital. Wherever the care setting, the overall aim is to meet the needs of the child and their family and to maintain the equilibrium of life as far as possible. Seamless care follows the child from one environment to another and recognizes the skills and expertise of the multidisciplinary team. Recently there has been a commitment by many agencies to work collaboratively with families and with each other. For example, Together for Short Lives (2018) has campaigned for many years about the need for services to be coordinated around the individual needs of each family, taking account of their views and recognizing the central role and expertise that parents have in the care of their children.

The term 'collaboration' is now largely replaced by the term 'co-production'.

Notwithstanding, there appears to be little consensus on the meaning of co-production. However, within children's palliative care the palliative care workforce, volunteers and communities, generally understands the term as involvement in the delivery of care. Therefore, policy makers as pivotal to successful collaboration (Bryson et al. 2014) consider co-production.

Families are often overwhelmed by the number of professionals involved with them. Carter et al.'s (2015) study demonstrated the fundamental importance of key worker staff who were able to provide aspects of support not usually provided by statutory agencies: *encompassing and embracing* families through supporting needs and promoting resilience; *befriending and bonding* through developing knowledge, trusting relationships and a sense of closeness; and *accompanying and enduring* by 'being with' families in different settings, situations and crises and by enduring alongside the families.

Each family's needs are individual and may change over the trajectory of their child's illness. Therefore, a wide range of services will be required in order to provide flexible care that complements each family's own skills and the contribution of primary care teams.

EMPOWERING PARENTS

Since the early 1980s, a tremendous amount has been written about working with parents who have a child with a disability. Authors such as Murray (2000) have described the importance of working collaboratively in practice. Although Hornby's 1999 theoretical model was originally designed for educational settings, Brown (2020) suggests that with some adaptations the Hornby model is relevant to professionals working with families who have a sick child.

The diamond in Figure 10.1 represents parental needs and the contributions that parents can make to their child's care. The model also demonstrates how some parents will need greater guidance, whilst others are able to make extensive contributions. For example, all parents need professionals who can communicate with them, and some may need individual counselling.

INFORMATION ABOUT THEIR CHILD

All parents have a wealth of knowledge about their child. Indeed, they *are* the experts about their child's behaviour, likes and dislikes, and daily care, including medical care. Professionals need to work with parents in order to be able to tap into this knowledge. They will also need to possess excellent communication and listening skills in order to enter into meaningful conversations with families.

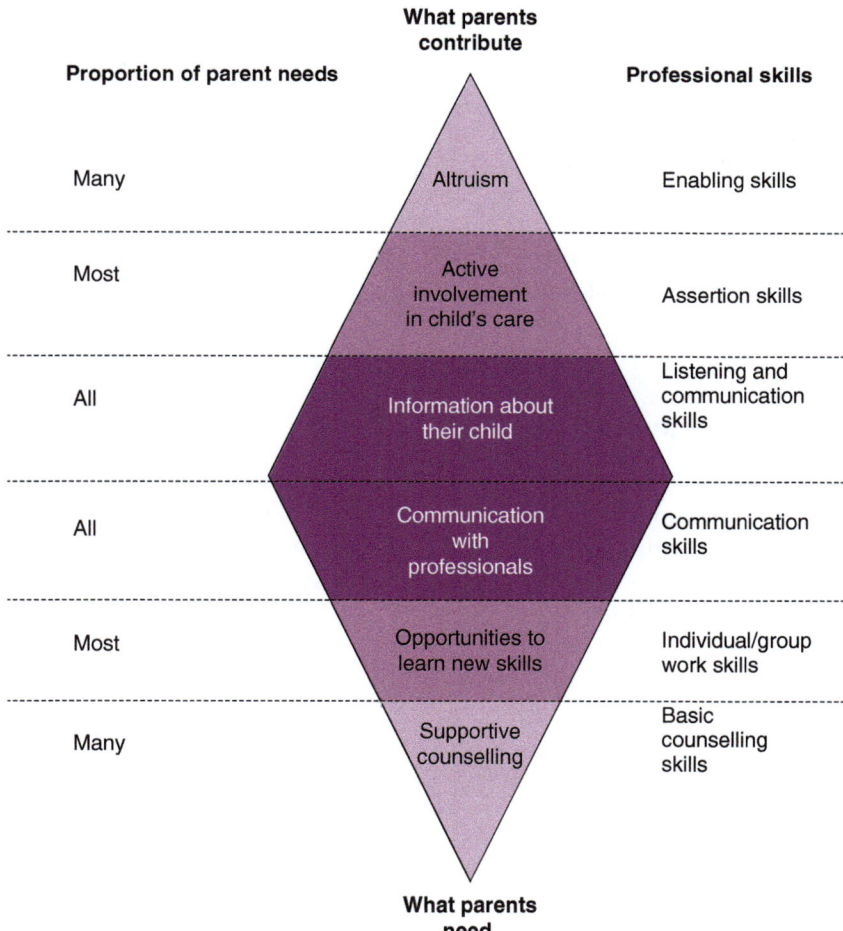

FIGURE 10.1 Meeting parent's needs – the supportive role of professionals (based on Hornby 1999).
Source: Brown (2007). Reproduced with kind permission.

Mack and Sisk (2021) argue that communication is the primary tool for helping families to accept and to acknowledge the limitations posed by their child's life-limiting condition. Therefore, effective communication forms the bedrock of practice in children's palliative care (Aoun et al. 2020; Mack & Sisk 2021).

Additionally, Larsson et al. (2018) make a plea for children and young people to be recognized as experts in defining their needs and to be actively involved in the co-creation of new knowledge rather than involved as subjects in research where there is a reliance on the views of parents, caregivers, and other stakeholders. Notwithstanding, despite increasing expectations that children and young people are involved as partners in health research and the design of services there remains considerable uncertainty about how to optimally provide opportunities for involving them.

INVOLVING PARENTS IN THEIR CHILD'S CARE

Many parents develop complex skills in their child's care, including medical procedures, symptom control, and pain management. Professionals are often astounded by the expertise of parents. They need to encourage and empower parents to make decisions on behalf of, or with, their child, whilst also being available to give advice and support when it is needed. A flexible working partnership involves listening to parents' needs and helping them to be assertive, in order to communicate their ideas, needs, and concerns, so that they are able to gain the best care for their child. Professionals also need to be assertive with colleagues from within and outside their own service in order to act as advocates for families.

ALTRUISM

Many families with a sick child seem to possess the capacity to reach out and to support other parents, taking comfort from shared experience. At Acorns children's hospices this is lived out in practice in groups such as men's groups, Asian mothers' groups, grandparent groups and user involvement groups. Other parents, both bereaved and non-bereaved, speak at professional conferences and open days, or write in journals and newsletters. It should be recognized, however, that parents should never be exploited but enabled by professionals to make the contribution that is right for them:

> *I felt less isolated when I was able to chat to other mums. The common ground we shared was nothing to do with where we lived or what kind of employment we were in. At a basic level it was about having a very poorly child.*
>
> *(anonymous)*

OPPORTUNITIES TO LEARN NEW SKILLS

Most parents welcome opportunities to learn new skills in caring for their child. Sometimes parents prefer to develop new capacities through attending groups, but more often skills are acquired through modelling care and medical procedures carried out by professionals. Whatever the setting, in addition to learning, parents will benefit from being able to share their own ideas and to raise their concerns, a process that can be facilitated by professionals who have developed teaching and group-work skills.

SUMMARY	Resource allocation in the future is likely to be determined by efficacy and on cost effectiveness, with the result that where efficacy is lacking, funds will not be provided. The care of sick children and their families is at a critical stage in its evolution. Amongst the challenges will be the necessity for rigorous assessment of the quality of everyday practice matched to the needs of individual family members so that services are worthy of being deemed to be excellent and the relationship between professionals and families truly demonstrates collaborative partnership in practice.

FURTHER READING

Aldridge, J. & Carragher, P. (2021) Teamwork. In: Hain, R. & Goldman, A. (eds). *Oxford Textbook of Palliative Care for Children*, 3rd edn. Oxford: Oxford University Press.

Aldridge, J. & Sourkes, B. (2021) The psychological impact of life-limiting conditions on the child. In: Hain, R. & Goldman, A. (eds). *Oxford Textbook of Palliative Care for Children*, 3rd edn. Oxford: Oxford University Press.

Contro, N. & Zimmerman, J. (2021) Assessment of the child and family. In: Hain, R., and Goldman, A. (eds). *Oxford Textbook of Palliative Care for Children*, 3rd edn. Oxford: Oxford University Press.

Dussel, V. & Jones, B. (2021) Impact on the Family. In: Hain, R. & Goldman, A. (eds). *Oxford Textbook of Palliative Care for Children*, 3rd edn. Oxford: Oxford University Press.

Grunauer, M., & Hynson, J. (2021) Planning Care. In: Hain, R. & Goldman, A. (eds). *Oxford Textbook of Palliative Care for Children*, 3rd edn. Oxford: Oxford University Press.

REFERENCES

Aoun, G., Fenella, J., Gill, M. & Phillips, B. (2020) The profile and support needs of parents in pediatric palliative care: Comparing cancer and non-cancer groups. *Palliative Care and Social Practice*. doi: 10.1177/2632352420958000.

Bally, J., Burles, M., Smith, N., Holstander, L., Mpofuc, C., Hodgson-Viden, H. & Zimmer, M. (2020) Exploring possibilities for holistic family care of parental caregivers of children with Life-limiting or Life-threatening illnesses. *Journal of Qualitative Social Work*, **20**(5), 1356–1373.

Bevan, A. & Bedells, E. (2016) Roles of nurses and parents caring for hospitalized children. *Nursing Children and Young People*, **28**(2), 24–28.

Bohannon, J. (1990) Grief responses of spouses following the death of a child: A longitudinal study. *Omega Journal of Death and Dying*, **22**(2), 109–121.

Bowlby, J. (1980) *Attachment and Loss: Loss, Sadness and Depression*. London: Tavistock Institute.

Broberg, A. (2000) A review of interventions in the parent-child relationship informed by attachment theory. *Acta Paediatrica*, **89**(434), 37–42.

Brown, E. (2007) *Supporting the Child and the Family in Paediatric Palliative Care*. London: Jessica Kingsley.

Brown, E. (2020) SOFT UK support volunteer training handbook. www.soft.org.uk. [Accessed 28 February 2023]

Brown, E., Muckaden, M. & Mndende, N. (2021) Culture, spirituality, religion and ritual. In: Hain, R., and Goldman, A. (eds). *Oxford Textbook of Palliative Care for Children*, 3rd edn. Oxford: Oxford University Press.

Bryson, J., Crosby, B. & Bloomberg, L. (2014) Public Value Governance: Moving beyond traditional public administration and the new public management. *Public Administration Review*, **74**(4), 445–456.

Carter, B., Edwards, M. & Hunt, A. (2015) Being a presence: The ways in which family support workers encompass, embrace, befriend, accompany and endure with families of a life-limited child. *Journal of Child Healthcare*, **19**(3), 304–319.

Casey, A. (1988) A partnership with the child and family. *Senior Nursing*, **8**(4), 8–9.

Collins, A., Burchell, J., Remedios, C. & Thomas, K. (2020) Describing the psychosocial profile and unmet support needs of parents caring for a child with a life-limiting condition: A cross-sectional study of caregiver-reported outcomes. *Palliative Medicine*, **34**(3), 358–366.

Coyne, I., Amery, A., Gibson, F. & Kiernan, G. (2016) Information-sharing between healthcare professionals, parents and children with cancer. More than a model of information exchange. *European Journal of Cancer Care*, **15**(1), 141–156.

Fraser, L., Gibson-Smith, D., Jarvis, S., Norman, P. & Parslow, R. (2020) Estimating the current and future prevalence of life-limiting conditions in children in England. sagepub.com/journals-permissions. doi:10.1177/0269216320975308 journals.sagepub.com/home/pmj.

Goldman, A., Hain, R., Liben S. (2012) *Oxford Textbook of Palliative Care for Children*. Oxford University Press.

Hinton, D. & Kirk, S. (2017) Living with uncertainty and hope: A qualitative study exploring parents' experiences of living with childhood multiple sclerosis. *Chronic Illness*, **13**(2), 88–89.

Hornby, G. (1999) *Improving Parental Involvement*. London: Continuum International Publishing Group.

Jaaniste, T., Coombs, S., Donnelly, T., Kelk, N. & Baston, D. (2017) Risk and resilience factors related to the death of a child with a Life-limiting condition. *Children*, **4**(11), 96. doi: 10.3390/children4110096. (Accessed 29 08 2021).

Jones, B., Contro, N. & Koch, K.D. (2014) The duty of the physician to care for the family in pediatrics palliative care: Context, communication and caring. *Pediatrics*, 133, 8–15.

Knapp, S. & Wurm, G. (2019) Theorizing family change: A review and reconceptualization. *Journal of Family Theory and Review*, **11**(2), 212–229.

Langner, M. & Langner, R. (2021) Decision-making with children, young people and parents. In: Hain, R., and Goldman, A. *Oxford Textbook of Palliative Care for Children*. Oxford: Oxford University Press.

Larsson, I., Staland-Nyman, C., Svedberg, P., Nygren, J. & Carlsson, I. (2018) Children and young peoples' participation in developing interventions in health and well-being: A scoping review. *British Medical Council Health Research*, **18**, 507–527.

Mack, J. & Sisk, B. (2021) Communication. In: Hain, R. & Goldman, A. *The Oxford Textbook of Palliative Care for Children*, 3rd edn. Oxford: Oxford University Press.

Matthews, T. & Marwit, S. (2004) Complicated grief and the trend towards cognitive behavioral therapy. *Death Studies*, **28**(9), 849–863.

Mitchell, S., Bennett, K. & Morris, A. (2019) Achieving beneficial outcomes for children with life-limiting and life-threatening conditions receiving palliative care and their families: A realist overview. *Palliative Medicine*, **34**(3), 387–402.

Murray, J. (2000) Understanding sibling adaptation to childhood cancer. *Issues in Comprehensive Pediatric Nursing*, **23**, 39–47.

O'Connor, S. (2019) Family-centered care of children and young people in the acute hospital setting: A concept analysis. *Journal of Clinical Nursing*, **28**, 3353–3367.

Smith, N., Nicole, R., Bally, J., Holtslander, L., Peacock, S., Spurr, S., Hodgson-Viden, H., Mpofu, C., & Zimmer, M. (2018) Supporting parental-caregivers of children living with life-threatening or life-limiting illnesses: A Delphi study. *Journal for Specialists in Palliative Nursing*, **23**(4), e12226.

Smith, J., Chafe, R. and Audas, R. (2020) Managing the Wait. *Parents' experience in accessing diagnostic and treatment services for children and adolescents. Health Services Insights.* **13**, 1–10.

Stroebe, M. (2015) Family matters in bereavement: Towards an integrative interpersonal coping model. *Perspectives in Psychological Science*, **10**(6), 873–879.

Stroebe, M. (2021) A Study of Security and Separation: An unexpected forerunner of attachment theory? *OMEGA Journal of Death and Dying*. **84** (1) 146–56.

Strudley-Brown, E. (2021) (in press) Understanding and responding to Adverse Childhood Experiences (ACEs) in practice. In: Richards, H. & Malomo, M. (eds). *Developing Your Professional Identity – A Guide for Working with Children and Families*. London: Critical Publishing.

Tatterton, M. (2019) How grandparents experience the death of a grandchild with a Life-limiting condition. *Journal of Family Nursing*, **25**(1), 109–127.

Together for Short Lives (2018) *A Core Pathway for Children with Life-limiting and Life-threatening Conditions*, 3rd edn. Bristol: Together for Short Lives.

Turnas, S. (2020) Skilling and motivating staff for co-production. In: Loeffler, E. & Bovairs, T. (eds). *The Palgrave Handbook of Co-production of Public Services and Outcomes*. London: Palgrave Macmillan. 491–506.

Ufer, L., Moore, J., Hawkins, K., Geinbel, G., Entwistle, D. & Hoffman, D. (2018) Care Co-ordination: Empowering families and promise in practice to facilitate medical home use among children and youth with special health care needs. *Maternal and Child Health Journal*, **22**, 648–659.

Wolfelt, A. (2021) *Understanding Your Grief – Ten Essential Touchstones for Finding Hope and Healing in Your Heart*, 2nd edn. Fort Collins, Colorado: Companion Press.

Reflective Account

Ian and Nicola Markwell

CHAPTER 11

INTRODUCTION

Ryan was born on Christmas Day 2000, after a fast journey down the motorway to the maternity hospital. He was born 15 weeks premature, weighed in at 1 pound 11 ounces (762 g) and was delivered by Caesarean section. Since the time that Nicola had realised that she was having contractions at home, things all happened so quickly that we did not have time to think of names. When we were shown into the neonatal unit to see him for the first time, we were introduced to him as Joseph, but by that time we had already decided on Ryan as a name and quickly got it corrected. Ryan was not actually due until April 2001, and as we sat and watched him in the incubator over that Christmas period, it was hard to comprehend what would be in front of us over the coming months and years.

MEDICAL HISTORY – THE FIRST NINE MONTHS

As Ryan was born at 25 weeks, he was ventilated for 60 days and developed chronic lung disease (see Figure 11.1). His early weeks in hospital were very difficult, as he lost weight, was given phototherapy for jaundice and was tube fed. Over these weeks, the aim of the medical and nursing staff was to reduce Ryan's dependence on ventilation and they made steady progress towards this goal.

Nevertheless, it soon became apparent that Ryan would be difficult to extubate. On one occasion we had a difficult situation, when Ryan extubated himself and the medical staff found it difficult to re-intubate him.

After this episode, it was concluded that he had sub-glottic stenosis, and therefore the best way to reduce his dependence on the ventilator would be for him to have a tracheostomy. This was successfully completed on the 21 February 2001, and within a matter of days Ryan's dependence on the ventilator had stopped, although he remained on low flow oxygen for the remainder of his time in hospital.

Gradually, Ryan started to gain weight and improve to the point that the medical staff started to talk about discharging him, but this was on the assumption that we would take him home attached to an oxygen cylinder which was connected to his tracheostomy tube. Although this was initially a very daunting prospect, the medical staff, nurses, and technicians prepared us well for what was involved in handling the oxygen cylinders and managing Ryan's care, whilst on oxygen. We therefore started to prepare to bring him home, and he was finally discharged from hospital in May 2001.

Unfortunately, this was not the end of the medical problems as within a week of discharge, we were back in intensive care due to Ryan aspirating on his food and milk and a significant reduction in his lung function to the point that he stopped breathing at home. It was a long week in intensive care, but fortunately Ryan made a full recovery and was discharged again, after a revision of his medication. Over the next period of months, Ryan was in and out of hospital on a regular basis, only remaining at home for 1–2 weeks at a time. We seemed to be going round in a vicious circle. Ryan had a gastro-oesophageal reflux and he was aspirating milk into his lungs which were already badly damaged, causing severe chest infections, which required hospitalisation. To try and treat this, the medical options were thickened milk and food, to try and prevent the reflux and other medication to try and empty the contents of his stomach quickly.

Eventually, it was concluded that the best solution would be to conduct a fundoplication, which is a surgical procedure where the top of the stomach is tightened to prevent the stomach contents from refluxing back and entering the windpipe. This was completed in September 2001, and it was soon clear that the issue with the reflux had been solved. The cycle of hospital visits was broken for now.

Care Planning in Children and Young People's Nursing, Second Edition. Edited by Sonya Clarke and Doris Corkin.
© 2024 John Wiley & Sons Ltd. Published 2024 by John Wiley & Sons Ltd.

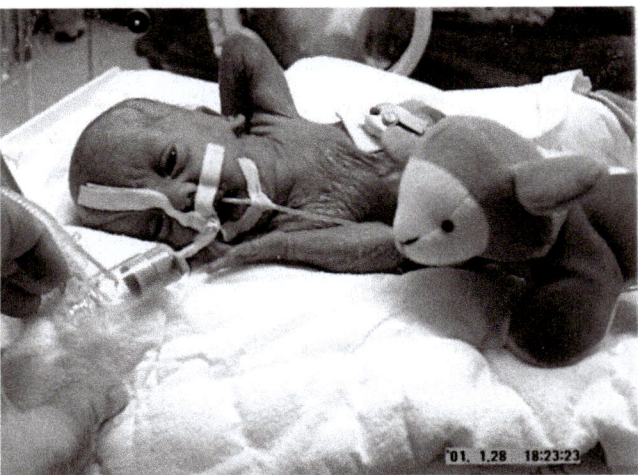

FIGURE 11.1 Ryan in neonatal unit.

PLANNING CARE

From September 2001, Ryan's care was primarily managed at home. He had a tracheostomy tube, which needed changing weekly and required regular suction. In order to maintain Ryan's breathing he required low-flow oxygen via a cylinder 24 hours a day and he also received nebulisers four times a day. His feeds were thickened with carobel and he was given domperidone medication daily to help prevent the reflux (despite the fundoplication).

In order for us to care properly for Ryan at home we had to transform his bedroom and other parts of the house into what looked like a small 'medical' centre. The essential equipment and facilities which we needed were:

- Two full size oxygen cylinders (one upstairs and one downstairs)
- One small handheld oxygen cylinder for use in the car or when on trips out
- Two suction machines (one portable and one electric)
- Nebuliser medication and equipment (Figure 11.2)
- Tracheostomy tubes and humidifiers Oxygen saturation monitor (Figure 11.2).

The treatment of Ryan's medical issues changed as he became older:

- His dependence on bottled oxygen: gradually over the first three months, we were able to slowly reduce the level of oxygen which Ryan required, whilst still maintaining his oxygen saturation levels. It got to the stage where we could remove the bottled oxygen and from that point forward he only required oxygen when suffering reduced lung performance due to chest infections.

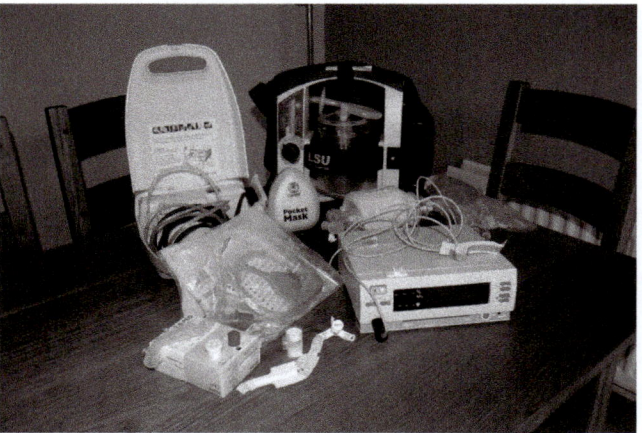

FIGURE 11.2 Ryan's equipment at home.

- The presence of the tracheostomy tube: this was the most obvious sign of Ryan's medical problems. From a medical perspective this was a source of chest infections – it required regular suction, led to difficulties in Ryan learning to talk and, as he became older, it led to an element of social awkwardness.
- He was very susceptible to chest infections, and from time to time he required hospitalisation and treatment with intravenous antibiotics.
- The presence of his fundoplication meant that he could not vomit, and on one occasion, when he had a serious gastro – intestinal infection, this led to emergency treatment in hospital, as he could not get rid of the infection.

As Ryan began to be regularly assessed through the community nursing system, a number of other medical or developmental issues emerged:

- Ryan was diagnosed as having reduced hearing due to the presence of glue ear, and had vents put in to correct this. He was quite susceptible to ear infections because of the issues with his ears.
- Ryan was assessed as being developmentally delayed and therefore required additional assistance, although he was able to enter mainstream school.
- Ryan was slow to begin to learn to talk because of the presence of his tracheostomy tube, as the air bypassed his mouth and nose. He began to learn to talk, by dropping his chin over the entrance to his tube, thereby forcing the air through his mouth and nose and in this way could talk. Despite this mechanism, which Ryan developed himself, he could not make some specific word sounds and could not speak for long periods without pausing to take a breath.

Each of these issues tended to be dealt with by a different group of people, either community or hospital based, and it was one of our main frustrations, particularly in the early days of Ryan's care at home, that there did not seem to be one person charged with Ryan's overall care.

HOSPITAL TO HOME

With Ryan's medical history and treatment, we have spent a significant portion of time in hospitals. Particularly over the first nine months of Ryan's life, we seemed to spend half of our lives in hospital. This meant that we came to know quite a few of the medical staff fairly well. As Mum, Nicola, was qualified in adult nursing, she seemed to slip easily into the ward routine, particularly those wards where Ryan was cared for over longer periods of time.

Ryan's hospital notes seemed to grow and grow, and with each new visit to hospital we found that when Ryan was admitted to a new ward in the hospital we always ended up repeating Ryan's life story to a new doctor or nurse. At home we had become very used to handling Ryan's various medical needs, such as tracheostomy care, suction and nebulisers, and at times seemed to be more aware of how to treat him than some of the hospital staff. This usually led to them backing off slightly from providing 'front-line' care in those aspects and allowing us to take the lead in those areas. This usually worked well for both parties, as the hospital staff could then concentrate on treating Ryan's condition, which had led to that particular hospital admission.

Although on the whole the medical staff were very good, it is also true to say that the hospital visits allowed us to come into contact with other non-medical people, who were able to give us additional advice which led to our care of Ryan in the home becoming that little bit easier. Hospital technicians quite often had little hints and tips on how to operate or use some of the equipment which was necessary to have in the home. This allowed us to resolve some of the problems, which gave us sleepless nights from time to time, such as a poor signal on an oxygen monitor. During hospital visits, we also met other parents who were trying to cope with a similar set of circumstances to ours, and it was always quite therapeutic to compare notes with each other. This was particularly true of the treatment of children with a tracheostomy, where the medical staff rely on other more experienced parents to provide guidance to those who are faced with managing a child with a tracheostomy. This was a service which we have felt the benefits of, having participated as experienced tracheostomy carers ourselves.

LIVING WITH RYAN AND HIS TRACHEOSTOMY

Ryan had his tracheostomy tube inserted in February 2001, and up until July 2008 there were three unsuccessful attempts to remove Ryan's tracheostomy tube in Northern Ireland. On each occasion, Ryan encountered difficulties breathing without the tracheostomy tube for more than 48 hours and so the tracheostomy tube was reinserted. This meant that we became used to dealing with a child with a tracheostomy, even though Nicola would have admitted that this was one of the tasks which she hated most whilst she was doing her nurse training. The main issues with tracheostomy care were:

- The tracheostomy tube required replacement with a new tube on a weekly basis.
- Ryan had difficulty coughing up mucus and therefore required suction at home. This needed to be more frequent when Ryan had a cold or chest infection.
- We had to be careful with his clothing and mindful of the activities which Ryan could do, to ensure that the tracheostomy tube was never covered and that he did not participate in activities which could have led to materials entering his tube, for example swimming or playing in the sand pit. Anything which had the potential to block Ryan's tube would essentially have blocked his airway and therefore would have been a serious risk to his health.

We both received training on tracheostomy care from the medical and nursing staff, but once we were in the home environment and became used to doing the various tasks routinely, we realised that the training that we had been given was not necessarily the most practical, and was really derived from textbooks. One very simple example of this was the emphasis, which some staff in the hospital placed on linen tracheostomy tapes, which could be tied around Ryan's neck and which were supplied as standard with each tracheostomy tube. However, over time we learnt that Velcro tapes were available, and although we were aware of the potential safety risks (can easily open), Velcro was in fact a more practical and comfortable solution to keeping Ryan's tracheostomy tube in place.

The various aspects of tracheostomy care also needed to be emphasised to the staff at the local school, prior to Ryan becoming a pupil, and this was backed up by training for Ryan's teachers in how to deal with him should a difficulty be encountered at school. This training was delivered by Mum Nicola. It is fair to say that the school staff willingly participated in the training, and this gave us great comfort in ensuring that Ryan was in safe hands whilst at school.

As indicated above, the path to removing Ryan's tracheostomy tube was not a smooth one, and led to intense frustration on our part, as the only surgeon based in Northern Ireland who could perform these types of operations retired, and it was not obvious if (or when) a replacement would take up the post. This meant that there was minimal medical assistance locally, and after several years of frustration with the lack of progress, we eventually wrote to our MP to bring the matter to his attention. Thanks to his intervention, and with the help of senior consultants in Northern Ireland, we managed to get a referral to a children's hospital in England.

We journeyed over to England to attend our first appointment with a feeling of trepidation over what might be in front of us, but were met with a very experienced and highly competent team, dealing with children with tracheostomies. The medical team in England took ownership of Ryan's care, in terms of his tracheostomy tube and history of sub-glottic stenosis, and within a matter of months an operation was successfully performed to surgically correct his condition and remove his tracheostomy tube. To summarise our experience, after an initial assessment appointment, we arrived in England on a Monday and when leaving the children's hospital the following Monday, Ryan was discharged without his tracheostomy tube and no ill effects. After one year at home that is still the case.

PARENTS AS CARERS

As Ryan has developed and grown, and his medical conditions have steadily improved; the role which we have played as parents has gradually changed from one of full-time carers to a normal parent–child relationship. In the early days, when Ryan was hospitalised, our life was made up of daily visits to the neonatal unit to visit Ryan, and this was despite having to care for his two older sisters, aged three and five years at the time. Upon reflection, it was difficult to sit beside him in the incubator, particularly when we were not allowed to hold him, and when he gripped your hand through the incubator glove port it was a whole different experience.

After his discharge from hospital, we became Ryan's main carers, with Mum Nicola giving up her career to devote 100% of her time to Ryan and the girls. The first few months of his time at home were very stressful, as we had a lot of medical equipment in the home and had to carry an oxygen cylinder *everywhere* that we went, including trips to the shops, to visit family and friends, and on holidays. Over this time, there were very regular spells of hospitalisation, and several ambulance or fast car journeys, as on occasions we found that his condition deteriorated very quickly. On the whole these hospital spells brought some respite to our lives, as it was not necessary for one of us to stay in hospital with Ryan and we were able to recharge the batteries.

In our experience, the caring situation resulted in varying degrees of depersonalisation brought about by:

- Lack of sleep
- Loss of privacy and personal space
- Loss of freedom of choice in personal and family matters
- Loss of leisure activities, including holidays, and social isolation

Although a lot could be said about any of the problems listed above, perhaps the most difficult to cope with was the combination of disturbed sleep and inadequate sleep. This was particularly applicable for us in the early days when Ryan was discharged from hospital, or on occasions when he was unwell at home. It is not surprising that there is a sense of unreality about the world which we live in when we are acting as the primary carers.

The fear and stress of caring does not arise solely from the physical act of caring. Relationships can become strained and this can lead to the possible breakdown of marriage due to the loss of time spent together by husband and wife. One person may have to give up their job to become the primary carer at home and this can also bring an additional financial burden on the family budget.

However, the caring role can also arise due to the complex nature of the support systems which exist in the community, that is, it may become difficult to determine who to turn to for assistance in the various agencies. In our case, this took quite some time to organise, as the community children's nursing service had just been established. After unsuccessfully trying several avenues, it was finally with the help of our MP, that we were able to have a children's nurse to stay in our home and care for Ryan overnight.

This was still only for one day over several weeks, and although it did give us the required respite for a short period, we soon came to the conclusion that it was not worth the hassle of sorting out the house and medication, organising the girls, and having someone else in our home, for just a few hours' respite. There was a sense that we had lost ownership of our home, the professional carer could go home after her shift, while we had to return to our role as primary carers as soon as the children's nurse left the house.

As Ryan became older, the trips to hospital became less frequent, but when he was admitted this proved to be quite challenging as the management of the rest of the family placed additional stresses on us as parents. For each of these stays in hospital, one of the parents had to stay, and in these periods we went through a cycle where the parent staying in hospital lived in an unreal situation of boredom and quick bites of something to eat as Ryan was having treatment. Ryan himself grew to dislike these trips to hospital and hated being left alone.

SIBLINGS AND EXTENDED FAMILY

To fully understand the impact that Ryan's medical conditions and treatment have had on his sisters, you need to consider it from their perspective. They woke up on Christmas Day in 2000 to find that their mum gone and to be told that they had a new baby brother. Although they were both very excited at that time, this excitement soon changed as our new pattern of living emerged. They did not actually get to visit their new baby brother until 17 March 2001, and spent parts of every weekend from then to September 2001, either in hospital visiting him, or with relatives as we visited him. The girls were quite accepting of Ryan's tracheostomy and the various medicines which we had to dose him with, and they treated him like any other little brother.

When Ryan's problems with reflux were resolved in September 2001, everyone was relieved that we could settle into some semblance of a normal family life, albeit interrupted occasionally by Ryan's follow-up visits to hospital. When this happened the girls could have become quite annoyed and afraid for him, but generally when they were allowed to see him in hospital and they could see that he was improving, they were quite accepting of the reality of the situation.

Until Ryan's premature birth, the girls had enjoyed a relatively normal family life and although this was occasionally seriously disrupted, as we went through the ups and downs of Ryan's hospitalisation and treatment, the girls never displayed any resentment towards him; their reaction has rather been to be very protective of him, and display a relatively mature concern for his wellbeing.

OUR SON RYAN

Within a matter of days of Ryan's premature birth, it was apparent that he was a determined character, as he moved around the incubator as much as he could and extubated himself a couple of times, much to the consternation of the medical staff. Our view has consistently been that it is this element of his character which has helped him get over the various medical hurdles that he has had to overcome.

When Ryan was at home, he was a very quiet baby due to the presence of the tracheostomy and he never really cried, as the air escaped through his tracheostomy, rather than going through his mouth and nose. He never really crawled, but developed a way of moving around the floor on his side, which he became quite good at.

As Ryan grew up, he developed quite well socially and mixes well with his own age group and with other children and adults, and he is a very happy little boy, despite his medical history.

Furthermore, Ryan's reaction to his intermittent stays in hospital over the years has been what you might expect from a child, in that he did not like to be left alone, and when he had started to recover he was keen to get home. One of the most traumatic times for Ryan, in recent years, was when he was preparing to go to England to have his tracheostomy removed. The entire family was concerned as to how successful the operation would be, and the emotions were running very high in the days before the trip, to such an extent that Ryan himself became more aware of the significance of this operation. Fortunately, the operation was successful and it has seen Ryan take another step forward in terms of improving his speech and reducing his dependence on nebulisers. Ultimately the medical staff believe that it will help his chronic lung disease in the longer term.

RYAN'S EDUCATION

One of the key challenges which we have faced as Ryan has developed and grown has been the question as to whether he could be placed in mainstream schooling, given his medical and developmental needs. Fortunately, we already had a relationship with the local primary school as both of our other children attended the school and Mum Nicola was involved in the parent teacher association. This did assist us in the long run, but nevertheless we had to go through the necessary red tape to finally achieve a place for Ryan. The first steps towards school were through a visit by the educational psychologist to the playgroup which Ryan attended, to conduct an assessment of him. This led to the requirement to have a statutory assessment of Ryan's educational needs carried out by the local Education and Library Board. This resulted in a recommendation that Ryan could attend mainstream schooling with the presence of a classroom assistant for a few hours each day, but the extent of red tape involved was such that we only finally got this recommendation in October, with the school year commencing in September. It was thanks to the good relationship with the school that they permitted Ryan to attend from September.

Each year the validity of the statement was reviewed and an assessment made. We also faced an additional challenge when Ryan's tracheostomy was removed, as this was the primary medical need on which the statement was based and therefore we had to go through the whole process all over again to be reassessed from a developmental perspective. Fortunately, this also resulted in support being continued and that is where we are today.

GIVING SOMETHING BACK

We have been quite fortunate that we have had an opportunity to give something back to the nursing profession in that the community children's nursing sister, who assisted us in the early days at home, took up an educational post in Queen's University Belfast. Since then Nicola has been invited into the School of Nursing and Midwifery to present Ryan's journey to pre-registration second-year child branch nursing students. This yearly classroom tutorial is based on the 'lived experience' which we have had and does not rely on any reference to textbooks, thus giving the nursing students an insight into what it is really like to be the primary carer of a child with life-threatening needs in the community setting. Planning care for Ryan's complex healthcare needs initially brought a major upheaval into the lives of the whole family and this has led to a long-standing relationship with the main healthcare professionals. We are very pleased to be able to give something back to our healthcare system which has provided us with so much practical training over the years and supported the planning of care for our precious son.

This unique journey with our son Ryan has taught us as parents to think outside the box, to explore all possible avenues and to ensure we are fully informed, using specialist input where needed. Home was recognised as the best place to care for Ryan and he was only admitted to hospital if the care he required could not be provided within his home, despite the fact that, as you may appreciate, this proved to be extremely challenging at times for everyone involved. Nevertheless, we, his parents, and the whole family have ultimately been rewarded for our perseverance.

UPDATE – AUGUST 2022

When providing this update during August 2022, we wanted to cover the changes in Ryan's medical needs, his progress through the education system in Northern Ireland and the social side of his life today.

Since Ryan's tracheostomy was reversed in July 2008, we have never looked back as the chest infections and hospital visits, which he had been susceptible to previously, essentially stopped. His care was managed from that point forwards by the normal outpatient paediatric team in Northern Ireland. The level of medication, which Ryan required was also gradually reduced to the point, where he just required an inhaler twice a day. He managed this treatment himself as he got older, in the same way that other children and adults who are on inhalers do.

Ryan continued his education through mainstream school attending secondary school and the local regional college. He is currently completing a degree at the University of Ulster. The level of developmental support, which Ryan required through school, has gradually reduced over the years, to the point where the support from classroom assistants etc. was no longer required. Only remaining support, which he receives is some additional time to complete exams. It is fair to say that although Ryan was never top of the class from an educational perspective, the determination which he showed from an extremely early age is still there and has helped him immensely on his educational journey.

Socially, Ryan is no different than any other person in that he enjoys a wide range of activities including walking regularly, watching sport, family holidays, etc. His participation in more strenuous activities has been slightly curtailed by his reduced lung function, in that he would get out of breath quickly, but this has not impacted on his social life in any way. To all intents and purposes, Ryan's life today as a 21-year-old is the same as anyone else's. It is also important to note that as his life has become more normal, family life has also returned to a more normal routine without the background concerns in relation to Ryan's health.

Having reflected upon progress over the years it is clear that Ryan's medical and nursing interventions, alongside support in the community through education and Ryan's own determination, have enabled him to get to this point, where he is no different than any of his peers.

CHAPTER 12

The Mental Health and Wellbeing of Children and Young People

Deirdre O'Neill

KEY CONCEPTS

- Mental illness can occur across the life span.
- Early intervention and prevention are key for early detection of mental ill health.
- Undetected illness can lead to further problems into adulthood.
- Everyone who works with children and young people and his or her families and care givers have key roles and are responsible for the care they deliver.

INTRODUCTION

One in seven 10–19-year-olds experience a mental illness, which accounts for 13% of the global burden of disease within this age population (WHO 2022a). Individuals who suffer from mental illness have an increased likelihood of premature death. The World Health Organisation's (WHO 2022a) Comprehensive Mental Health Action Plan 2013–2030 states when compared to the general population, those who have a diagnosis of major depression and schizophrenia have a 40–60% greater chance of dying prematurely. Parity of both physical and mental health is crucial and an integrated approach to care is essential for this to be addressed. Factors which contribute to poorer health outcomes such as social, cultural, environmental, and exposure to adversities in childhood, all play a key role in this. Early intervention and prevention is key to reducing the risk of developing mental illness, this takes into account the entirety of and child and young person (CYP), their family environment, educational opportunities and contributing factors such as poverty, ethnic group or homelessness.

Significant gaps are evident for those who present with mental illness and receive care. For example, between 76–85% of people who have a severe mental illness receive no treatment in low-income countries compared to 35–50% for high-income countries (WHO 2022a). CYP have been significantly affected by the pandemic due to public health measures imposed through 'lock down' resulting in major mental health concerns. It has been reported that there has been a significant increase in crisis presentations to general CYP healthcare settings, which is placing further demands on services and staff. The exact cause of this is unknown however, it can be hypothesised that isolation, which is closely linked with depression, has been one of the main causing factors (Loades et al. 2020). Eating disorders are a common presentation in this age range with it being reported that in 2019, 6% of CYP inpatient beds are due to CYP with a mental illness (Hudson et al. 2021).

With increased demands and complex presentations of CYP, this indicates the need for all health, social and educational sectors to have further knowledge and understanding of potential mental health conditions, which are commonly presented in this population. Further understanding will therefore increase the likelihood that early intervention and prevention will allow for CYP to reach their full potential throughout the life span. It is also important to consider the health equalities for CYP and that social inequalities vary according to their social condition where they live and economic status (Rajmil et al. 2014). It has also been identified that socioeconomic environment and family environment are associated with mental health in childhood.

Given the gravity of mental illness within this population, it is crucially important to widen the conversations and address issues such as 'stigma' and the importance of allowing CYP to have 'a voice' (UNCRC 1989), which is heard, and more importantly validated. Compassionate nursing should be at the core of every nursing intervention and compassionate conversations are required to help aid assessments and develop a plan of care, which is individualised to meet the needs of the child, young person, their family, and support system. Along with physical health, parity of esteem

Care Planning in Children and Young People's Nursing, Second Edition. Edited by Sonya Clarke and Doris Corkin.
© 2024 John Wiley & Sons Ltd. Published 2024 by John Wiley & Sons Ltd.

is required and a comprehensive approach with the understanding that across the life span there will be periods whereby people may be unwell, and that recovery is achievable so that individuals are able to function in a healthy, positive way.

EARLY INTERVENTION AND PREVENTION

The development of mental health issues can start in early childhood with 75% of all mental health problems becoming evident by the age of 18 years (Department of Health 2015). Untreated mental health problems in childhood can lead to further long-term problems in adulthood such as an increase in unemployment and poorer physical health outcomes. For that reason, individuals are prevented from reaching their full potential.

Early intervention and prevention of mental health issues are key to reduce the risk of further problems developing in adulthood (UNICEF 2021, WHO 2022b). Mental health issues can present in numerous ways with some of the most common being depression, anxiety, and early symptoms of first onset of psychosis. Healey (2017) postulate that societal expectations and the need to succeed educationally can put added pressure on a young person, which can increase vulnerability and add stress, which may exacerbate or increase the likelihood of becoming unwell. Self-harm and suicide are also major public health concerns amongst adolescents with suicide being the second most common cause of death in young people world-wide (Hawton et al. 2012). Females are more likely to engage with self-harm behaviour. Alcohol and drug misuse during adolescence can increase suicidal thoughts and impulsivity, which are all of concern. Table 12.1 identifies the risk factors for self-harm and suicidal behaviour – this information should be communicated to all professionals who work with CYP.

MENTAL HEALTH IN THE CONTEXT OF COVID 19

There is considerable evidence to support the rise in mental health issues for CYP during the COVID-19 crisis in which the epidemic has led to further disparity between socioeconomic populations. The most vulnerable groups have had further increase in risk factors with families been negativity impacted and an increase in poverty. Rosen et al. (2021) postulate that risk factors for mental health are increased during times of hardship and crisis and the impact on school closures and lock down has intensified the risk further.

CASE STUDY EXAMPLE

On completing the Box Activity 12.2, consider the treatment plan required and interventions for 'Alex'.

Alex is a 12-year-old female who has attended ED due to a recent episode of self-harm by superficial cutting on her inner thighs. Alex initially attended her GP who advised Alex and her

Table 12.1 Key risk factors for self-harm and suicidal behaviour.

- Mental illness such as depression, anxiety, or psychosis
- Family history of self-harm
- Family history of suicide
- Previous self-harm
- Contact with others who engage in self-harm
- Expressed suicidal intent
- Access to means for self-harm or suicide
- Lack of social support

Source: (Hawton et al. 2012).

ACTIVITY 12.1 CYP EXPERIENCES OF ATTENDING ED WITH SELF-HARM

Consider the experiences of a CYP attending the Emergency Department (ED) services following an episode of self-harm:

- What concerns may be expressed by the CYP during the assessment process?
- What is your role as a CYP Nurse in addressing these concerns?
- What are the next steps following the assessment, which are key for recovery?

ACTIVITY 12.2 — REFLECTIVE RECORD

Using the above questions in Activity 12.1 as a guide, reflect on the role of the nurse and the wider interdisciplinary team. Secondly, consider additional key people who would be part of the support system of CYP such as the education sector that is, nursery schools, primary education, and post primary education sector.

mother to attend ED due to concerns raised at this time about overall mood. A referral at this point has been made to the Child and Adolescent Mental Health Services (CAMHS) – a service that provides assessment and treatment for young people and their families who are experiencing mental health difficulties.

Alex lives with her mother and younger sibling and is in year nine in the local secondary school. Recently there has been a decline in her overall mood and school teaching staff have reported poor concentration in class and Alex not completing work in class and at home. There have also been days missed at school. This has increased following the period of lock down during the COVID-19 pandemic. Alex and her mother report a close relationship. Alex also discloses poor appetite and having trouble sleeping. On observation, it is noted that she has poor eye contact and speaks in a low voice and finds it difficult to engage in conversation. Alex and her family have lived in the local area for eighteen months and prior to this they lived with their wider family including grandparents and others.

ASSESSMENT AND FORMULATION

Mental Health assessment indicates the following information, and the biopsychosocial model was applied in order to ensure a comprehensive overview of Alex and her family was considered along with collateral history. The biopsychosocial model first proposed by George Engle 40 years ago sits within the context of understanding illness in a holistic way. https://www.ncbi.nlm.nih.gov/pmc/articles/PMC1466742

When conducting a mental state assessment, it is important to consider how the information is formulated. It is also key to consider key aspects of the development stage of the child and young person and how this may inform the assessment process. When applied to Alex the following example of a mental state assessment of the main current concerns will inform the plan of care for Alex and her family. It is also important to consider the level of expertise and knowledge and to work within the framework of our knowledge and competencies: https://www.nmc.org.uk/globalassets/sitedocuments/standards/nmc-standards-for-competence-for-registered-nurses.pdf

HISTORY INCLUDING DEVELOPMENTAL MILESTONES

Alex was born four weeks premature and required speech and language intervention at the age of four due to delayed speech, which was highlighted by nursery staff following observations. A referral was generated by the GP and Alex remained on a waiting list for nine months before being seen. Alex attended for six months, and good progress was noted. No other concerns were reported in relation to development, and milestones were met with no delay. Alex's mother discussed her own mental health at this time and a diagnosis of post-natal depression was made and treatment via psychological intervention aided her recovery.

SLEEP

Alex, who reports a change in her sleeping for the last month, finds it difficult to get over to sleep at night, and wakes up earlier than normal. Alex has no history of sleep difficulties and has generally a good routine before sleeping. Alex now spends time on her laptop and phone before she goes to sleep and her mother is concerned that this is impacting her ability to sleep at night.

APPETITE

Decrease in appetite resulting in Alex having some weight loss alongside a lack of energy.

EDUCATION

Alex is in mainstream education and has recently developed poor concentration and attendance at school. This has impacted her overall academic performance. She has had difficulty making friends and feels isolated from her peers but speaks positively about relationships with teaching staff. The staff have highlighted their concerns to Alex's mother.

FAMILY RELATIONSHIPS

Alex describes a close relationship with her mother and siblings however; she does not feel her mother understands her worries and concerns. Alex misses the support of her grandparents.

MOOD

With the aid of 'scaling questions' used for assessing low mood, for example, visit PHQ-9 Depression Test Questionnaire | Patient Alex articulates low mood and particularly at night-time. Alex discloses bullying has been a recurring theme, and when questioned further this has significantly affected her thoughts and feelings; when this occurs Alex cuts her inner thigh with the use of razors and other sharp objects. Alex has used self-harm as a means of coping for the last six months and has not disclosed this to anyone. Alex denies thoughts of life not worth living and denies any suicidal ideations.

RISKS

Alex has low mood, which has impacted her sleep. Alex has adapted the use of self-harm as a means of coping and is at risk of continuing to use this when further difficulties arise. Alex is also at risk of developing infection in the wounded area and further risk of significant harm. Alex is not attending school regularly and this may affect her education attainment and maintaining relationship with others. Refer to Table 12.2 and Table 12.3.

Table 12.2 Care planning: assessment, formulation, and goals.

Reason for assessment	Alex is 12-year-old girl who presents with low mood and has lacerations on both inner thighs that require suturing.
Assessment of CYP needs (Biopsychosocial Model)	Alex requires further assessment from the child and adolescent mental health team due to reports of low mood. Currently Alex has good support from her mother and wider family system. Further assessment of this support is required to ensure her safety. Alex reports bullying as the main issue. Alex currently engages in self-harm as a means of coping and requires further education on positive coping skills.
CYP strengths	Alex is open throughout the assessment and is willing to accept help and support. A positive relationship with her mother is observed throughout the assessment and Alex was able to talk to her mother about her recent concerns.
Formulation (cross Sectional) Situation/Trigger Thoughts Feelings Physical reactions Behaviours Padeskey and Mooney (1990)	**Situation:** When I try to sleep at night, my body feels exhausted however, I cannot get over to sleep and try to distract myself with my phone. I then see comments, which have been written about me. **Thoughts:** My thoughts start to race, and I am thinking "Why me?" "When will this stop?" **Feelings:** I feel useless, why cannot I be like my peers and just laugh at the comments. I also feel guilty as the thoughts of harming myself are strong and I am worried about upsetting my mum. I feel so tired all the time. **Physical reactions:** My stomach hurts and I have a sore head. My breathing changes and it feels at times I cannot fill my lungs with air. I then start to feel dizzy and am afraid I might vomit. My legs ache and I am sore all over. **Behaviour:** I tell my mum I am not going to school the next day as I cannot face the people in my class as they will be laughing at me. I cannot concentrate in class, as I am so tired. The feelings are so intense and I have persistent urges to harm myself.
Value Directed Goals Short, medium, and long term	• *Short-term goals* identified by Alex are to improve her sleep and increase her dietary intake. • *Medium term goals* – Alex would like to reduce her self-harm and to learn other ways of managing her emotions. • *Long term goals* – Alex would like to be attending school full time and have an increase in her ability to concentrate.

Table 12.3 Interventions and rationale.

Interventions (Linked to short term goal)	Rationale
Alex to be referred to CAMHS for further assessment of her mood and commence psychological intervention	Alex has been experiencing low mood for several months and despite intervention from school counsellor, there has been no/little improvement. The episodes of self-harm have increased with medical intervention required. Overall mood requires ongoing assessment as this has now impacted on her ability to attend school and to participate in her daily activities.
Alex to complete a sleep diary and daily activity scheduling	This information will identify for Alex and her key workers how much sleep she is getting and general routines which will inform Alex further.

SUMMARY: PSYCHOLOGICAL INTERVENTIONS

Assessment and intervention of all young people who present with mental illness such as low mood and self-harm needs to be assessed accordingly. A key priority lies within the timing, in order to avoid further deterioration in mental state. Initial conversations by professionals who are not mental-health trained will significantly aid the process with further engagement with mental health services. Therefore, training for all non-mental health staff will help staff understand the causes for young people presenting in distress and in a crisis to services. Trauma informed practice could help guide professionals to understand the reasons for people engaging in self-harm and the impact of adverse childhood experiences. A variety of psychological interventions are available for CYP, with Cognitive Behavioural Therapy (CBT) being the recommended intervention (NICE 2019); this alongside family work are recommended based on the individual needs of the CYP. Other key factors, which will further indicate the level of intervention is the risk assessment outcomes, and if there are suicidal ideations, which the CYP is expressing.

The use of medication as first line treatment for mild depression is not recommended; however, if a CYP is presenting with moderate to severe depression, it is recommended that combined therapy (Fluoxetine and psychological therapy) may be required (NICE 2019). CYP should be under the care of a CAMHS team, receive regular reviews, and follow up for nonattendance at appointments. Most importantly, the CYP and their families should be consulted as to the evidenced based treatment approached and fully informed of expected outcomes with these approaches.

ADDTIONAL RESOURCES

CAMHS, Child and Adolescent Mental Health Services – HSE.ie

UNICEF (2021) The State of the World's Children. On My Mind–Promoting, Protecting and Caring for Children's Mental Health. Available at https://files.eric.ed.gov/fulltext/ED615261.pdf Acessed 5/1/23

REFERENCES

Department of Health (2015) Future in Mind. Promoting, Protecting and Improving Our Children and Young People's Mental Health and Wellbeing. assets.publishing.service.gov.uk/government/uploads/system/uploads/attachment_data/file/414024/Childrens_Mental_Health.pdf[Accessed 11 March 2023]

Hawton, K., Kate, D.S., Saunders, E. & O'Connor, R.C. (2012) Self-harm and suicide in adolescents. *The Lancet*, 379, 2373–2382.

Healey, J. Ed (2017) *Youth Mental Health*. Thirroul NSW: Spinney Press.

Hudson, L.D., Chapman, S., Street, K.N., Nicholls, D., Roland, D., Dubicka, B., Gibson, F., Mathews, G. & Viner, R.M. (2021). Increased admissions to paediatric wards with a primary mental health diagnosis: Results of a survey of a network of eating disorder paediatricians in England. *Archives of Disease in Childhood*, doi: 10.1136/archdischild-2021-322700.

Loades, M.E., Chatburn, E., Higson-Sweeney, N., Reynolds, S., Shafran, R., Brigden, A., Linney, C., Brigden, A., McManus, M.N., Borwick, C. & Crawley, E. (2020) Rapid systematic review: The impact of social isolation and loneliness on the mental health of children and adolescents in the context of COVID-19. *Journal of the American Academy of Child and Adolescent Psychiatry*, 59(11), 1218–1239.e3. doi: 10.1016/j.jaac.2020.05.009.

NICE (2019) Recommendations | Depression in children and young people: identification and management | Guidance | NICE [Accessed 5 1 2023].

Padesky, C.A. (1990) Schema as Self-Prejudice. *International Cognitive Therapy Newsletter*, 6, 6–7.

Rajmil, L., Herdman, M., Ravens-Sieberer, U., Erhart, M., Alonso, J. & The European KIDSCREEN group. (2014) Socioeconomic inequalities in mental health and health-related quality of life (HRQOL) in children and adolescents from 11 European countries. *International Journal of Public Health*, 59, 95–105. doi: 10.1007/s00038-013-0479-9.

Rosen, M.L., Rodman, A.M., Kasparek, S.W., Mayes, M., Freeman, M.M., Lengua, L.J. et al. (2021) Promoting youth mental health during the COVID-19 pandemic: A longitudinal study. *PLoS ONE*, **16**(8), e0255294. doi: 10.1371/journal.pone.0255294.

United Nations Convention for the Rights of the Child (1989). *Ratified by the United Kingdom Government in 1991*. Geneva: United Nations.

World Health Organisation WHO (2022a) Comprehensive Mental Health Action Plan 2013–2030. Available at Comprehensive Mental Health Action Plan 2013-2030 (who.int) [Accessed on 5 1 2023].

World Health Organisation WHO (2022b) Adolescent Mental Health. Available at Adolescent mental health (who.int) [Accessed 5 1 2023].

Care Planning – Pain Management

SECTION 2

Managing a Neonate in an Intensive Care Unit

CHAPTER 13

Clare Morfoot

SCENARIO

Molly was born prematurely at 32 weeks' gestation by normal vaginal delivery, following spontaneous rupture of membranes. At birth, Molly weighed 1.3 kg with an Apgar score (Calmes 2015) of 7 at one minute and 10 at five minutes. Following delivery, Molly had shallow, irregular respirations with a heart rate less than 100 beats per minute. She was dusky in colour with good tone. On the resuscitaire, Molly received continuous positive airway pressure (CPAP) via a facemask, which improved her heart rate but she continued to show increased work of breathing, with intermittent grunting and sternal recession. Molly's parents were able to see and touch Molly prior to transfer to the neonatal unit on CPAP.

On admission to the neonatal unit, Molly was moved to a closed incubator and commenced heated, humidified high-flow nasal cannula (HHFNC), as a means of non-invasive respiratory support (Fleeman et al. 2019; Hui Hong et al. 2021). An orogastric tube and peripheral venous cannula were sited. Molly's improving respiratory function and blood gases permitted weaning of the HHFNC and this was discontinued at 48 hours of age. The suboptimal progression of enteral feeding by 72 hours of age resulted in the insertion of a central venous long line to allow the administration of total parenteral nutrition (TPN), in line with national guidance (NICE 2020). Throughout the first three days of life, Molly required a number of painful invasive procedures, including an intramuscular injection, eight venous cannulations (including unsuccessful attempts) and ten heel pricks for newborn blood spot screening, blood gases, and glucose levels. Subsequently, Molly underwent further invasive procedures, although these gradually reduced in frequency, until she was discharged home.

QUESTIONS

1. Assessment: how would you assess whether Molly is in pain?
2. Planning: how would you prepare Molly and her family for painful invasive diagnostic procedures?
3. Implementation: what pain management strategies might you use to support Molly during painful invasive diagnostic procedures?
4. Evaluation: what might be the consequences of not managing Molly's pain effectively?

This chapter will focus on the non-pharmacological management of pain in the neonate. Although this scenario is based on a premature infant, the principles of care included within this chapter are also relevant to the term neonate. Pharmacological pain measures will not be addressed as these are covered in other relevant chapters.

ANSWERS TO QUESTIONS

Activity of living: communication.

Question 1. Assessment: How would you assess whether Molly is in pain?

Until the 1980s, neonates were regarded as incapable of experiencing pain due to the immaturity of their nervous system (Agakidou et al. 2021). However, it is now widely acknowledged that premature infants possess the neurological capacity to perceive pain (Anand & Hickey 1987; Simons & Tibboel 2006) with evidence of hypersensitivity to noxious stimuli when compared to adults (Fitzgerald & Beggs 2001; Ranger & Grunau 2015), due to the immaturity of descending inhibitory pathways, larger pain perception areas in the spinal cord and the volume of pain receptors lying closer to the skin.

Although many definitions of pain acknowledge its subjective, emotional, and sensory nature, the inclusion of an emotional component, means that they fail to accurately reflect the neonatal pain experience. In addition, it can be challenging to differentiate between discomfort, stress, and pain, particularly in the non-verbal infant (Olsson et al. 2021).

At 32 weeks' gestation, Molly is capable of feeling pain and it is essential that healthcare professionals observe Molly for specific pain indicators (Table 13.1), in order to adequately assess and treat her pain. Molly's response to pain may result in physiological, behavioural, metabolic, and hormonal changes (Witt et al. 2016).

Numerous neonatal pain assessment scales exist for different infant populations and types of pain, although not all of these are validated (Olsson et al. 2021). Most tools tend to focus on the observation of behavioural and physiological responses, with the evaluation of chemical indicators often reserved for research, since these require additional painful, invasive, diagnostic procedures to detect them. It is important to remember that the sick, preterm, sedated, paralysed, or ventilated infant may not be capable of demonstrating the anticipated behavioural responses to pain. A few examples of commonly cited and validated neonatal pain assessment tools include:

Premature Infant Pain Profile (PIPP)
This tool assesses seven items, including behavioural and physiological indicators, each scoring 0–3. The revised scale (PIPP-R) also incorporates contextual factors, such as gestational age and sleep state, thereby acknowledging that infants who are sleeping or extremely preterm may be unable to demonstrate a typical behavioural response (Stevens et al. 2014). This tool is validated for both premature and term infants for acute procedural and postoperative pain (Gibbins et al. 2014; Witt et al. 2016).

Neonatal Infant Pain Score (NIPS)
This is the second most cited tool within studies about procedural pain assessment (Olsson et al. 2021). The scale evaluates six behavioural and physiological indicators with a maximum score of seven. It is used for both preterm and term infants and is validated for acute procedural pain (Witt et al. 2016).

CRIES (Crying, Requires oxygen, Increased vital signs, Expression, Sleeplessness)
This tool assesses five behavioural and physiological indicators, each attracting a score of 0–2. It is validated for both premature and term infants for postoperative pain (Olsson et al. 2021; Witt et al. 2016).

The accurate assessment of pain is not only an important ethical consideration but also key to reducing the risk of significant short- and long-term deleterious consequences that are associated with continued exposure to pain (American Academy of Pediatrics Committee on Fetus and Newborn and Section on Anesthesiology and Pain Medicine 2016). Despite international recommendations emphasising the importance of neonatal pain assessment, a European multicentre study demonstrated that only ten percent of premature infants and a third of admissions to neonatal intensive care are assessed for pain (Anand et al. 2017). Lack of knowledge, concerns

Table 13.1 Examples of neonatal pain indicators.

Behavioural responses	Physiological parameters	Chemical changes
Facial expression e.g. grimace, cupped tongue, brow bulge, naso-labial furrow, open mouth, eye squeeze, pursed lips, taut tongue	↑↓ heart rate	↑ stress hormone production
Cry (may be silent if intubated)	↑↓ respiratory rate	↑ blood glucose
Body movement e.g. splayed digits, arching, hand swiping, clenching of fists and toes, limb withdrawal, rigidity, flaccidity	↑↓ oxygen saturations	↓ insulin
Changes in sleep/wake cycle, for example hyper-alert or lethargic, irritability	↑↓ blood pressure	

regarding the validity of pain assessment scales and the availability of guidelines all appear to influence the use of such tools (Carlsen Misic et al. 2021).

Question 2. Planning: How would you prepare Molly and her family for painful invasive diagnostic procedures?

Preparing Molly

During her admission to the neonatal unit, Molly will be exposed to significant environmental stressors, including noxious sound, light, smell, taste, and touch, at a time when she would otherwise be developing *in utero*. Failure to minimise the adverse impact of the neonatal environment or the stress and pain associated with invasive procedures may jeopardise Molly's neurodevelopment and adversely impact her long-term outcomes (Altimier & Phillips 2016). In contrast, the adoption of neuroprotective, family oriented, developmental approaches to neonatal care will promote more positive outcomes (Altimier & Phillips 2016).

The assessment of Molly's behavioural cues (Table 13.2) allows the healthcare professional to interpret how Molly is coping with the stressors of the environment (Als & Butler 2008; Warren & Bond 2010). For example, Molly may display avoidance behaviours, such as splayed digits or side swiping during attempts at blood sampling or cannulation. If such avoidance behaviours are observed, the environment must be modified and where possible, procedures should be delayed. During these invasive procedures, appropriate pain management strategies must be employed.

The timing of all procedures should be individualised and planned to ensure that Molly has adequate rest to promote growth and development. Procedures should coincide with other caregiving activities wherever possible. Invasive procedures should not be performed around Molly's feed times to avoid vomiting and the risk of aspiration.

Preparing Molly's Family

The neonatal unit is an extremely artificial and stressful environment, with many parents experiencing feelings of guilt, helplessness, anxiety, depression, and even post-traumatic stress disorder (Gibbs et al. 2016; Malin et al. 2020; O'Brien et al. 2018). Neonatal family integrated care is a concept that builds on the principles of family centred care to empower parents to share the delivery of a substantial part of their baby's care (Patel et al. 2017). The specific components of family integrated care may vary but commonly incorporate a range of inclusive and supportive strategies, such as timetabled parent education and coaching sessions, peer support by veteran parents, and access to a psychologist (O'Brien et al. 2018; Patel et al. 2017). Molly's parents may be invited to present a summary of her admission and current medical issues during multidisciplinary ward rounds and encouraged to deliver many aspects of her care, including tube feeds, oral feeds, bathing, kangaroo care, nappy changes, oral medication administration, and checking Molly's temperature (O'Brien et al. 2018). This collaborative model is associated with improved infant weight gain, reduced nosocomial infections, higher breastfeeding rates, reduced parental

Table 13.2 Examples of behavioural cues.

Avoidance behaviour	Approach behaviour
Sneezing	Hands together
Hiccoughing	Grasping
Yawning	Hands to face
Grimacing	Hands to mouth
Limp or stiff posture	Smooth movements
Sudden or jerky movements	Orientation to voice or sound
Trembling	Flexed posture
Finger splay	Relaxed expression
Arm swiping	Mouth making 'ooh' shape
Arm salute	Sucking
Crying	Smooth transition from sleep to wake
Looking away	Snuggling

stress, and anxiety and shorter length of stay (Givrad et al. 2021; O'Brien et al. 2018; Patel et al. 2017).

During Molly's admission, her parents are likely to feel vulnerable and, as a result, the retention and recall of information provided by healthcare professionals may be impaired (Williams et al. 2020). It is, therefore, important to utilise clear, consistent explanations, which must be repeated, if necessary. Medical jargon and abbreviations should be avoided. The reason for the procedure should be given, along with the potential risks and benefits, to ascertain consent. Verbal information must be supported by written or digital resources and all information should be available in the parents' first language, in line with the fifth principle of the BLISS Baby Charter, a practical guide to improving the delivery of family oriented neonatal care services (Bliss 2015).

The active involvement of parents throughout invasive procedures will promote enhanced neonatal pain practices (Ullsten et al. 2021) and Molly's parents should be offered the opportunity to support her in this way. However, some parents may prefer not to, and this decision should be respected. Although Molly's parents may choose to be present for one procedure, it should not be assumed that they wish to be included for every intervention.

Preparation of the Practitioner
It is imperative that the practitioner undertaking the procedure is the most appropriate person for the task. Consideration should be given to the practitioner's availability and level of competence. The healthcare professional should ensure that two people are available throughout the procedure: one to support Molly or her parents and one to undertake the procedure. Equipment and the environment should be prepared in advance, with consideration for health and safety. This may include a height-adjustable incubator and a functioning, mobile light source.

Aseptic non-touch technique should be employed at each stage of an invasive procedure, including effective handwashing, use of alcohol gel, and appropriate personal protective equipment. The number of attempts for invasive procedures, such as venepuncture and cannulation, should be limited to usually no more than three attempts and if unsuccessful, Molly must be allowed to recover and a more senior practitioner asked to undertake the procedure.

Question 3. Implementation: What pain management strategies might you use to support Molly during painful invasive diagnostic procedures?

There are several appropriate, non-pharmacological pain management strategies which may help Molly prepare for, cope with, and recover from painful or stressful procedures.

Comfort Holding and Positive Touch
The physical and thermal stimulation of positive touch can provide gentle disturbance, prior to an intervention, to signal an imminent procedure for Molly. The technique of comfort holding (also known as containment holding or facilitated tucking) involves the still holding of an infant in a flexed midline position, with one hand cupping the baby's head and the other cradling the lower limbs or feet to maintain flexion of the lower body (Figure 13.1). In this way, comfort holding facilitates the infant's ability to self-regulate, thereby promoting physiological stability (Gomes Neto et al. 2020). Comfort holding is also an effective method of non-pharmacological pain management during stressful or invasive procedures. The application of this still touch by parents or staff provides a valuable contrast to procedural related contact, causing a release of endogenous endorphins which moderate pain (Gomes Neto et al. 2020). The support and inclusion of Molly's parents to provide this comfort measure may empower them to participate in her general care.

Kangaroo Care and Rooming-in
Kangaroo care or skin-to-skin contact (Figure 13.2) describes the upright holding of an infant wearing only a nappy against the parent's bare chest (Johnston et al. 2017). Kangaroo care elicits a favourable reduction in physiological and behavioural pain responses to invasive procedures, such as heel prick or intramuscular injection, that is comparable to the effects of oral sucrose administration (Campbell-Yeo et al 2019; Shukla et al. 2018). In addition, kangaroo care decreases parental and infant salivary cortisol (Mörelius et al. 2015), a known marker of stress linked to insulin resistance, elevated cholesterol, and reduced immunity. Therefore, kangaroo care may be utilised by Molly's parents as an appropriate method of non-pharmacological pain control.

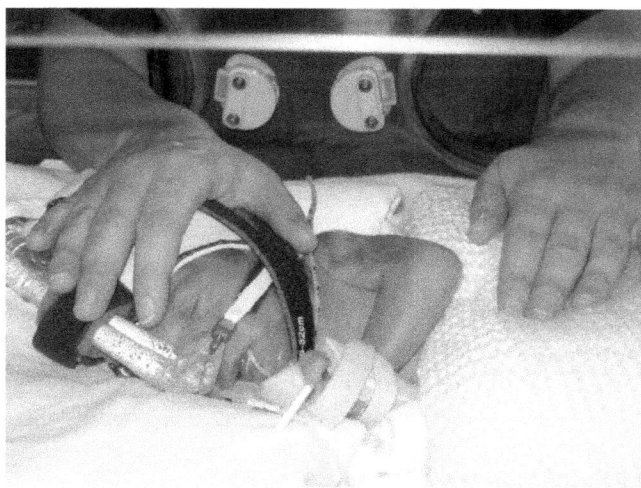

FIGURE 13.1 Comfort holding.

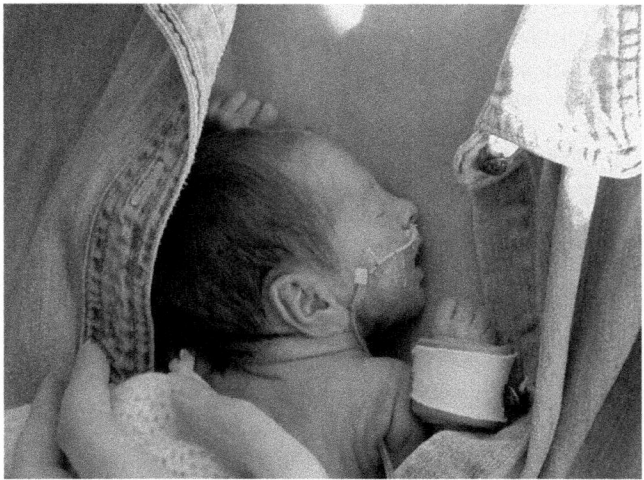

FIGURE 13.2 Kangaroo care.

The process of rooming in, where parents temporarily reside with their infant also reduces salivary cortisol levels in term newborns. Studies indicate that cortisol levels are significantly lower in those infants whose parents are present both day and night (De Bernardo et al. 2018). Thus, the provision of unrestricted unit access is key to ensuring that Molly's parents are coached and supported to deploy appropriate pain relieving strategies and to act as equal partners in her care. A number of pioneering neonatal units now offer dedicated shared spaces for parent and baby to remain together from admission to discharge, thereby promoting the true integration of the family (Givrad et al. 2021).

Auditory and Visual Exposure
The reduction of excessive noise and light will minimise the impact of environmental stressors, promoting homeostasis and better sleep for Molly (Givrad et al. 2021). The use of individual spotlights, padded incubator covers and eye protection, during invasive procedures, may all help to limit the number of stressful stimulants for her.

Although inappropriate and extreme noise may be detrimental to Molly, the moderated use of music therapy or parental voice may serve to mitigate physiological stress responses and promote positive neurodevelopment (Givrad et al. 2021; Scala et al. 2018). Music therapy is described as the systematic and individualised application of carefully chosen sounds by trained professionals to support physiological and neurological wellbeing (Maitre & Arnon 2020). The use of a short recording of a lullaby sung by the parent mixed with heart sounds, during retinopathy of prematurity screening, has been shown to reduce neonatal pain scores and shorten the procedural recovery time for eye examinations lasting more than eighty seconds (Corrigan et al. 2020). Similar physiological and behavioural benefits were noted when music is played for short periods before and after blood sampling (Shabani et al. 2016).

Non-nutritive Sucking, Sucrose, and Breastmilk
Non-nutritive sucking refers to the promotion of sucking behaviours without nutritional gain and may involve a pacifier, gloved finger, or empty breast with or without small volumes of breastmilk or sweet solution. The administration of oral sucrose/glucose or breastmilk produces a release of endogenous endorphins. Each of these strategies is reported to reduce physiological and behavioural pain responses following minor procedures, including intramuscular injections, hip examination, retinopathy of prematurity screening, and blood sampling, although debate continues about the most efficacious approach and whether combining these modalities brings additional benefit (Campbell et al. 2014; Olsson et al. 2019; Shukla et al. 2018; Tanyeri-Bayraktar et al. 2019; Wu et al. 2021). Further uncertainty remains about the potential long-term effects and the optimal strength, volume, and frequency of sucrose administration (Shukla et al. 2018; Tanyeri-Bayraktar 2019).

Although the use of pacifiers may be considered therapeutic and offer protection against sudden infant death, the reported risk of nipple confusion impacting breastfeeding success may, nevertheless, generate controversy for both staff and parents alike (Alm et al. 2016; Lubbe & ten Ham-baloyi 2017). Local guidelines and parental wishes regarding the use of pacifiers must always be followed.

Question 4. Evaluation: What might be the consequences of not managing Molly's pain effectively?

It is important to acknowledge that Molly will not only have pain responses that are immediate (seconds to minutes), but also some that are persistent (days to weeks) and others that are prolonged, outlasting her hospital stay (Fitzgerald & Beggs 2001). The pain experienced by Molly, during her time in the neonatal unit may result in long-lasting deleterious consequences. This early exposure to pain and stress can produce neurodevelopmental, behavioural, cognitive, motor, and psychosocial effects (Shukla et al. 2018; Walker 2019). Some children are known to become increasingly sensitised or preoccupied with pain, while other sequelae include depression and anxiety, deficits in learning, poor motor performance, behavioural problems, attention deficits, impulsivity and poor adaptive behaviour (Givrad et al. 2021; Maitre & Arnon 2020; Shabani et al. 2016; Stevens et al. 2014; Walker 2019).

REFERENCES

Agakidou, E., Konstantia, T., Stathopoulou, T., Thomaidou, A., Farini, M., Kontou, A., Karagianni, P. & Sarafidis, K. (2021) Changes in physicians' perceptions and practices on neonatal pain management over the past 20 years. A survey conducted at two time-points. *Frontiers in Pediatrics*, **9**, doi: 10.3389/fped.2021.667806.

Alm, B., Wennergren, G., Möllborg, P. & Lagercrantz, H. (2016) Breastfeeding and dummy use have a protective effect on sudden infant death syndrome. *Acta Paediatrica*, **105**, 31–38. doi: 10.1111/apa.13124.

Als, H. & Butler, S. (2008) Newborn individualized developmental care and assessment program (NIDCAP): changing the future for infants and families in intensive and special care nurseries. *Early Childhood Services*, **2**(1), 1–20.

Altimier, L. & Phillips, R. (2016) The neonatal integrative developmental care model: Advanced clinical applications of the seven core measures for neuroprotective family-centered developmental. *Newborn and Infant Nursing Reviews*, **16**, 230–244.

American Academy of Pediatrics (AAP) Committee on Fetus and Newborn and Section on Anesthesiology and Pain Medicine (2016) Prevention and management of procedural pain in the neonate: an update. *Pediatrics*, **137**(2), e20154271. doi: 10.1542/peds.2015-4271.

Anand, K.J.S., Eriksson, M., Boyle, E.M., Avila-Alvarez, A., Andersen, R.D., Sarafidis, K., Polkki, T., Matos, C., Lago, P., Papadouri, T., Attard-Montalto, S., Ilmoja, M., Simons, S., Tameliene, R., van Overmeire, B., Berger, A., Dobrzanska, A., Schroth, M., Bergqvist, L., Courtois, E., Rousseau, J. & Carbajal, R. (2017) Assessment of continuous pain in newborns admitted to NICUs in 18 European countries. *Acta Paediatrica*, **106**, 1248–1259. doi: 10.1111/apa.13810.

Anand, K.J.S. & Hickey, P.R. (1987) Pain and its effects in the human neonate and fetus. *The New England Journal of Medicine*, **317**, 21.

BLISS (2015) *Bliss Baby Care Charter (Principle 5)*. London: BLISS. Available at https://bliss.org.uk.

Calmes, S.H. (2015) Dr. Virginia Apgar and the Apgar score: How the Apgar score came to be. *Anesthesia & Analgesia*, **120**(5), 1060–1064. doi: 10.1213/ANE.0000000000000659.

Campbell, N., Cleaver, K. & Davies, N. (2014) Oral sucrose as an analgesia for neonates: how effective and safe is the sweet solution? A review of the literature. *Journal of Neonatal Nursing*, **20**, 274–282.

Campbell-Yeo, M., Johnston, C.C., Benoit, B., Disher, T., Caddell, K., Vincer, M., Walker, C.D., Latimer, M., Streiner, D.L. & Inglis, D. (2019) Sustained efficacy of kangaroo care for repeated painful procedures over neonatal intensive care unit hospitalization: a single-blind randomized controlled trial. *Pain*, 1–9. doi: 10.1097/j.pain.0000000000001646.

Carlsen Misic, M., Anderson, R.D., Strand, S., Eriksson, M. & Olsson, E. (2021) Nurses' perception, knowledge, and use of neonatal pain assessment. *Paediatric and Neonatal Pain*, **3**, 68–74. doi: 10.1002/pne2.12050.

Corrigan, M.J., Keeler, J.R., Miller, H.D., Khallouq, B.A. & Fowler, S.B. (2020) Music therapy and retinopathy of prematurity screening: using recorded maternal singing and heartbeat for post exam recovery. *Journal of Perinatology*, **40**, 1734–1735. doi: https://pubmed.ncbi.nlm.nih.gov/32681063 [Accessed 11 March 2023].

De Bernardo, G., Riccitelli, M., Giordano, M., Proietti, F., Sordino, D., Longini, M., Buonocore, G. & Perrone, S. (2018) Rooming-in reduces salivary cortisol level of newborn. *Mediators of Inflammation*, 2018 Mar 8 Article ID 2845352, 1–5. Doi: 10.1155/2018/2845352. PMID: 29706798; PMCID: PMC5863308.

Fitzgerald, M. & Beggs, S. (2001) The neurobiology of pain: developmental aspects. *Neuroscientist*, **7**, 246–257.

Fleeman, N., Dundar, Y., Shah, P.S. & Shaw, B.N.J. (2019) Heated humidified high-flow nasal cannula for preterm infants: an updated systematic review and meta-analysis. *International Journal of Technology Assessment in Health Care*, **35**, 298–306. doi: 10.1017/S0266462319000424.

Gibbins, S., Stevens, B.J., Yamada, J., Dionee, K., Campbell-Yeo, M., Lee, G., Caddell, K., Johnston, C. & Taddio, A. (2014) Validation of the premature infant pain profile – revised (PIPP-R). *Early Human Development*, **90**, 189–193. doi: 10.1016.j.earlhumdev.2014.01.005.

Gibbs, D.P., Boshoff, K. & Stanley, M.J. (2016) The acquisition of parenting occupations in neonatal intensive care: A preliminary perspective. *Canadian Journal of Occupational Therapy*, **83**(2), 91–102. doi: 10.1177/0008417415625421.

Givrad, S., Dowtin, L.L., Scala, M. & Hall, S.J. (2021) Recognizing and mitigating infant distress in Neonatal Intensive Care Unit (NICU). *Journal of Neonatal Nursing*, **27**, 14–20.

Gomes Neto, M., da Silva Lopes, I.A., Araujo, A.C., Oliveira, L.S. & Saquetto, M.B. (2020) The effect of facilitated tucking position during painful procedure in pain management of preterm infants in neonatal intensive care unit: A systematic review and meta-analysis. *European Journal of Pediatrics*, **179**, 699–709.

Hong, H., Xiao-xia, L., Jing, L. & Zhang, Z.-Q. (2021) High-flow nasal cannula versus nasal continuous positive airway pressure for respiratory support in preterm infants: A meta-analysis of randomized controlled trials. *The Journal of Maternal-Fetal & Neonatal Medicine*, **34**(2), 259–266. doi: 10.1080/14767058.2019.1606193.

Johnston, C., Campbell-Yeo, M., Disher, T., Benoit, B., Fernandes, A., Strenier, D., Inglis, D. & Zee, R. (2017) Skin-to-skin care for procedural pain in neonates. *Cochrane Database of Systematic Reviews*, Article CD008435 doi: 10.1002/14651858.CD008435.pub3.

Lubbe, W. & ten Ham-Baloyi, W. (2017) When is the use of pacifiers justifiable in the baby-friendly hospital initiative context? A clinician's guide. *BMC Pregnancy Childbirth*, **17**, 130. doi: 10.1186/s12884-017-1306-8.

Maitre, N.L. & Arnon, S. (2020) Music therapy for neonatal stress and pain – music to our ears. *Journal of Perinatology*, **40**, 1734–1735.

Malin, K.J., Johnson, T.S., McAndrew, S., Westerdahl, J., Leuthner, J. & Lagatta, J. (2020) Infant illness severity and perinatal post-traumatic stress disorder after discharge from the neonatal intensive care unit. *Early Human Development*, **140**, doi: 10.1016/j.earlhumdev.2019.104930.

Mörelius, E., Örtenstrand, A., Theodorsson, E. & Frostell, A. (2015) A randomised trial of continuous skin-to-skin contact after preterm birth and the effects on salivary cortisol, parental stress, depression, and breastfeeding. *Early Human Development*, **91**(1), 63–70. doi: 10.1016/j.earlhumdev.2014.12.005.

National Institute for Health and Care Excellence (NICE) (2020) *Neonatal Parenteral Nutrition. NICE Guideline (NG 154)*.

O'Brien, K., Robson, K., Bracht, M., Cruz, M., Lui, K., Alvaro, R., da Silva, O., Monterrosa, L., Narvey, M., Ng, E., Soraisham, A., Le, X.Y., Mirea, L., Tarnow-Mordi, W. & Lee, S.K. (2018) Effectiveness of family integrated care in neonatal intensive care units on infant and parent outcomes: a multicentre, multinational, cluster-randomised controlled trial. *Lancet*, Feb 7. doi: 10.1016/S2352-4642(18)30039-7.

Olsson, E., Ahl, H., Bengtsson, K., Vejayaram, D.N., Norman, E., Bruschettini, M. & Eriksson, M. (2021) The use and reporting of neonatal pain scales: A systematic review of randomized trials. *Pain*, **162**(2), 353–360. doi: 10.1097/j.pain.0000000000002046.

Olsson, E., Pettersson, M., Eriksson, M. & Ohlin, A. (2019) Oral sweet solution to prevent pain during neonatal hip examination: A randomised controlled trial. *Acta Paediatrica*, **108**, 626–629.

Patel, N., Ballantyne, A., Bowker, G., Weightman, J. & Weightman, S. (2017) Family integrated care: changing the culture in the neonatal unit. *Archives of Disease in Childhood*, **103**, 415–419.

Ranger, M. & Grunau, R.E. (2015) How do babies feel pain? *eLife*, **4**, e07552. doi: 10.7554/eLife.07552.

Scala, M., Seo, S., Lee-Park, J., McClure, C., Scala, M. & Palafoutas, J. (2018) Effect of reading to preterm infants on measures of cardiorespiratory stability in the neonatal intensive care unit. *Journal of Perinatology*, **38**(11), 1536–1541.

Shabani, F., Nayeri, N.D., Karimi, R., Zarei, K. & Chehrazi, M. (2016) Effects of music therapy on pain responses induced by blood sampling in premature infants: a randomized cross-over trial. *Iranian Journal of Nursing and Midwifery Research*, **21**, 391–396.

Shukla, V., Chapla, A., Uperiya, J., Nimbalkar, A., Phatak, A. & Nimbalkar, S. (2018) Sucrose vs. skin to skin care for preterm neonatal pain control – a randomized control trial. *Journal of Perinatology*, **38**, 1365–1369.

Simons, S.H.P. & Tibboel, D. (2006) Pain perception, development and maturation. *Seminars in Fetal and Neonatal Medicine*, **11**, 227–231.

Stevens, B.J., Gibbins, S., Yamada, J., Dionee, K., Lee, G., Johnston, C. & Taddio, A. (2014) The premature infant pain profile – revised (PIPP-R). Initially validation and feasibility. *The Clinical Journal of Pain*, **30**(3), 238–243.

Tanyeri-Bayraktar, B., Bayraktar, S., Hepokur, M. & Kuran, G. (2019) Comparison of two different doses of sucrose in pain relief. *Pediatrics International*, **61**, 797–801.

Ullsten, A., Andreasson, M. & Eriksson, M. (2021) State of the art in parent-delivered pain-relieving interventions in neonatal care: a scoping review. *Frontiers in Pediatrics*, **9**, 651846. doi: 10.3389/fped.2021.651846.

Walker, S.M. (2019) Long-term effects of neonatal pain. *Seminars in Fetal and Neonatal Medicine*, **24**(4), doi: 10.1016/j.siny.2019.04.005.

Warren, I. & Bond, C. (2010) *A Guide to Infant Development in the Newborn Nursery*, 5th edn. London: Winnicott Baby Unit.

Williams, L., I'Anson, J., Malarkey, M., Purcell, A., Vries, N. & McKinlay, C. (2020) Information sharing in neonatal intensive care: parental perceptions and preferences. *Journal of Paediatrics and Child Health*, **56**(7), 1121–1125.

Witt, N., Coynor, S., Edwards, C. & Bradshaw, H. (2016) A guide to pain assessment and management in the neonate. *Current Emergency and Hospital Medicine Reports*, **4**, 1–10. doi: 10.1007/s40138-016-0089-y.

Wu, H., Zhang, J., Ding, Q., Wang, S. & Li, J. (2021) Effect analysis of embracing breast milk sucking to relieve pain of neonatal heel blood sampling: a randomised controlled trial. *Annals of Palliative Medicine*, **10**(4), 4384–4390.

Continuous Patient- and Nurse-Controlled Opiate Analgesia and Ketamine Infusions

CHAPTER 14A

Sharon Douglass and Michelle Whitehouse

SCENARIO

Sadie is a 15-year-old girl who was diagnosed with Crohn's disease three years ago. Conservative management is no longer effective; therefore, she has been admitted electively for formation of a colostomy. A colostomy is when the colon (large intestine) is connected to the abdominal surface. It usually protrudes above skin level on the abdomen to help reduce the risk of skin irritation from faeces.

Before the procedure, the stoma nurse specialist or surgeon will talk to the child or young person (CYP) and family about the surgery and the stoma placement on the abdomen. Usually, the stoma would be low down on the left side, but final placement is dictated by where the affected part of the bowel is. Bowel contents travel through part of the colon, where the body absorbs some of the remaining water. Depending on where the stoma is, faeces that passes through the stoma may be semi-formed or fully formed, depending on the placement of the stoma.

Colostomy surgery can be performed either as a laparoscopic or an open procedure. Sadie is having a laproscopic procedure (keyhole), which minimises the interruption of all tissue and muscle layers. In addition, previous frequent acute exacerbations of her Crohn's disease have resulted in thickening of the intestinal wall with swelling and scar tissue (Crohn's and Colitis UK 2021).

It is essential to take into consideration any child's underlying condition when planning postoperative pain management. In Sadie's case non-steroidal anti-inflammatory drugs (NSAIDs) such as ibuprofen and diclofenac are contra-indicated as one of the side effects is gastric irritation, which is already a symptom of Crohn's disease. Therefore, suitable analgesia includes paracetamol, opiates, ketamine, and local anaesthetics to provide comprehensive multimodal pain management.

The route of administration must also be considered and in the immediate postoperative period, the oral route would not be appropriate for the following reasons: being nil by mouth, potential presence of a paralytic ileus, nasogastric tube on free drainage, nausea, and vomiting.

Also, Crohn's is known to have a negative impact on absorption in the body and the development of scar tissue. The Association of Paediatric Anaesthetists of Great Britain and Ireland (APAGBI 2012) recommend use of regular intravenous paracetamol alongside an advanced analgesic technique such as an intravenous opiate patient-controlled analgesia (PCA) infusion. When the anaesthetist visits Sadie and her family pre-operatively they discuss the options and decide on a Fentanyl PCA infusion. Refer to Box Activity 14.1.

ACTIVITY 14.1

Recommended reading:

Association of Paediatric Anaesthetists of Great Britain and Ireland (2012) *Good Practice in Postoperative and Procedural Pain.* http://www.apagbi.org.uk

Crohn's & Colitis UK (2021) Living with a stoma information leaflet. http://www.crohnsandcolitis.org.uk accessed 14.9.2021.

Twycross, A., Dowden, S., Bruce, E. & Blackwell, L.B. (2013) *Managing Pain in Children: A Clinical Guide.*

*Especially guidelines regarding pain assessment, management, and pharmacology.

Care Planning in Children and Young People's Nursing, Second Edition. Edited by Sonya Clarke and Doris Corkin.
© 2024 John Wiley & Sons Ltd. Published 2024 by John Wiley & Sons Ltd.

QUESTIONS

1. What is the difference between a patient-controlled analgesia (PCA) infusion, nurse-controlled analgesia (NCA) infusion and a continuous Ketamine infusion?
2. What opiates are used and what are the common side effects and key points to consider when administering opiates?
3. Reflecting on the nursing process and a model of care, how would the children's nurse prepare this young person, Sadie, and her family for having an PCA infusion?
4. What general aspects of nursing management would you need to address when considering PCA analgesia for Sadie?
5. Discuss the postoperative nursing care Sadie will require whilst a PCA infusion is in progress.

ANSWERS TO QUESTIONS

Question 1a. What is a PCA?

Patient Controlled Analgesia

Patient controlled analgesia (PCA) is a technique that gives the CYP control over the amount of analgesia they receive, delivered via a lockable-programmed pump. A background continuous infusion dose may be prescribed to help maintain a therapeutic level of drug in the bloodstream which aids good analgesic effect. If the CYP experiences pain they are able to activate the bolus system by pressing the button on a handset attached to the pump, which allows a small bolus dose of drug to be administered intravenously.

Parents/carers/siblings should be advised about the dangers of pressing the button for the CYP. Only the child knows how much pain they are experiencing and therefore only the child should press the button. This is a safety feature of the machine as the child becomes sedated; they are unable to press the button successfully.

Question 1b. What is an NCA?

Nurse Controlled Analgesia (NCA)

A nurse-controlled analgesia (NCA) infusion provides background continuous analgesia with the options for additional boluses to be administered if required. The system is suitable for any CYP, regardless of age or cognitive ability. Infants and young children (less than 6yrs of age) would usually be prescribed and NCA along with CYP lacking the manual dexterity or cognitive ability to use a PCA.

Two registered nurses can deliver an immediate pre-determined bolus dose if the child is assessed to be in moderate to severe pain or prior to painful procedures or episodes. This can avoid delays from waiting for a doctor to administer a bolus dose, or the continuous infusion to be increased slowly over a period of one hour. The advantages of using an NCA rather than a continuous opioid infusion are that the programme allows an analgesic regime to be prescribed which is more flexible and may provide a better quality of analgesia.

Question 1c. What is a continuous Ketamine infusion?

Ketamine Continuous Infusion

Ketamine has historically been used as an anaesthetic drug but in recent years has proved to be a good analgesic when used in lower doses. The mode of action is different to the action of opioid drugs such as Morphine or Fentanyl, and therefore the use of Ketamine in combination with Morphine or Fentanyl can optimise pain management and reduce the dose of opiate needed, therefore helping to reduce opiate side effects (Chumbley 2010; Hadi et al. 2012). The Ketamine infusion is a continuous infusion with no bolus facility; the rate can be increased or decreased according to the CYP analgesic need.

Ketamine can be particularly beneficial postoperative pain management for CYP who are having complex surgery known to require more analgesia (e.g. major abdominal, orthopaedic, and spinal surgery). In addition, Ketamine as an effective alternative when opiates need to be avoided, for example:

- CYP with opiate sensitivity or allergy
- CYP requiring medication which increases central nervous system depression in combination with an opiate
- CYP with inflammatory bowel disease (Lewin & Veleyos 2020).

Question 2. What opiates are used and what are the common side effects and key points to consider when administering opiates?

Morphine

Morphine is the standard, first line choice of opioid used in PCA infusions. Morphine reaches a peak effect in four to five minutes, which is why the lockout interval is five minutes, preventing the child from receiving further boluses before the analgesia has time to be effective.

Fentanyl is a synthetic opioid, related to pethidine but with similar properties to morphine. It is short acting but has relatively long elimination half-life because of the rapid distribution in the body. Fentanyl has a rapid onset and is metabolised in the liver and metabolites excreted in the urine. It can be given IV, buccal, transdermal, or epidurally.

Fentanyl is reported to have less histamine release than Morphine and has a better side effect profile than Morphine. However, side effects of bradycardia and transient hypotension can occur following rapid IV administration and rarely occurs with a PCA or NCA bolus. Moderate to severe acute pain can be managed with a Fentanyl PCA/NCA. Fentanyl is used if the patient is experiencing inadequate analgesia or unmanageable side effects with a Morphine PCA/NCA.

FENTANYL

- Side effects include nausea and vomiting, pruritus, sedation, constipation, urinary retention, respiratory depression, and must be managed effectively.
- When initiating strong opioids, always ensure appropriate anti-emetics (e.g. ondansetron) and laxatives are prescribed.
- Patients will need to be carefully weaned from opiates if being used for long periods to avoid withdrawal abstinence syndrome.
- Weak opiates such as codeine should not be used to treat pain in children under the age of 12 years, or in *any* patient who has undergone tonsillectomy or adenoidectomy (or both) or has symptoms of obstructive sleep apnoea (APAGBI 2013; MHRA 2013). Codeine is no longer routinely used and the opiate of choice for oral analgesia is Morphine Sulphate.

KEY POINTS

- *Morphine should be used with caution* in patients with neuromuscular disorders and severe cardiac or respiratory conditions and renal impairment, due to increased risk of toxicity.
- Patients with *eGFR < 50mL/kg/min/1.73m^2* are at significant risk of Morphine accumulation. As a result, Morphine should be used with extreme caution in this patient group.

CAUTIONS

Activity of living: maintaining a safe environment.

Question 3. Reflecting upon the nursing process and a model of care, how would the children's nurse prepare this young person, Sadie, and her family for having a PCA infusion?

Assess: ensure that both Sadie and her parents/carers have an appropriate level of knowledge and understanding regarding PCA analgesia. This is essential to ensure that they can make an informed decision when approached for consent.

Plan: the children's nurse must ensure that Sadie and her parents are given appropriate pre-operative preparation at ward level. This will involve explaining the physical and psychological impact of the surgery, postoperative recovery, and observations, and interventions associated with the analgesic technique used. All planned care should adopt an appropriate model of nursing, for example the Roper-Logan-Tierney Model (Holland et al. 2008, with Casey 1988).

Implement pre-operative interventions:

Pre-operative assessment – achieved through attending a pre-admission clinic (if available, or a discussion and demonstration pre surgery if possible).

Verbal information should be supported with written information leaflets, which the family may take home to read and digest the information at a later time. These can also be used to prepare Sadie further pre-operatively.

Discuss with Sadie and her family the importance of regular pain assessment, demonstrate available pain assessment tools, negotiate on the most appropriate and offer a demonstration on its use. The 0–10 Visual Analogue Scale would be appropriate for a 15-year-old young person, where 0 is 'no pain' and 10 is the 'most imaginable pain' (RCN 2009).

Discuss potential pain management options:

- Patient controlled analgesia (PCA)
- Regular intravenous paracetamol and step-down medication

Wherever possible demonstrate the use of the equipment which will deliver the analgesic technique. First, this enables recognition postoperatively, which reduces levels of anxiety, but more importantly it allows the nurse to assess whether the correct level of understanding and manual dexterity is present to ensure effective delivery of analgesia is achievable.

Evaluate all nursing interventions and documentation.

Question 4. What general aspects of nursing management would you need to address when considering PCA analgesia for Sadie?

Selection criteria for the CYP person

The CYP needs to be identified and assessed as suitable for this technique:

- The cognitive ability to understand the relationship between pushing the button and medication being delivered.
- To be aware that the expected outcome is pain relief and not necessarily the complete absence of pain.
- Should have the manual dexterity to push the button of the device.
- Equipment should be available and demonstrated on the ward, and parents advised not to press the button for their child.

Patient suitability – establish whether any contraindications are present:

These pre-requisites should be met before discussion and the informed consent of Sadie/carer obtained.

When analgesia is required for moderate or severe pain for 24 hours or more.

The workload of the ward allows the child to be observed closely.

Potential complications to consider and monitor for

- Problems related to equipment
- Equipment malfunction
- Operator error
- Tampering
- Inappropriate patient or non-patient use

- Side-effects related to opioids
- Adverse drug reaction

Equipment required

- Oxygen available at the bedside
- Resuscitation equipment available on the ward/department
- Naloxone available
- Lockable infusion pump
- PCA opioid prescription and observation chart
- 50 mls B/D plastipak syringe
- Giving set with anti-reflux/anti-siphon valve
- Pulse oximeter if advised by the anaesthetist
- Opiate intravenous (IV) giving set label

ACTIVITY 14.2

Reflect upon ward policy and procedures regarding safety issues.

Activity of living: maintaining a safe environment (Holland et al. 2008).

Question 5. Discuss the postoperative nursing care Sadie will require whilst a PCA infusion is in progress

See Table 14a.1.

Table 14a.1 Proposed answer plan.

Action	Rationale
Assess and plan post-operative interventions	
1. Sadie should be identified and prepared for the technique pre-operatively by the anaesthetist, children's pain nurse specialist, and the child's nurse.	To ensure that Sadie and her family/carer understands the technique and appropriately trained staff are available to care for Sadie postoperatively.
2. Sadie and her family/carer should be given the PCA infusion information sheet.	To ensure that they understand and are able to absorb the information and ask questions at their own pace.
3. PCA infusion pump and appropriate administration set with an anti-syphon valve shoule be sent to theatre with Sadie. Ensure previous rates on the machine are zeroed.	To ensure an appropriate infusion pump is available prior to surgery.
Implement, document, and evaluate all nursing interventions – this is a continuous cycle	
4. On collecting Sadie from theatre recovery ensure that: • The machine is working and ensure the giving set is labelled with appripriate stickers for the infusion running, i.e. opiate stickers for morphine or fentanyl infusion. • The rate of the infusion complies with the prescription. • The drug complies with the prescription. • Both the recovery and the ward registered nurses record the readings on the infusion pump and ensure pump is locked. • The cannula site is secure with a transparent dressing. • Venous access is available and patent.	• To ensure continuity of the analgesia. • To ensure all staff are aware that an opiate infusion is in progress. • To ensure the prescription, infusion rate, and solution are the same as the prescription to prevent errors. • To prevent the cannula from dislodging and ensure the site can be observed at all times. • To facilitate resuscitative measures if unwanted side effects occur.

(Continued)

Table 14a.1 (Continued)

Action	Rationale
Assess and plan post-operative interventions	
5. One hourly observations of the following must be recorded throughout the duration of the infusion. • Continuous oxygen saturation monitoring. • Respiratory rate, heart rate, sedation score, pain score, and oxygen saturation level every 15 minutes in recovery until condition stabilises, then half hourly for two hours and hourly thereafter. • After discontinuation of the PCA one hourly observations must be recorded for a further four hours.	To ensure Sadie is receiving effective pain management. To monitor for side effects/potential complications: • Excessive sedation – caution with the use of oral Diazepam in patients with a opiate infusions. • Respiratory depression • Hypotension • Nausea and vomiting • Pruritis (itching) • Urinary retention • Inadequate pain relief • Adverse drug reaction To ensure that the drug has been eliminated from the body.
6. Monitor for side effects such as pruritis and nausea and vomiting (APAGBI 2012 and 2016) and adverse reactions. Ensure the appropriate medications are prescribed and administered and the side effects are appropriately managed. Record any unwanted side effects in Sadie's records and inform the anaesthetist.	To counteract any unwanted side effects or adverse reactions promptly. To ensure that Sadie receives appropriate analgesia. To ensure that staff are aware of unwanted side effects or adverse reactions for future reference.
7. Administer concurrent analgesia as prescribed e.g. regular IV Paracetamol. When a continuous opiate infusion is in progress then no other opiates or central nervous system (CNS) depressants should be administered. ** unless the CYP is prescribed these for an underlying condition e.g. anticonvulsants, and opiates for complex pain. In this case extra caution must be taken and the opiate dose may need to be reduced.	To ensure that Sadie receives regular, combined analgesia. To avoid potential CNS depression with concurrent use of sedative medications e.g. oral opiates, Diazepam.
8. Read and record the amount of infusion hourly, including tries and good tries. If there is a large disparity between good and total tries assess for any issues with understanding, technique, pump function, and administration (kinks, clamps, blocked, or dislodges cannula).	To facilitate an accurate record of the analgesia Sadie receives. To ensure this mode of analgesia is providing effective analgesia and is being utilised appropriately by Sadie.
9. A clear dressing will be used over the cannula site and the site should be checked with each set of observations.	To ensure connections are secure. To observe for leakage, infection, or signs of extravasation (Matras et al. 2012).
10. Nurse Sadie in a comfortable position and check skin integrity and pressure areas at least once per shift. If appropriate depending on the postoperative instructions regarding mobilising, Sadie may be helped to sit in a chair by the bed with the support of nurses or physio when appropriate.	To reduce the risk of pressure sores or DVT's developing due to immobility or poor skin integrity.
11. Monitor and record accurate fluid balance and inform the medical team if there are any concerns.	To ensure that Sadie does not have urinary retention which can be a side effect of opiates in addition to postoperative dehydration.
12. Ensure that concurrent analgesia is prescribed prior to discontinuing the PCA. When disposing of the PCA syringe, the volume of wasted drug must be recorded and signed for by two registered nurses and the remaining opiate solution disposed of as per local controlled drug policy.	To ensure that the transition from intravenous analgesia to oral analgesia is smooth and an appproprate analgesic step down regime has been prescribed to ensure continued effective pain management and a positive patient experience.

REFERENCES AND READING

Association of Paediatric Anaesthetists of Great Britain and Ireland (2012) *Good practice in postoperative and procedural pain.* https://www.apagbi.org.uk/guidelines [Last accessed 20 April 2020].

Association of Paediatric Anaesthetists of Great Britain and Ireland (2013) *Codeine and paracetamol in paediatric use.* https://www.apagbi.org.uk/sites/default/files/inline-files/Codeine%20revised%20final%20November%202013%20.pdf. [Accessed 11 March 2023]

Association of Paediatric Anaesthetists of Great Britain and Ireland (2016) *Guidelines on the prevention of postoperative vomiting in children.* https://www.apagbi.org.uk/sites/default/files/inline-files/2016%20APA%20POV%20Guideline-2.pdf [last accessed 20 04 2020].

Casey, A. (1988) A partnership with child and family. *Senior Nurse*, **8**(4), 8–9.

Chumbley, G. (2010) Use of ketamine in uncontrolled acute and procedural pain. *Nursing Standard*, **25**(15–17), 35–37 https://crohnsandcolitis.org.uk/info-support/become-a-member?gclid=EAIaIQobChMI0rCE8_XT_QIVBcbtCh3MPQMNEAAYASAAEgJrt_D_BwE Crohn's and Colitis.

Hadi, B., Daas, R. & Zelko, R. (2012) A randomized, controlled trial of a clinical pharmacist intervention in microdiscectomy surgery – Low dose intravenous ketamine as an adjunct to standard therapy. *Saudi Pharmaceautical Journal.* doi:10.1016/j.jsps.2012.08.002. [Accessed 11 March 2023]

Holland, K., Jenkins, J., Soloman, J. & Whittam, S. (2008) *Applying the Roper Logan Tierney Model in Practice*, 2nd edn. Edinburgh: Churchill Livingstone.

Lewin, S. & Velayos, F. (2020) Day-by-day management of the inpatient with moderate to severe inflammatory bowel disease. *Gastroenterol Hepatol (N Y)*, **16**(9), 449–457.

Matras, P., Poulton, B. & Derman, S. (2012) Pain physiology and assessment, ,patient controlled analgesia, epidural and spinal analgesia, nerve block catheters. FHA Surgical Acute Pain Nursing Shared Work Team. Medicines and Healthcare Products Regulatory Agency (2013) *Codeine for analgesia: Restricted use in children because of reports of morphine toxicity.* https://www.gov.uk/drug-safety-update/codeine-for-analgesia-restricted-use-in-children-because-of-reports-of-morphine-toxicity. [Accessed 11 March 2023].

CHAPTER 14B

Epidural Analgesia

Sharon Douglass and Michelle Whitehouse

SCENARIO

John is a 15-year-old boy who was diagnosed with Crohn's disease three years ago. Conservative management is no longer effective; therefore, he has been admitted electively for a right hemi-colectomy; the aim being to improve John's quality of life.

A hemi-colectomy can be performed either as a laparoscopic or an open procedure. It involves the tying of the right colic artery, ileo-colic artery, and also, if needed, the right branch of the middle colic artery (Hope et al. 2020). John is having an open procedure, which involves interruption of all tissue and muscle layers. In addition, previous frequent acute exacerbations of his Crohn's disease have resulted in thickening of the intestinal wall with swelling and scar tissue. Crohn's also causes ulcers (fistulas) that tunnel through the affected area into the surrounding tissues. Therefore, this surgery may involve significant handling of the bowel and surrounding organs. As a result, this procedure is potentially very painful and will require *multi-modal and advanced analgesic techniques*.

It is essential to take into consideration any child's underlying condition when planning postoperative pain management. In John's case non-steroidal anti-inflammatory drugs (NSAIDs) such as ibuprofen and diclofenac are contra-indicated as one of the side effects is gastric irritation, which is already a symptom of Crohn's disease. Therefore, suitable analgesia includes paracetamol, opiates, and local anaesthetics.

The route of administration must also be considered and in the immediate postoperative period, the oral route would not be appropriate for the following reasons: being nil by mouth, potential presence of a paralytic ileus, nasogastric tube on free drainage, nausea, and vomiting.

Also, Crohn's is known to have a negative impact on absorption in the body. After major surgery such as a hemi-colectomy the Association of Paediatric Anaesthetists of Great Britain and Ireland (APAGBI 2012) recommend use of intravenous paracetamol alongside an advanced analgesic technique such as an epidural infusion and/or an intravenous opiate patient-controlled analgesia (PCA) infusion. When the anaesthetist visits John and his family pre-operatively they discuss the options and decide on an epidural infusion. Refer to Box Activity 14b.1.

ACTIVITY 14B.1

Recommended reading:

Association of Paediatric Anaesthetists of Great Britain and Ireland (2012) *Good Practice in Postoperative and Procedural Pain*. http://www.apagbi.org.uk

Twycross, A., Dowden, S., Bruce, E. & Blackwell, L.B. (2013) *Managing Pain in Children: A Clinical Guide*.

Especially guidelines regarding pain assessment, management, and pharmacology.

QUESTIONS

1. What is epidural analgesia?
2. Reflecting upon the nursing process and a model of care, how would the children's registered nurse prepare this young person, John, and his family for having an epidural infusion?
3. What general aspects of nursing management would you need to address when considering epidural analgesia for John?
4. Discuss the postoperative nursing care John will require whilst an epidural infusion is in progress.

ANSWERS TO QUESTIONS

Question 1. What is epidural analgesia?

Epidural analgesia is the administration of local anaesthetic drugs with or without other analgesic medications into the epidural space via a fine bore catheter. The local anaesthetic reversibly blocks the transmission of peripheral nerve impulses by inhibiting the entry of sodium ions into the nerve cells, preventing depolarisation, and the nerve transmission being passed on from cell to cell (Taylor & McLeod 2020).

A continuous epidural infusion of a local anaesthetic in combination with low dose opiate reversibly blocks pain transmission along the pain pathway and offers unique benefits in the relief of acute and peri-operative pain. Used to its full potential, it can offer children pain-free post-surgical recovery and is associated with a reduction in postoperative and post trauma morbidity, particularly in the high-risk patient (e.g. children with respiratory disease, poor lung function, and complex disability).

Epidural analgesia can provide excellent effective, long-lasting pain relief both intraoperatively and postoperatively, blunting the stress response to surgery and reducing the need for other analgesic medications (Twycross et al. 2013). High quality analgesia with minimal sedation allows better lung expansion and improves the patient's ability to cough and clear secretions. In older patients there is a decrease in the risk of deep vein thrombosis. The reduced quantity of opiate drugs used in combination with the local anaesthetic can decrease the degree of paralytic ileus after abdominal surgery and may also decrease or abolish the incidence of nausea and vomiting, which are recognised side effects of opiates (Twycross et al. 2013).

Activity of living: maintaining a safe environment.

Question 2. Reflecting upon the nursing process and a model of care, how would the children's registered nurse prepare this young person, John, and his family for having an epidural infusion?

Assess: ensure that both John and his parents/carers have an appropriate level of knowledge and understanding regarding epidural analgesia. This is essential to ensure that they can make an informed decision when approached for consent.

Plan: the children's registered nurse must ensure that John and his parents are given appropriate pre-operative preparation at ward level. This will involve explaining the physical and psychological impact of the surgery, postoperative recovery, and observations, and interventions associated with the analgesic technique used. All planned care should adopt an appropriate model of nursing, for example the Roper-Logan-Tierney Model (Holland et al. 2008, with Casey 1988).

IMPLEMENT/ PRE-OPERATIVE INTERVENTIONS

- Pre-operative assessment – achieved through attending a pre-admission clinic (if available).
- Verbal information should be supported with written information leaflets, which the family may take home to read and digest the information at a later time. These can also be used to prepare John further pre-operatively.
- Discuss with John and his family the importance of regular pain assessment, demonstrate available pain assessment tools, negotiate on the most appropriate and offer a demonstration on its use. The 0–10 Visual Analogue Scale would be appropriate for a 15-year-old young person, where 0 is 'no pain' and 10 is the 'most imaginable pain' (RCN 2009).
- Discuss potential pain management options:
  - Patient controlled analgesia (PCA)
  - Continuous epidural infusion
  - Intravenous paracetamol and step-down medication

Wherever possible demonstrate the use of the equipment which will deliver the analgesic technique. First, this enables recognition postoperatively, which reduces levels of anxiety, but more importantly it allows the registered nurse to assess whether the correct level of understanding and manual dexterity is present to ensure effective delivery of analgesia is achievable.

N.B. Although epidural analgesia is the advanced technique chosen, John and his family still need to be prepared for patient-controlled analgesia which may be used in conjunction with or to replace the epidural infusion.

Evaluate all nursing interventions and documentation.

Question 3. What general aspects of nursing management would you need to address when considering epidural analgesia for John?

PRE-REQUISITES

These pre-requisites should be met before discussion and the informed consent of John/carer obtained. Also refer to Box Activity 14b.2.

1. Patient suitability – establish whether any contraindications are present:
   a) Local skin infection
   b) Systemic infection
   c) Coagulation disorders
   d) Known allergy to local anaesthetics
   e) Patient/parent refusal
   f) Spinal deformities
   g) Neurological disease
   h) Raised intracranial pressure
   i) Extreme obesity

2. Patient safety – establish the following:
   a) Bed availability – in line with local trust guidelines (e.g. either on PCCU, HDU or on a ward where John can be closely observed).
   b) The workload of the ward allows the child to be observed closely.
   c) Minimum trained staff numbers in line with local trust guidelines.
   d) Minimum of one epidural trained registered nurse per shift. This must be a registered nurse who has completed the appropriate theoretical and practical training and has been assessed competent in line with local trust guidelines.
   e) Intravenous access must be available at all times.

ACTIVITY 14B.2

Reflect upon ward policy and procedures regarding safety issues.

Activity of living: maintaining a safe environment (Holland et al. 2008)

Question 4. Discuss the postoperative nursing care John will require whilst an epidural infusion is in progress

See Table 14b.1.

Table 14b.1 Proposed answer plan.

Action	Rationale
Assess and plan post-operative interventions	
1. John should be identified and prepared for the technique pre-operatively by the anaesthetist, pain registered nurse specialist, and child's registered nurse.	To ensure that John and his family/carer understand the technique and appropriately trained staff are available to care for John postoperatively.
2. John and his family/carer should be given the epidural information sheet.	To ensure that they understand and are able to absorb the information and ask questions at their own pace.
3. Epidural infusion pump and yellow tubing should be sent to theatre with John. Ensure previous rates on the machine are zeroed.	To ensure an appropriate pump is available prior to surgery.

Table 14b.1 (Continued)

Action	Rationale

Implement, document, and evaluate all nursing interventions – this is a continuous cycle

Action	Rationale
4. On collecting John from theatre recovery ensure that: (a) The machine is working. Place 'Epidural drugs in use' sign on the machine and ensure the giving set is labelled with yellow epidural stickers. (b) The rate of the infusion complies with the prescribed regime. (c) The drug complies with the prescription. (d) Both the recovery and ward registered nurses record the readings on the infusion pump and ensure pump is locked. (e) The catheter site is secure with a transparent dressing. (f) Venous access is available and patent.	To ensure continuity of the analgesia. To ensure all staff are aware that an epidural infusion is in progress. To ensure the prescription, infusion rate, and solution are the same as the prescription to prevent errors. To comply with the National Patient Safety Agency Alerts (2009). See also http://www.apagbi.org.uk. To prevent the catheter from dislodging and to ensure the site can be observed at all times. To facilitate resuscitative measures if severe side effects occur. To facilitate changing to a patient-controlled analgesia infusion (PCA) if the epidural fails or as step down from the epidural infusion. To enable medication to be given to manage unwanted side effects.
5. One hourly observations of the following must be recorded throughout the duration of the infusion and after removal of the epidural catheter until normal sensation returns to the site of the anaesthetised area (usually approximately six hours). (a) Continuous oxygen saturation monitoring. (b) Record respiratory rate, heart rate, sedation score, pain score, and oxygen saturation level every 15 minutes in recovery until condition stabilises, then half hourly for two hours and hourly thereafter. (c) Blood pressure, sensory level, and motor block must be recorded hourly for the first four hours then every four hours thereafter. If these observations remain within limits written on the prescription sheet. (d) Recording of blood pressure, sensory level, and motor block must revert back to hourly or more frequent in the following circumstances: (i) The sensory block is higher than prescribed. (ii) John becomes hypotensive. (iii) A change has been made to the infusion rate. (iv) The motor block score is 3. (v) The pain score is 3 (severe). (vi) The sedation score is 3.	To ensure John is receiving effective pain management. To ensure that the block is working, and the level is not above that prescribed by the anaesthetist. To monitor side effects/potential complications: 1. Excessive sedation – **caution should be taken with the use of oral Diazepam in patients with a Clonidine epidural in progress** 2. Respiratory depression 3. Hypotension 4. Nausea and vomiting 5. Pruritus (itching) 6. Urinary retention 7. Altered lower limb function 8. Unilateral block 9. Inadequate pain relief 10. Horner's syndrome (a rare complication with a triad of symptoms – meiosis, ptosis, and anhidrosis) (Cowie et al. 2015). To ensure that the drug has been adequately eliminated from the body. John's motor function and level of motor block is assessed by using the Bromage scale: Score 0 (none) – full flexion of the knees Score 1 (partial) – just able to move knees Score 2 (almost complete) – able to move feet only Score 3 (complete) – unable to move knees or feet (Department of Anaesthesia and Pain Management, RCH, Melbourne 2007, cited in Twycross et al. 2013).
6. Side effects of the infusion should be appropriately managed, noted in John's records, and the anaesthetist informed.	To ensure that staff are aware of adverse reactions to the drug for future reference. To ensure that John receives appropriate analgesia. To counteract any adverse effects promptly.
7. Administer concurrent analgesia as prescribed e.g. regular IV Paracetamol. When a continuous epidural infusion with an opiate added e.g. fentanyl is in progress then no other opiates or central nervous system (CNS) depressants should be administered.	To ensure that John receives regular, combined analgesia. To avoid potential CNS depression with concurrent use of sedative medications e.g. oral opiates, Diazepam.
** unless the CYP is prescribed these for an underlying condition e.g. anticonvulsants, and opiates for complex pain. In this case extra caution must be taken and the opiate dose may need to be reduced.	

Table 14b.1 (Continued)

Action	Rationale
8. Read and record the amount of infusion hourly.	To facilitate an accurate record of the analgesia administered.
9. A clear dressing will be used over the catheter insertion site and the site should be checked at least once each shift.	To ensure connections are secure. To observe for leakage or infection (Matras et al. 2012).
10. Nurse John in a comfortable position and check skin integrity and pressure areas at least once per shift. If appropriate depending on the postoperative instructions regarding mobilising. John may be helped to sit in a chair by the bed with the support of two registered nurse when his motor score is 0–1.	To reduce the risk of pressure sores developing due to immobility, poor skin integrity or altered lower limb function. Low concentration solutions of levobupivacaine produce complete sensory blockade and are associated with a very low incidence of motor block.
11. Monitor and record accurate fluid balance and inform the medical team if there are any concerns N/B. CYP with lumbar epidurals are usually catheterised in theatre.	To ensure that John does not have urinary retention which can be a side effect of an epidural infusion and opiates in addition to postoperative dehydration.
12. If the epidural infusion contains an opiate, Monitor for side effects such as pruritus and nausea and vomiting (APAGBI 2012 and 2016) and adverse reactions. Ensure the appropriate medications are prescribed and administered and the side effects are appropriately managed. Record any unwanted side effects in John's records and inform the anaesthetist.	To counteract any unwanted side effects or adverse reactions promptly. To ensure that John receives appropriate analgesia. To ensure that staff are aware of unwanted side effects or adverse reactions for future reference.
13. The anaesthetist or registered nurse with appropriate competencies is responsible for the removal of the epidural catheter and the completion of the audit sheet on the prescription protocol.	To monitor the state of the catheter on removal (Matras et al. 2012).

REFERENCES AND READING

Association of Paediatric Anaesthetists of Great Britain and Ireland (2012) Good practice in postoperative and procedural pain. https://www.apagbi.org.uk/guidelines [Last accessed 09.05.2023].

Association of Paediatric Anaesthetists of Great Britain and Ireland (2016) Guidelines on the prevention of postoperative vomiting in children. https://www.apagbi.org.uk/sites/default/files/inline-files/2016%20APA%20POV%20Guideline-2.pdf [Accessed 11 March 2023].

Casey, A. (1988) A partnership with child and family. *Senior Nurse*, **8**(4), 8–9.

Cowie, S., Gunn, L. & Madhavan, P. (2015) Horner's syndrome secondary to epidural anaesthesia following posterior instrumented scoliosis correction. *Asian Spine Journal*, Feb **9**(1), 121–126. Published online 2015 Feb 13. https://pubmed.ncbi.nlm.nih.gov/25705345 [Accessed 11 March 2023].

Holland, K., Jenkins, J., Soloman, J. & Whittam, S. (2008) *Applying the Roper Logan Tierney Model in Practice*, 2nd edn. Edinburgh: Churchill Livingstone.

Hope, C., Reilly, J., Lund, J. & Andreyev, H. (2020) Systematic review: The effect of right hemicolectomy for cancer on postoperative bowel function. *Support Care Cancer*, **28**(10), p4549–4559.

Matras, P., Poulton, B. & Derman, S. (2012) Pain physiology & assessment, patient controlled analgesia, epidural & spinal analgesia, nerve block catheters. FHA Surgical Acute Pain Nursing Shared Work Team.

National Patient Safety Agency (2009) Patient Safety Alert Patient Safety Alerts NPSA/2009/PSA004A and NPSA/2009/PSA004B Safer spinal (intrathecal), epidural and regional devices – Part A and Part B. https://www.oaa-anaes.ac.uk/assets/_managed/cms/files/NPSA/2009%20NPSA%20_Safer-spinal%20supporting%20info_10215.pdf [Accessed 11 March 2023].

Royal College of Anaesthetists (2009) The 3rd National audit project of the royal college of anaesthetists – Major complications of neuraxial block in the United Kingdom report and findings 2009. https://www.bjanaesthesia.org.uk/article/S0007-0912(17)34049-7/pdf [Accessed 11 March 2023].

Taylor, A. & McLeod, G. (2020) Basic pharmacology of local anaesthetics. *BJA Education*, **20**(2), 34–41.

Twycross, A., Dowden, S. & Stinson, J. (2013) *Managing Pain in Children: A Clinical Guide for Nurses and Health Care Professionals*. Wiley Blackwell.

Care of Children and Young Persons with Special Needs

SECTION 3

Young Person with a History of Epilepsy

CHAPTER 15

Joanne Blair

CASE STUDY

Robert is a highly motivated, mature 17-year-old who is studying for his AS levels. Last year, he achieved excellent grades at GCSE, and intends studying mechanical engineering at university next year. He plays rugby, enjoys Adventure Scouting, is currently undertaking the Duke of Edinburgh Gold award, and is also learning to drive.

Robert has an unremarkable medical history, though six months ago he was admitted to hospital for a second time with severe concussion following injury in a rugby match when the scrum collapsed. Recently, he has been complaining of feeling tired at times and having tingling and slight twitching in his right arm and hand. He has attributed this to the additional pressures of schoolwork and leaning on his arm while studying. He had not mentioned this to his parents.

One afternoon at rugby training Robert was feeling more tired than usual. He was finding it difficult to concentrate on the game and unusually struggled to keep up with his team mates. After missing several easy catches, which he blamed on the pins and needles in his right hand and a sore arm, Robert suddenly fell to the ground, his body stiffened, and then started shaking uncontrollably. His concerned coach quickly responded by calling for an ambulance. By the time it arrived Robert was sitting up, but was obviously disorientated. Information regarding this collapse was relayed to the paramedics and Robert was transported immediately to hospital accompanied by a friend, while his coach contacted his parents.

On arrival at the emergency department his worried parents were immediately taken to see Robert. While being examined, his body suddenly stiffened again and began to shake violently. His now distraught parents were ushered out of the cubicle by a nurse as the doctor dealt with the situation.

While waiting, Robert's friend explained to them what had happened earlier. Eventually, the doctor came and spoke to them all. She explained that Robert had what appeared to be an epileptic seizure but he was now resting comfortably and she was admitting him to the neurological unit for further specialist investigations.

THE EPILEPSIES

Defined by Sun et al. (2021) as a neurological disorder caused by abnormal brain activity, epilepsy has been noted as one of the most common neurological disorders in childhood, with potential to impact on physical, psychological, and social health (Fisher et al. 2005). Referred to as a disorder rather than a disease, epilepsy is a complex spectrum of symptoms which can manifest in up to 40 different types of seizure activity (Fisher et al. 2005). The main characteristic of epilepsy is recurrent, unprovoked seizures due to the presence of excess electrical activity in the brain, which causes a temporary disruption in the normal nerve impulses passing between brain cells (Epilepsy Research UK 2010; Glasper & Richardson 2020). Hauser and Banerjee (2008) further add that the recurrent seizures are separated by more than 24 hours. In some cases, it is possible for one person to have several types of seizure. Refer to Activity 15.1 for additional definitions.

ACTIVITY 15.1

The websites below offer useful definitions of epilepsy. Access at least one and differentiate between seizures and epilepsy.

www.epilepsy.org.uk/info/whatisepilepsy.html
https://epilepsyresearch.org.uk/about-epilepsy/what-is-epilepsy
http://www.jointepilepsycouncil.org.uk/understanding-epilepsy-induced-seizures

Care Planning in Children and Young People's Nursing, Second Edition. Edited by Sonya Clarke and Doris Corkin.
© 2024 John Wiley & Sons Ltd. Published 2024 by John Wiley & Sons Ltd.

NICE 2021 estimate the prevalence of epilepsy in the UK to be 5–10 cases per 1000 people and it is thought to affect approximately 63,400 children and young people under the age of 18 years in the UK (Joint Epilepsy Council (JEC) 2011). Those who have other neurological problems, for example a learning disability, show a higher incidence with risk of developing epilepsy increasing with the severity of learning disability (Whittaker 2004). Epilepsy is most commonly diagnosed during the first year, after a child has had two or more unprovoked seizures (Camfield & Camfield 2006) and although normally diagnosed in childhood, it can affect people of any age as a result of trauma to the brain such as injury or infection (Ricci & Kyle 2009).

The causes of epilepsy fall into three categories (National Society for Epilepsy (NSE) 2010a; Wolraich et al. 2008):

- Idiopathic epilepsy: has no apparent cause, but a genetic defect is thought to be involved. It is known that epilepsy can be inherited. In some cases, single or combinations of two or more genes can be involved, and environmental factors cannot be underestimated.

- Symptomatic epilepsy: has a definite cause, for example meningitis, birth trauma, anoxia, or congenital abnormalities, for example hydrocephalus.

- Cryptogenic epilepsy: has a likely cause, but for which nothing definite can be found.

According to Scheffer et al. (2007) there is growing evidence of the role of genes in symptomatic and cryptogenic epilepsies. Gene defects do not lead directly to epilepsy, but can affect the excitability of the brain, making it more susceptible to seizures. Each of us is born with a genetically inherited seizure threshold. Those with low thresholds are more susceptible to having a seizure when exposed to certain circumstances or *triggers*, for example sleep deprivation. Conversely, those with higher thresholds are less likely to have a seizure in similar circumstances. According to the NSE (2009a) anyone has the potential to have a seizure given the right circumstances, or a strong enough stimulus (Whittaker 2004).

Seizures are a clinical manifestation or symptom of epilepsy associated with a disturbance of the electrical activity in the brain; however, it is important to note that not all seizures are due to epilepsy. They may also be associated with other non-epilepsy conditions, such as infections of the central nervous system, hypoglycaemia, syncope, hyponatraemia, and hypoxia, which can disturb the neuronal environment. Dissociative seizures (previously known as pseudo seizures and also known as functional seizures or psychogenic seizure) are thought to be a severe reaction to emotional or psychological distress. Due to the unconscious nature of these and their similarity to epileptic seizures, these can initially be misdiagnosed as epilepsy. Whilst all seizure types may have much in common, they differ in their cause, and therefore must be investigated in order to make an accurate diagnosis.

QUESTIONS

1. Outline what is meant by pre-ictal, ictal, post-ictal and inter-ictal phases.

2. Access the following website and describe the classification of seizures.

   https://www.epilepsy.com/article/2016/12/2017-revised-classification-seizures

3. As a nurse involved in Roberts' care you speak to his friend who witnessed the seizure to gather a complete picture of the event. What information are you seeking from him?

4. Apart from the example given earlier, list six triggers that may cause a susceptible person to have a seizure.

5. Discuss the impact a diagnosis of epilepsy might have on Robert.

ANSWERS TO QUESTIONS

Question 1. Describe what is meant by pre-ictal, ictal, post-ictal, and inter-ictal phases?

The pre-ictal phase refers to the period immediately before a seizure. This phase may include an aura.

The ictal phase refers to the actual seizure and associated activity.

The post-ictal phase refers to the period following the seizure when the individual is recovering and may be confused or sleepy. This recovery phase is often longer than the ictal phase.

The inter-ictal phase refers to the period of time between seizures after the individual has recovered from the post-ictal phase.

Question 2. Describe the classification of seizures

The NSE (2010b) classifies seizures into two main groups. This classification was carried out by the International League against Epilepsy (ILAE 1981), based on the manifestation of seizure activity. The ILAE carried out a further review and reclassification of epilepsy, the purpose of which was to provide a clearer description of an individual's seizure thus enabling doctors to prescribe treatment more specific to an individual's needs (Scheffer et al. 2017). This followed on from recommendations made during a public consultation in 2013. Classifications are outlined in Boxes 15.1 and 15.2.

PARTIAL SEIZURES

Partial seizures (focal or localised seizures), affect a small area of the cerebral cortex, for example a single lobe. Consciousness is not usually lost, but can be altered, as typically the motor or sensory areas are affected (Glasper & Richardson 2020); thus the symptoms can vary depending on which part of the brain is involved. There are two types of partial seizure as shown in Box 15.1.

In some people, a partial seizure can extend as the electrical activity spreads to involve both cerebral hemispheres. Such seizures are referred to as *partial seizures, secondarily generalized* resulting in loss of consciousness.

GENERALISED SEIZURES

Generalised seizures involve both hemispheres of the cerebral cortex and are characterised by bilateral synchronous electrical discharges from the onset. Consciousness is usually lost. The main types are described in Box 15.2.

Classification of seizures by type alone in many instances ignores other important clinical manifestations, such as age of onset, triggers, genetics, EEG readings, or presence of a learning disability. Taking all these into consideration, we can define a particular epilepsy syndrome, for example West syndrome, Lennox-Gastaut syndrome, Angelman syndrome, Rett syndrome, and Ohtahara syndrome, which can present during childhood.

In the hours or days preceding a seizure (*prodromal period*) some people may experience mood or behavioural changes manifesting as insomnia, anxiety, depression, or aggression. These are harbingers of a forthcoming seizure, but are not part of it (Panayiotopolus 2010). They should not be

BOX 15.1 TYPES OF PARTIAL SEIZURE

	Manifestations
Simple partial seizure	Occurs without loss of consciousness or awareness. The person may experience sensory or motor symptoms such as: • Tingling or numbness in a limb • Limpness, stiffening or twitching in a limb • Déjà vu (feelings that events have happened before) or jamais vu (events that never happened before) • Sensory abnormalities affecting vision, hearing, taste, and smell
Complex partial seizure	This seizure is accompanied by altered consciousness, which may be displayed as unusual behaviour such as: • Pulling and plucking at clothing • Repetitive vocal sounds • Turning of head and eyes • Lip smacking, chewing, or swallowing • Not responding to verbal commands • Being unaware of surroundings or preceding events Complex partial seizures account for 20% of all seizures experienced by people with epilepsy.

BOX 15.2 GENERALISED SEIZURES

Type of generalised seizure	Manifestations
Absence seizures	Mainly affects children.
	Can occur several times a day – child abruptly stops activity.
	Causes a loss of awareness of surroundings for up to 20 seconds.
	Child may appear to stare vacantly into space, sometimes mistaken for day-dreaming.
	There may be fluttering of eyes or lip-smacking.
	Child's school performance may be affected.
Myoclonic seizures	Causes sudden twitching of the limbs or trunk. Sometimes the whole body can be involved.
	Usually last less than a second.
	Consciousness is not usually lost; however, if the legs are involved, the person may fall to the ground.
Clonic seizures	May be similar twitching as in myoclonic jerks.
	Can continue for several minutes.
	Consciousness may be lost.
Atonic seizures	Sudden loss of muscle tone causing the body to go limp.
	The person suddenly collapses to the ground.
Tonic seizure	Muscles suddenly stiffen causing the person to lose balance and fall to the ground.
	Can occur during sleep.
Tonic-clonic seizure	The seizure passes through two stages:
	Tonic stage
	• Loss of consciousness, usually without warning.
	• Sudden generalised muscle contraction causing the body to stiffen and fall to the ground, the person may also cry out.
	• Teeth are clenched.
	• Pallor, with cyanosis due to apnoea.
	• Pupil dilation and eye rolling.
	• This stage lasts approximately 10–30 seconds.
	Clonic stage
	• Twitching or jerking of the arms, legs, and head due to alternating contraction and relaxation of muscles. These gradually reduce in frequency.
	• There can be frothing from the mouth as a result of excess salivation, which sometimes is bloodstained if the patient has bitten his tongue or cheek.
	• Hyperventilation can occur.
	• Sweating and increased pulse.
	• Incontinence can occur.
	• This stage can last approximately 30–60 seconds.
	The seizure normally lasts up to three minutes, after which consciousness returns but the person may sleep afterwards.
	The patient usually has no recollection of the seizure but may complain of headache or muscle soreness afterwards.
	This type of seizure accounts for approximately 60% of all seizures experienced by people with epilepsy.

confused with *auras*, which occur minutes to seconds before a seizure, and are considered part of the seizure. Auras differ in individuals but manifest themselves in symptoms similar to a simple partial seizure which becomes secondarily generalised (David 2009). Normally it is not possible to prevent the seizure from occurring; however, it is possible in some cases to act on the warning signs.

Establishing a correct diagnosis is important to ensure appropriate treatment. To achieve this, accurate history taking is important; additionally, a number of investigative procedures will be performed to confirm the diagnosis and rule out other possible causes.

Question 3. As a nurse involved in Robert's care you speak to his friend who witnessed the seizure to gather a complete picture of the event. What information are you seeking from him?

In order to achieve an accurate diagnosis, it is crucial to obtain an accurate history of events. This is best given by parents, carers, or witnesses to the events, as depending on the event, the patient is often unaware of what happened, though they may be able to assist with events during the prodromal period, or after the seizure event.

The friend who was with him at the time might be able to provide some of the following information.

Background information:
- How hard has Robert been working on his school work? Does he spend a lot of time on hobbies/interests?
- How did he obtain his rugby injury that resulted in hospitalisation?
- Has he been complaining of feeling more tired than usual or unwell in anyway?

Immediately before the event (prodromal period or aura?):
- He was complaining of being very tired that evening.
- He had to be coaxed to come out.
- He complained of pins and needles in his right hand and a sore arm.
- He missed a lot of easy shots.

During the event (ictal period):
- He suddenly fell to the ground, his body stiffened, and began shaking.
- Location and time of seizure.
- Were there any injuries?
- Was consciousness lost?
- How long did the body stiffening last?
- How long did the shaking last?
- Did he bite his tongue?
- Was he incontinent?
- Did his colour change?
- How long did the seizure last?

After the event (post-ictal period):
- Did he sleep – if so, for how long?
- Was he confused/disorientated?

Any information, no matter how apparently insignificant, can help in determining an accurate diagnosis.

Question 4. List six triggers that may cause a susceptible person to have a seizure

- *Fatigue* – late nights, over-exertion, insomnia.
- *Stress* – school, studying, work, peers, etc.
- *Medication* – missing or over-medicating with anti-epileptic drugs (AED) or other prescription or non-prescribed medication. Some prescribed medications, for example antidepressants, can lower the seizure threshold, while aspirin can enhance phenytoin (https://bnfc.nice.org.uk).
- *Alcohol* – binging or intoxication, especially if taking some AEDs.

- *Drug abuse* – recreational drugs can have both direct and indirect effects (e.g. cocaine can cause seizures). Some drugs can cause sleep deprivation or cause the person to forget to take AED.
- *Infection* – in some susceptible children a raised temperature can induce a seizure (not to be confused with a febrile convulsion).
- *Hormone changes* – particularly in females in relation to their menstrual cycle.
- *Environmental stimulants* – in those with rare reflex epilepsy certain individual stimulants can cause a seizure, for example flickering lights, noise, music, reading, or tone of voice. Photosensitive epilepsy is the most common form. Reflex epilepsy affects 4–7% of people with epilepsy (Panayiotopoulos 2010).

This list is not exhaustive and potential triggers may not be captured here. It is also important to note that for some people there may be no identifiable trigger for their seizures.

A diagnosis of epilepsy was eventually confirmed, based on Robert's presenting history and results from the diagnostic procedures. Robert and his parents were informed of the diagnosis.

ACTIVITY 15.2

Follow the link to the NICE guidelines and outline the assessment strategies used to provide a potential diagnosis of epilepsy. https://www.nice.org.uk/guidance/cg137/chapter/1-Guidance#investigations

Consider five evaluation/diagnostic tools (e.g. electroencephalograph) that could be used to confirm Robert's condition, including an appropriate rationale for their use.

During his stay in hospital Robert's care was planned based on the initial assessment data completed on admission. It involved the setting of priorities, establishing goals, determining nursing interventions, and documenting care plans. The main objectives in managing his care were to include preventing injury during a seizure, preventing or reducing seizure activity by the administration of suitable anti-epileptic drugs (AEDs), and providing information and support to Robert and his family. Refer to box Activity 15.3.

In order to reduce the likelihood of seizures and the risk of complications, patients are usually commenced on anti-epileptic drugs (AEDs) in the first instance. There is a wide variety of such medications available today, and treatment strategies are based on individual requirements.

ACTIVITY 15.3

With reference to the activities of living, '*maintaining a safe environment*' and '*working & playing*' (Roper et al. 2004), complete the nursing care plan below to meet the needs of Robert and his family.

A/L	Nursing Assessment	Nursing Problem	Goal/ objective	Nursing interventions	Rationale
Maintaining a safe environment	Robert has had several seizures				
	Robert is a newly diagnosed patient with epilepsy				
	Robert and his family know little about epilepsy				
Working & Playing	Robert and his family know little about epilepsy				

ACTIVITY 15.4

Using the online *British National Formulary for Children* (BNFC), https://bnfc.nice.org.uk complete a panel similar to the following for three AEDs.

Drug	Action	Dosage	Side effects
Sodium valproate			
Topiramate			
Carbamazepine			

Question 5. How might a diagnosis of epilepsy impact Robert?

As a teenager used to feeling fit and healthy and increasingly independent, the adjustment to life with a serious medical condition could prove difficult. Robert enjoys sport and outdoor pursuits and may feel less able to participate in these due his diagnosis. Learning to drive will need to be postponed until he has been deemed medically fit to continue with his lessons. Chang et al. (2016) explored children's experiences of epilepsy and identified a number of recurring themes in their study. These included a fear of loss of bodily function, a loss of privacy, increased feelings of vulnerability and a loss of normality. The potential psychological impact of such a diagnosis must be anticipated and addressed within Roberts' care plan. Optimal seizure control can only be worked towards if Robert takes his medications as prescribed and follows the advice provided. If Robert is fully informed about this (effects/side effects of medication, impact of skipping doses, the need to avoid alcohol and get sufficient rest, for example), and involved in the decision-making process he is more likely to adhere to the guidance. Enabling Robert to have control over his condition from the beginning will empower him to make well informed decisions.

Parenting a teenager can be challenging and having a teen with a serious medical condition can increase parental anxiety. The need to protect their child from all potential risks may cause increased stress within the household. Jones and Reilly (2016) suggested that parental anxieties are linked with the child's quality of life, and if a child has a higher quality of life then parental anxiety is lower. In Robert's case, if he is able, with parental support, to manage his epilepsy and retain his level of independence alongside continuing with his studies and sports, it is hoped he will maintain his quality of life and continue to pursue his ambition of studying mechanical engineering at university. Refer to box Activity 15.5.

People with epilepsy have a 2–3 times higher mortality rate than the general population (Nashef & Langan 2003). Although seizures are generally self-limiting, one major seizure event which can put a patient's life at risk is a state called status epilepticus. This is a medical emergency requiring prompt treatment to prevent a fatality. Another cause of fatality is sudden unexpected death in epilepsy (SUDEP). Although rare, there is a suggestion that young adult males may be more at risk of SUDEP (NSE 2019). Refer to box Activity 15.6.

ACTIVITY 15.5

Considering Robert's lifestyle, with reference to *The Epilepsies: Diagnosis and Management of the Epilepsies in Children and Young People in Primary and Secondary Care* (NICE 2012), ascertain what *specific* information Robert and his family might require to help them live with this condition. See also:

https://epilepsyontario.org/?s=wellness+and+quality+of+life and https://epilepsysociety.org.uk/living-epilepsy/young-people-and-epilepsy

ACTIVITY 15.6

Refer to https://www.cdc.gov/epilepsy/communications/features/sudep.htm and obtain a definition of status epilepticus and SUDEP.

It is important to note that for some children, AEDs alone are not sufficient to reduce seizure frequency and, depending on the type of epilepsy, some have to consider other adjunctive techniques (NICE 2004) to gain control. Such therapies that you may read about include surgery, ketogenic diet and vagus nerve stimulation.

REFERENCES

Camfield, P.R. & Camfield, C.S. (2006) Pediatric epilepsy: an overview, Chapter 40. In: Swaiman, K., Ashwal, S. & Ferriero, D. (eds). *Pediatric Neurology Principles and Practice*, 4th edn. Philadelphia: Mosby Elsevier.

Chong, L., Jamieson, N.J., Gill, D., Singh-Grewal, D., Craig, J.C., Ju, A., Hanson, C.S. & Tong, A. (2016) Children's experiences of epilepsy: A systematic review of qualitative studies. *Pediatrics*, **138**(3).

Commission on Classification and Terminology of the ILAE (1981) Proposal for revised clinical and electro-encephalographic classification of epileptic seizures. *Epilepsia*, **22**, 489–501.

David, R.B. (2009) *Clinical Pediatric Neurology*, 3rd edn. New York: Desmos Medical Publishing.

Epilepsy Research UK (2010). *What is Epilepsy?* https://epilepsyresearch.org.uk/about-epilepsy/?gclid=EAIaIQobChMImaerlbG6_QIVDdDtCh2sBQPnEAAYASABEgL0J_D_BwE [Accessed 1 March 2023].

Fisher, R.S., van Emde Boas, W., Blume, W. et al. (2005 April) Epileptic seizures and epilepsy: definitions proposed by the International League Against Epilepsy (ILAE) and the International Bureau for Epilepsy (IBE). *Epilepsia*, **46**(4), 470–472. doi: 10.1111/j.0013-9580.2005.66104.x. PMID: 15816939.

Glasper, A. & Richardson, J. (2020) *A Textbook of Children's and Young People's Nursing*. Edinburgh: Churchill Livingstone, Elsevier.

Hauser, W.A. & Banerjee, P.N. (2008) Epidemiology of epilepsy in children, Chapter 9. In: Pellock, J.M., Dodson, W.E. & Bourgeois, B.F.D. (eds). *Pediatric Epilepsy: Diagnosis and Therapy*, 3rd edn. New York: Demos Medical Publishing.

Joint Epilepsy Council (2011) *About Epilepsy*. http://internalmedicineteaching.org/pdfs/Epilepsy-stats.pdf [Accessed 10 June 2010].

Jones, C. & Reilly, C. (2016) Parental anxiety in childhood epilepsy: a systematic review. *Epilepsia*, April; **57**(4), 529–537. doi: 10.1111/epi.13326. Epub 2016 Feb 11. PMID: 26864870.

Nashef, L. & Langan, Y. (2003) Sudden unexpected death in epilepsy (SUDEP). Review article. *Advances in Clinical Neurosciences and Rehabilitation (ACNR)*, **2**(6), 6–8.

National Institute for Clinical Excellence (2012) *The Epilepsies. The Diagnosis and Management of the Epilepsies in Adults and Children in Primary and Secondary Care*. London: NICE.

(2004). NICE guidance on epilepsy recommends specialist diagnosis. *BMJ*, **329**. doi: 10.1136/bmj.329.7473.995-a.

National Society for Epilepsy (2009a). *Epilepsy. An Introduction to Epilepsy – What Is It?* Chalfont St Peter: National Society for Epilepsy.

National Society for Epilepsy (2019) Sudden Unexplained Death in Epilepsy (SUDEP) (online). https://epilepsysociety.org.uk/living-epilepsy/sudden-unexpected-death-epilepsy-sudep [Accessed 1 March 2023].

Panayiotopoulos, C.P. (2010) *A Clinical Guide to Epileptic Syndromes and Their Treatment*, 2nd edn. London: Springer.

Ricci, S.S. & Kyle, T. (2009) *Maternity and Pediatric Nursing*. Philadelphia: Lippincott Williams & Wilkins.

Roper, N., Logan, W.W. & Tierney, A.J. (2004) *The Roper, Logan and Tierney Model of Nursing: Based on Activities of Living*. Philadelphia: Churchill Livingstone Elsevier.

Scheffer, I.E., Berkovic, S., Capovilla, G., Connolly, M.B., French, J., Guilhoto, L., Hirsch, E., Jain, S., Mathern, G.W., Moshe, S.L., Nordli, D.R., Perucca, E., Tomson, T., Wiebe, S., Zhang, Y.H. & And Zuberi, S.M. (2017) ILAE classification of the epilepsies: Position paper of the ILAE Commission for Classification and Terminology. *Epilepsia*, **58**(4), 512–521. *2017*.

Scheffer, I.E., Dibbens, L., Berkovic, S.F. & Mulley, J.C. (2007) What is the role of genetics in epilepsy? In: Sisodiya, S., Cross, J.H., Blumcke, I. et al. Genetics of epilepsy: Epilepsy research foundation workshop report. *Epileptic Discord*, **9**(2), 194–236.

Sun, M., Ruan, X., Li, Y., Wang, P., Zheng, S., Shui, G., Li, L., Huang, Y., Zhang, H.. (2021). Clinical characteristics of 30 COVID-19 patients with epilepsy: A retrospective study in Wuhan. *International Journal of Infectious Diseases*, **103**, 647–653. ISSN 1201-9712, doi: 10.1016/j.ijid.2020.09.1475.

Whittaker, N. (2004). Epilepsy. In: Whittaker, N. (eds). *Disorders and Interventions*. New York: Palgrave Macmillan.

Wolraich, M.L., Dworkin, P.H., Drotar, D.D. & Perrin, E.C. (2008) *Developmental-behavioral Pediatrics: Evidence and Practice*. Philadelphia: Mosby Inc.

WEBSITES FOR FURTHER READING

https://www.who.int/news-room/fact-sheets/detail/epilepsy
https://www.nhs.uk/conditions/epilepsy
www.epilepsy.org.uk/info/driving

Nut Allergy – Anaphylaxis Management

CHAPTER 16

Susie Wilkie

SCENARIO

Katie is a four-year-old child who lives with her parents in a five-bedroom house in a semirural location. She has a three-year-old brother and her mother is 25 weeks pregnant, expecting her third child. Katie was diagnosed with atopic eczema at the age of one month, and asthma at the age of two years.

Whilst attending a family wedding reception, Katie becomes distressed. Her eyes have swollen, and she says her 'tummy aches', and subsequently she vomits. Katie's concerned parents notice she appears to have a nettle rash on her face. Her parents take her home, and she gradually starts to feel better.

The next day her parents contact their GP, who arranges for Katie to be referred to a specialist allergy clinic to be tested for suspected nut allergy. There is a four-month waiting period.

QUESTIONS

1. How prevalent is nut allergy in children?
2. Explain the current approaches to diagnosing nut allergy.
3. Discuss the current approaches to management of nut allergy at home/school.
4. What is anaphylaxis?
5. Describe the emergency treatment of anaphylaxis.

ANSWERS TO QUESTIONS

Question 1. How prevalent is nut allergy in children?

Foods have been known to cause adverse reactions in susceptible individuals for almost 2000 years. Both Hippocrates and Galen reported allergic reactions to milk. One of the earliest references to food allergy is found in the often quoted aphorism:

> 'One man's meat is another man's poison'
>
> *Lucretious, BC 55, cited by Vojdani et al. (2014)*

According to Du Toit (2015), peanut allergy in children has doubled within the last 10 years in Western countries. National Institute for Health and Care Excellence (NICE) Clinical Knowledge Summaries (CKS) (2018) placed the figure as high as 1 in 50 children being affected. Whilst Conrado et al. (2021) reported UK data to show a significant increase in hospital admissions for anaphylaxis during the period 1998 to 2018, it also shows a decrease in fatality rates. The age of onset is decreasing, with children often being diagnosed in the first year of life.

Possible causes

The reason for the significant increase in this allergic disease remains unclear, although it is thought to be influenced by increased exposure to widespread use of peanuts in food manufacture. The hygiene hypothesis also asserts that too hygienic an environment may set the stage for allergic disease later in life as immunity is not being challenged in affluent homes. The emergence of nut allergy also appears to relate directly to the increase in prevalence of allergic asthma and eczema, in predominantly western populations.

Care Planning in Children and Young People's Nursing, Second Edition. Edited by Sonya Clarke and Doris Corkin.
© 2024 John Wiley & Sons Ltd. Published 2024 by John Wiley & Sons Ltd.

Drug trials have been positive with treatments being developed to aid peanut desensitisation, for what has long been considered a lifelong condition, finding that up to 50% could tolerate a small amount of exposure reducing risk of severe anaphylaxis (NICE 2022).

Allergy to peanuts and other types of nuts and seeds is the most serious form of food allergy, characterised by more severe symptoms than other food allergies, wherein sensitivity is often extreme, with minute amounts of the allergen being capable of triggering a rapid and severe type 1 allergic response. The course of anaphylaxis is by nature rapidly progressive, and failure to recognise the severity of these reactions and to administer adrenaline promptly, significantly increases the risk of a fatal outcome.

Question 2. Explain the current approaches to diagnosing nut allergy

Diagnosis is based on clinical history, along with skin prick test, or quantisation of allergen-specific immunoglobulin E (IgE), and oral food challenges, when indicated in a specialist allergy clinic.

IgE specific blood tests venepuncture

Assess: as the children's nurse caring for the needs of the child and family whilst undergoing these tests in an allergy clinic, what approaches would you consider appropriate to help the child cope with the anticipated skin prick test and venepuncture?

How would you support the family in terms of the anxiety whilst undergoing these procedures and awaiting confirmation of diagnosis in the clinic?

Details of how a skin prick test is carried out can be found at the following link for NHS website information on allergies and diagnosis:
www.nhs.uk/conditions/food-allergy/diagnosis

Plan/implement:

- Give family information in advance of procedure.
- Explore with the family any previous experience the child has had of injections or venepuncture. This can provide valuable information for planning the procedure.
- Work in conjunction with a play specialist where possible. For younger children, consider providing a teddy or medical kit for the child to 'practise' with, to gain some familiarity and element of control.
- Provide choices – would they prefer to sit on the parent's lap, be sitting up, use the right or left hand, choose their sticking plaster.
- Ensure provision of adequate pain relief – local anaesthetic cream or ethyl chloride spray.
- Encourage child to have had a good fluid intake – if they are well hydrated this promotes easier venous access.
- Ensure child keeps warm – to promote vasodilatation and easier venous access.
- Consider using age-appropriate distraction during the procedure – read from a book, sing a favourite song, count backwards or blow bubbles.
- Comfort and praise child.

Supporting parents: this is an uncertain and anxious time. Give parents information on an ongoing basis and provide opportunities for clarification. Receiving the diagnosis for some parents can be like a bombshell and has the potential for profound changes in family life.

The technique involves using either a needle or lancet to puncture the epidermis through an extract of a food by specifically trained staff. The test site is examined after 10–20 minutes. A local weal and flare response indicates the presence of food specific IgE antibody. The preferred site is either along the inner forearm or on the child's back.

Question 3. Discuss the current approaches to management of nut allergy at home/school

Most studies and guidance recommend complete avoidance of the allergen once identified. This may appear relatively straightforward, but as Anagnostou and Clarke (2015) suggest, avoidance is easier to advocate than to undertake. There is the potential risk of inadvertent cross contamination in food manufacture, children sharing food, etc. The literature is replete with accidental exposure to the very allergen they are trying to avoid (Brough et al. 2014).

Adults responsible for the care of children are therefore advised to diligently read food labels. This level of constant vigilance creates the conditions for living under the threat of inadvertent exposure and consequent severe reaction.

In addition, parents and other adult carers need to be taught how to recognise the signs of anaphylaxis, and to administer adrenaline (epinephrine) via auto injector (i.e. Epipen®, Jext®) when necessary and to be able to give basic life support/CPR (Resuscitation Council 2021).

The groups of adult carers who will need to be advised on Katie's nut allergy management will include her parents, nursery/school staff and other family members. A management plan will be required for Katie's school/nursery.

For specific guidance on managing medicines in schools, nurseries and similar settings, visit www.allergyinschools.org.uk and www.medicalconditionsatschoolOrg.uk. In 2017, The Human Medicines Regulations (2012) was amended to allow schools in the UK to purchase and hold spare adrenaline auto injector for use in a child with known anaphylaxis who has had a failure of their own pen or it cannot be located.

Question 4. What is anaphylaxis?

Anaphylaxis is a severe, life-threatening, generalised or systemic hypersensitivity reaction. There is an exaggerated response to an allergen, characterised by rapidly developing, life-threatening airway and/or breathing and/or circulation problems usually associated with skin and mucosal changes.

When the specific allergen has been ingested it can react in widespread areas of the body with basophiles of the blood and the mast cells located immediately outside the small blood vessels, giving rise to a widespread allergic reaction throughout the vascular system and in closely associated tissues.

The large quantities of histamine released into the circulation causes widespread peripheral vasodilatation as well as increased permeability of the capillaries and marked loss of plasma from the circulation. This leads to potentially catastrophic circulatory shock within minutes, unless treated with epinephrine to oppose the effects of histamine.

Also released from the cells are leukotrienes, which cause spasm of the smooth muscle of the bronchioles, giving rise to asthma-like symptoms.

Urticaria results from antigen entering specific skin areas causing local reactions. Locally released histamines cause:

1. Local vasodilatation, inducing an immediate red flare.
2. Increased local permeability of capillaries that leads to swelling of the skin, known as hives.

Angioedema is deep swelling around the eyes, lips, and sometimes the mouth and throat.

Refer to Box activity 16.1 for more information on Katie.

Your priority is to recognise that she is seriously unwell, and that this is potentially an anaphylactic reaction. Call for help. Treat the greatest threat to life first. Initial treatment should not be delayed by the lack of complete history or definite diagnosis.

Recognition of an anaphylactic reaction

The Resuscitation Council Guidelines (2021) state that anaphylaxis is likely when all of the following three criteria are met:

- Sudden onset and rapid progression of symptoms.
- Life threatening **A**irway and/or **B**reathing and/or **C**irculation problems.
- Skin and/or mucosal changes (flushing, urticaria, angioedema).

ACTIVITY 16.1

Whilst at school Katie says the back of her throat is tickling, and her voice is becoming hoarse. She says she feels poorly, is frightened, wheezy and is losing consciousness. Katie has some swelling around the lips.

You are called to help. What are your priorities in this situation, and how would you assess Katie?

Please note, generalised urticaria, angioedema, rhinitis, gastro-intestinal symptoms (e.g. vomiting, abdominal pain) would not be described as an anaphylactic reaction, because the life-threatening features, such as airway problem, respiratory difficulty, and hypotension are not present.

The emergency treatment for suspected anaphylaxis should be based on general life support principles using ABCDE approach (Resuscitation Council 2021).

A Airway problems:

- Airway swelling, tongue, throat, patient feels their throat is closing up
- Hoarse voice
- Stridor – indicating upper airway obstruction

B Breathing problems:

- Shortness of breath
- Wheeze
- Becoming tired
- Confusion (caused by hypoxia)
- Cyanosis (late sign)
- Respiratory arrest

C Circulation problems:

Signs of shock – pale, clammy the child will look and feel unwell:

- Increased pulse rate – tachycardia
- Low blood pressure – feeling faint, dizzy, collapse – DO NOT STAND CHILD UP
- Decreased level of consciousness
- Cardiac arrest

D Disability problems:

There may be altered neurological status due to decreased brain perfusion; there may be confusion, agitation, and loss of consciousness and the child is usually anxious, panicky, and can experience an 'impending sense of doom'.

E Exposure:

- Skin and/or mucosal changes often the first feature (present in over 80% of anaphylactic reactions)
- Can be subtle or dramatic
- May be erythema – a patchy, or generalised, red rash
- Urticaria (also called hives, nettle rash, wheals or welts anywhere on the body)
- Angioedema – swelling of deep tissues, for example eyelids, lips, sometimes mouth, and throat

Differential diagnosis – life-threatening conditions

- Asthma (particularly in children)
- Septic shock (hypotension with petechial/purpuric rash)

Differential diagnosis – non-life-threatening

- Vasovagal episode
- Panic attack

- Breath-holding episode
- Idiopathic, non-allergic urticaria or angioedema

NB: SEEK HELP EARLY IF THERE ARE ANY DOUBTS ABOUT THE DIAGNOSIS

Question 5. Describe the emergency treatment of anaphylaxis

- Act immediately.
- Call for an ambulance.
- Do not make child vomit following ingestion.
- Loosen tight clothing, take a history from anyone present.
- Locate Epipen®/Jext® and be prepared to administer.

Patient positioning

All patients should be placed in a comfortable position, taking into account the following:

- Patients with airway and breathing problems may prefer to sit up as this will make breathing easier.
- Lying flat with legs raised is helpful for patients with low blood pressure. If feeling faint DO NOT stand them up – this can induce cardiac arrest.
- If breathing and unconscious they should be placed on their side in recovery position.

Administration of Epipen®/Jext®

Adrenaline (epinephrine) is the most important drug for the treatment of an anaphylactic reaction. It works by:

- Constricting the small blood vessels, causing a rise in blood pressure
- Relaxing smooth muscle in the lungs, improving breathing by dilating bronchial airways
- Stimulates the heart contractility
- Reverses peripheral vasodilatation, reducing oedema/swelling around the face and lips
- Suppresses histamine and leukotriene release, reducing the severity of the IgE mediated allergic reaction

The intramuscular (IM) route is used by most healthcare providers; intravenous (IV) can only be administered by specialists, such as intensivists or anaesthetists.

Adrenaline is administered into the muscle via a pre-loaded syringe (such as Epipen® or Jext®), which provides a single dose of epinephrine.

Using an adrenaline auto injector Epipen®/Jext® (Figure 16.1)

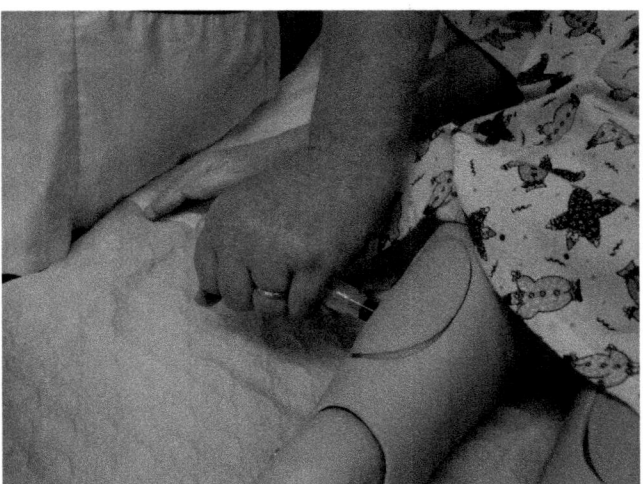

FIGURE 16.1 Adrenaline auto injector.

The injection is administered intramuscularly into the middle of the outer/front thigh. It can be given through clothing.

- Remove the injector from the packaging.
- Remove the safety cap (blue coloured if Epipen®, yellow coloured if Jext®).
- Hold the injector firmly in your fist, 10 cm away from outer thigh, with the black tip (Jext®) or orange tip (Epipen®) at right angles to the thigh.
- Epipen®: press orange tip firmly into thigh for three seconds (there should be a click).
- Jext®: press black tip firmly into the thigh and hold for 10 seconds (there should be a click).
- Remove the pen and massage the area for ten seconds.
- Stay with the child and be prepared to administer basic life support.
- Check heart rate and repository rate, and if no improvement occurs be prepared to give a second dose after five minutes.
- The child will need to be transferred to hospital via ambulance.

These are the current recommended dosages for intramuscular adrenaline supplied by Resuscitation Council 2021:

Adult or child over 12 yr	500 micrograms IM (0.5 ml)
Child 6–12 yr	300 micrograms IM (0.3 ml)
Child 6 months–6 years	150 micrograms IM (0.15 ml)
Child less than 6 months	100–150 micrograms IM (0.5 ml)

For video demonstrations of this please visit www.epipen.co.uk and www.jext.co.uk

After use
Auto injectors are now designed with a shield that covers the needle following discharge of the pen which reduces the chances of accidental needle injury. Adrenaline has a potent peripheral vasoconstrictive action, and accidental injection may cause acute ischemia of the end arteries of a distal digit. Reer to Box Activity 16.2.

There is no legal issue for a person administering adrenaline that is either prescribed for a specific person or in administering adrenaline to an unknown person in such a lifesaving situation, that said there are specific exemptions in The Human Medicines Regulations 2012. However, the nurse involved must practice within the Nursing & Midwifery Council (NMC) code of conduct (2018) and must therefore be competent in being able to recognise the anaphylactic reaction and administer adrenaline using an auto-injector. Furthermore, it would be sensible for trusts/employers to ensure that such a provision is included in their first aid or anaphylaxis guidelines (Resuscitation Council 2021).

ACTIVITY 16.2

As a children's nurse working in an acute hospital, if you come across a child outside hospital having an anaphylactic reaction, are you allowed to use their adrenaline auto-injector to give them IM adrenaline?

REFERENCES

www.epipen.co.uk [accessed August 2022].

www.jext.co.uk [accessed August 2022].

www.nhs.uk/conditions/food-allergy/diagnosis [accessed August 2022].

www.medicalconditionsatschool.org.uk [accessed August 2022].

Anagnostou, K. & Clarke, A. (2015) The management of peanut allergy. *Arch Dis Child*, **100**, 68–72.

Brough, H.A., Turner, P.J., Wright, T., Fox, A.T., Taylor, S.L., Warner, J.O. & Lac, G. (2014) Dietary management of peanut and tree nut allergy: what exactly should patients avoid? *Journal of Clinical and Experimental Allergy*, **45**(5), 859–871.

Conrado, A.B., Ierodiakonou, D., Gowland, M.H., Boyle, R.J. & Turner, P.J. (2021) Food anaphylaxis in the United Kingdom: analysis of national data, 1998-2018. *British Medical Journal*, **372**(251), 1–10.

Du Toit, G. & Roberts, G. (2015) Randomised trial of peanut consumption in infants at risk for peanut allergy. *The New England Journal of Medicine*, **372**(9), 803.814.

The Human Medicines Regulations (2012) Available at: https://www.legislation.gov.uk/uksi/2012/1916/contents/made [Accessed in August 2022].

NICE CKS (2018) Food Allergy: prevalence. Available at: https://cks.nice.org.uk/topics/food-allergy/background-information/prevalence [accessed August 2022].

NICE (2022) Palforzia for treating peanut allergy in children and young people. Available at: www.nice.org.uk/guidance/ta769 [accessed August 2022].

Nursing & Midwifery Council (2018) *The Code; Professional Standards of Practice and Behaviour for Nurses, Midwives, and Nursing Associates*. Available at: www.nmc.org.uk/globalassets/sitedocuments/nmc-publications/nmc-code.pdf [accessed August 2022].

Resuscitation Council UK (2021) Anaphylaxis. Available at: https://www.resus.org.uk/sites/default/files/2021-04/Anaphylaxis%20Summary%20Document.pdf [accessed August 2022].

Vojdani, A., Kharrazian, D. & Mukherjee, P.S. (2014) The prevalence of antibodies against wheat and milk proteins in blood donors and their contribution to neuro-immune reactivities. *Nutrients*, 2014, **6**, 15–36.

CHAPTER 17

Closed Head Injury

Carol McCormick
(acknowledging Katie Dowdie)

SCENARIO

Leah, a ten-year-old girl, who weighed 28 kg, lived at home with her parents, Noel and Jane, and had a six-year-old brother James.

Leah travelled on the bus each day to school. On a cold frosty November day, Leah as usual caught the bus to school with her brother, James.

Leah chose to sit at the back of the bus beside her school chum.

The school bus continued its journey along the busy road and then prepared to turn right into Leah's school entrance. Due to the frosty conditions the lorry travelling behind the bus braked quickly but unfortunately skidded into the back of the bus. Leah was propelled forward hitting her head of the seat in front and sustained a head injury.

The ambulance was called and Leah was stabilised at the scene.

Leah was then admitted via the accident and emergency department to the paediatric intensive care unit for further management of her closed head injury.

QUESTIONS

1. What is a closed head injury?
2. When using the Mead model, how would the children's nurse safely maintain the airway of a child with a Glasgow Coma Scale (GCS) below 8?
3. Why is pain relief and sedation an important aspect of the care of a child with a closed head injury?
4. (a) Use the Glasgow Coma Scale to assess Leah's neurological status.
   (b) What other observations would you carry out?
5. How would the children's nurse ensure adequate fluid balance?

ANSWERS TO QUESTIONS
Question 1. What is a closed head injury?

A closed head injury (CHI) is defined as non-penetrating injury to the brain and occurs when the head accelerates and then rapidly collides with another object (Steffen' Albert 2010). Trauma causes injury to the brain as a result of a blow to the head, or sudden, violent motion that causes the brain to impact against the skull. No object penetrates through the skull to the brain tissue itself.
Brain injury is classified into phases: primary injury and secondary injury.

The primary injury is the initial brain insult as a result of traumatic impact.

According to Moppett (2007), oedema, capillary leakage, and systemic inflammatory response is associated with secondary injury. Furthermore, secondary injury is worsened by hypoxia and hypotension (Pigula et al. 1993).

Coup is injury on site of impact and contre-coup is injury on opposite side of impact. This is shown in Figure 17.1.

Care Planning in Children and Young People's Nursing, Second Edition. Edited by Sonya Clarke and Doris Corkin.
© 2024 John Wiley & Sons Ltd. Published 2024 by John Wiley & Sons Ltd.

Please refer to Table 17.1.

Table 17.1 Mead model.

A Respiratory
B Cardiovascular
C Pain/sedation
D Neurology
E Nutrition/hydration
F Elimination
G (i) Skin/wound care
G (ii) Mobility
G (iii) Hygiene
H (i) Psychological and social/culture
H (ii) Circumstantial

Please see Chapter 1 for further reading.
Adapted from: McClune and Franklin (1987).

Question 2. When using the Mead model, how would the children's nurse safely maintain the airway of a child with a Glasgow Coma Scale below 8?

Respiratory and cardiovascular needs should be looked at (McClune & Franklin 1987). Any child presenting with a Glasgow Coma Scale (GCS) <8 is classified as a severe head injury (Moppett 2007; Weinstein 2006). The most important initial interventions are:

- Control of the airway and cervical spine
- Breathing and circulation

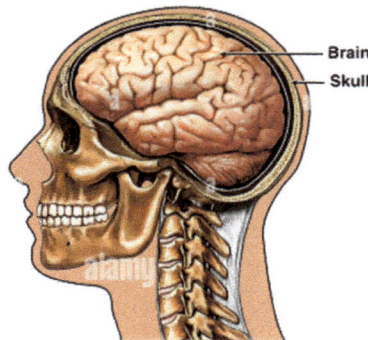
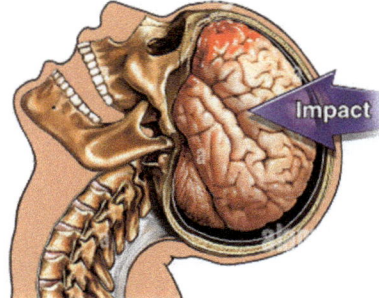
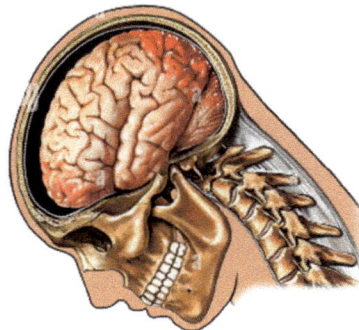
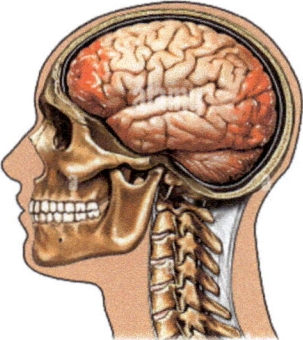

FIGURE 17.1 Coup and contre-coup injury (collection of L. Henry). Reproduced from Best Practice (https://bestpractice.bmj.com/search?q=Coup+and+contre-coup+injury+ – practice/monograph/967/resources/images.html) with kind permission.

Physical needs

Respiratory

Assess: continue to assess Leah's level of consciousness and ability to maintain her:
Airway, Breathing, and Circulation (ABC).

- Observe her colour – is Leah's skin pink, pale, dusky, or cyanosed?
- Check Leah's chest movement – assess rate, depth, and rhythm.
- Are there any abnormal breathing sounds, for example stridor?
- Have an understanding of the different types of abnormal respiratory pattern, for example apnoea, hyperventilation/hypoventilation.
- Monitor respiration rate, oxygen requirements, method of administration, and pulse oximetry.

Cardiovascular

Assess: this assessment has some overlap with the respiratory assessment:

- Is Leah's skin pink and warm to touch, or pale, mottled, and cool to touch?
- Are her peripheries warm or cold?
- What is Leah's capillary refill time (normal CRT is 2–3 secs)?
- Has intravenous (IV) access been established?
- Monitor/record heart rate (HR), blood pressure (B/P) (systolic diastolic and mean), respiratory rate, pulse oximetry (SaO_2), and temperature.
- Understand the significance of the HR, BP, central, and peripheral perfusion.

It is important to know the cardiovascular stability of the child prior to intubation as the choice of drugs used for induction and intubation can have adverse effects.

These assessments are carried out very quickly and the child is then prepared for intubation and ventilation.

Plan: preparation for child

- Prepare emergency/airway trolley for intubation (Table 17.2).
- Gather required drugs (Table 17.3).

Table 17.2 Emergency/airway trolley for intubation.

- Oral and nasal ET tube (required size + a size smaller)
- Introducer and bougie
- Laryngoscope and appropriate blade
- Magill's forceps appropriate size
- Yankauer sucker
- Nasogastric tube and drainage bag
- Elastoplast tape pre-cut
- Dressed applicators
- Friars' Balsam and gallipot
- Sterile lubricating gel and gauze

At the bedside:

- Oxygen and suction supply
- Facemask with bagging set
- Suction catheters
- Equipment to monitor vital signs

Table 17.3 Common drugs used for intubation (see BNFc 2023).

- Thiopentone sodium

Intravenous anaesthetic used for induction of anaesthesia.

Side effects: apnoea, hypotension, arrhythmias, laryngeal spasm. In excessive doses, hypothermia and reduction in cerebral function.

- Ketamine

Induction and maintenance of anaesthesia for short procedures.

- Atracurium

Neuromuscular blocking drug, also known as muscle relaxant.

Side effects – skin flushing, hypotension, tachycardia.

- Suxamethonium

Depolarising neuromuscular blocking drug. Used if fast action and brief duration of action is required.

- Propofol

Intravenous anaesthetic used for induction of anaesthesia.

Side effects: hypotension, tachycardia, less common – thrombosis, pulmonary oedema, hyperkalaemia, cardiac failure.

- Atropine

Antimuscarinic drug used in the treatment of bradycardia.

Side effects: tachycardia, dilatation of the pupils, dry mouth, nausea, and vomiting, confusion.

- Adrenaline

Direct acting sympathomimetic agent. Used in CPR, acute anaphylaxis, low cardiac output. Side effects: nausea, vomiting, tachycardia, arrhythmias, hypertension, cold peripheries.

- Morphine

Opioid analgesia used to relieve moderate to severe pain.

Side effects: nausea, vomiting, constipation, hypotension, respiratory depression.

- Midazolam

Benzodiazepine used for sedation.

Side effects: gastro-intestinal disturbances, hypotension, heart rate changes, laryngospasm, respiratory depression.

- Sodium chloride 0.9%

Used for drug/line flush.

Implement:

- Leah will be admitted to paediatric intensive care Unit (PICU); it is the nurse's responsibility to assist intubation and establishment of central venous access – one nurse to record observations and fluid balance.

NB The combination of drugs used will be decided by the anaesthetist, based on the clinical condition of the child.

- Continue to administer 100% oxygen via bag and mask and apply suction when necessary.
- Apply electrocardiograph (ECG) electrodes, B/P cuff and SaO_2 probe to ensure continuous trend of cardiovascular status and oxygenation.
- Pass nasogastric tube (NG), aspirate and attach to drainage bag to prevent aspiration of stomach contents and lung soiling.
- The endotracheal tube (ET) is passed via the nose or orally if basal skull fracture is suspected, and secured firmly with elastoplast.
- Anaesthetist/doctor will auscultate chest for equal air entry and bilateral chest movement.
- Essential to confirm position of tubes (ET & NG) by X-ray.

- Record size and length of ET tube at the lips or nose on observation chart. This is important as it is essential to check regularly for any movement of the position of the ET tube.
- The ET tube is suctioned to assess the type and amount of secretions and a specimen obtained for virology, culture, and sensitivity.
- The ventilator is set by the medical staff determined by the arterial blood gas (ABG) result and connected to the ET tube by the intensive care nurse.

Once the airway is established ongoing nursing care involves optimising respiratory function and being aware of potential complications. All ventilator settings are recorded hourly to ensure adequate ventilation and patient safety. Blood gases are checked regularly to ensure ventilation is adequate and ventilator settings changed accordingly. What we should be looking at in the ABG is PaO_2- to ensure oxygen level is adequate to prevent hypoxia. Cerebral hypoxia causes more oedema, leading to raised intracranial pressure (ICP) which further damages brain tissue as described by Williams (2000).

Monitor $PaCO_2$ to prevent hypocapnia/hypercapnia, as this can cause undesirable changes in ICP and cerebral perfusion pressure (CPP).

Leah's airway must be kept patent and she will have suction of her ET tube as indicted by her haemodynamic, respiratory, and cerebral stability. Gentle chest physiotherapy can be performed *if* the ICP and CPP are stable. This will prevent stasis of secretions leading to infection, therefore making ventilation more difficult, in turn having an undesirable effect on cerebral perfusion.

Ensure ventilator tubing is positioned to prevent tugging or dragging of the ET tube to prevent displacement or kinking causing loss of or obstruction of the airway. Keep ventilator tubing free from water and ensure water traps are emptied. Once spinal clearance has been documented it will be possible to nurse Leah on alternate sides keeping her head in midline. This also assists in prevention of infection and aids expansion of the lungs. Observation from a cardiovascular perspective will concentrate on HR, BP, and SaO_2.

Leah will have continuous monitoring in place with observations recorded hourly. Hypoxia is the most common cause of cardiovascular instability, as mentioned previously. Hypotension is a common complication due to the effects of other treatments such as analgesia, sedation, muscle relaxants, and barbiturate therapy. Management is aimed at using correct volume of IV fluids based on BP, central venous pressure (CVP), urine output and fluid balance.

In addition, an inotrope such as dopamine (BNF_C 2009) may be required to ensure adequate BP in order to optimise CPP (Table 17.4). Thiopentone lowers metabolism and therefore decreases HR, BP, temperature and may affect pupil reaction. It is important to recognise what may be drug related or a sudden deterioration in Leah's condition. Treatment of head-injured children can be

Table 17.4 Drugs which may be used.

- IV fentanyl

Opioid analgesia used to treat moderate to severe pain.

Side effects: abdominal pain, vasodilatation, apnoea, agitation, tremor, laryngospasm.

- Dopamine

Inotropic sympathomimetic. Cardiac stimulant acts on beta receptors in cardiac muscle and increases contractility to increase cardiac output.

Side effects: nausea and vomiting, peripheral vasoconstriction, hypertension, tachycardia.

- IV or oral paracetamol

Non-opioid analgesia used for mild to moderate pain. Also antipyretic properties. Side effects: rare, but rashes thrombocytopenia, leucopenia, neutropenia, hypotension also reported on IV infusion.

Important: liver and renal damage following overdosage.

- Oral or rectal chloral hydrate

Hypnotic, mainly used for sedation.

Side effects: gastric irritation, nausea and vomiting, abdominal distension, headache, dependence.

extremely complex; therefore, the children's nurse must understand the significance of the observations in order to recognise complications so that changes can be initiated early in management.

Evaluate: use the Mead model of nursing (McClune & Franklin 1987). This framework uses a continuum of care, from being highly dependent moving towards independence.

Question 3. Why is pain relief and sedation an important aspect of care of a child with a closed head injury?

Physical needs

Pain/sedation

In the acute phase of severe head injury, children require sedation and analgesia to prevent unplanned extubation and facilitate ventilation. To ensure invasive lines remain *in situ* and to rest the brain and reduce stimulation, it is important to understand the GCS, as children with low scores can feel pain and become stressed.

Nursing interventions and care are essential for prevention of secondary complications and to promote recovery. However, they can also cause adverse effects, such as raised ICP, reduced CPP, hypoxemia, and bradycardia. Therefore it is essential that analgesia and sedation is adequate.

Please refer to BNFc (2009) regarding drugs above and become aware of possible side effects of each.

Implementation: Leah will be commenced on a morphine intravenous infusion for pain and midazolam infusion for sedation. Atracurium is a neuromuscular blocking agent (NBA), and may be used if Leah has a raised ICP. It is particularly helpful in preventing a cough response to suction, which would further increase ICP. Muscle relaxants do not have sedative or analgesic properties and are not intended to be used without opioids and sedation (Martin et al. 1999). Thiopentone is an anaesthetic agent and lowers cerebral metabolism and therefore ICP. This drug causes myocardial depression and vasodilation necessitating inotropic support (BNFc 2023).

Evaluation: how can we assess if Leah is pain free and adequately sedated?

- Look at the HR and BP, is there an increase?
- Is it associated with nursing interventions, or at rest?
- Are there tears and dilatation of the pupils?
- Is there flushing/blotching of the skin? (for example red face)

Evaluation in this group of patients is challenging:

- Is it pain?
- Is it a seizure?

If Leah's analgesia and sedation is adequate you would expect her HR and BP to remain fairly static or show a slight increase in response to interventions but then quickly settle. An unprovoked increase in HR and BP may be associated with seizure activity, usually combined with a drop in SaO_2 and increase in pupil size. Muscle relaxants can make assessment difficult. Manifestations of pain may include tearing and pupillary dilation.

Record pain score hourly

There are a variety of pain tools available for use such as FLACC (depending on age of child and dependency level (see Appendix 3 for Chapter 14, RCN Guidelines).

However, a comprehensive clinical assessment remains the most valuable method of evaluating sedation until the development of a tool is developed in this particular patient population.

Question 4(a) Use the Glasgow Coma Scale (GCS) to assess Leah's neurological status. See Figure 17.2.

Neurology

Assess: according to Williams (2000) the level of consciousness has two parts: arousal and awareness. Leah's GCS will be recorded at least hourly and the assessment is divided into:

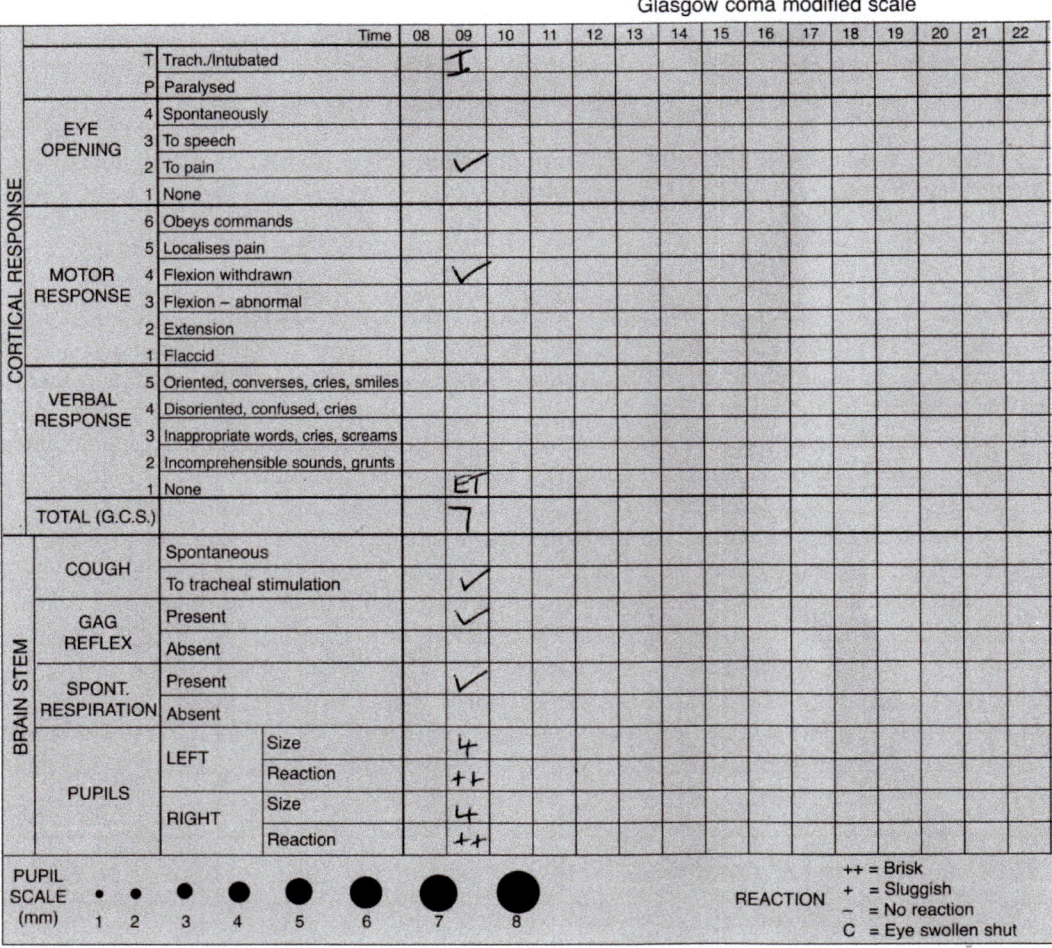

FIGURE 17.2 Royal Belfast hospital for sick children: Paediatric intensive care observation sheet.

1. Cortical response: eye opening, motor response, and verbal response.
2. Brain stem: cough, gag reflex, and spontaneous breathing.

CORTICAL RESPONSE

Eye opening (GCS top score is 4)
Check if Leah is able to open her eyes spontaneously (4/4), if not then call out her name, initially softly and then louder (3/4); if there is still no eye opening then apply peripheral painful stimuli by applying pressure with a pen to the lateral outer aspect of the second or third finger (2/4); see Figure 17.3 (Waterhouse 2005).

Gently open Leah's eyes to assess pupil size, reaction and equality. Use a + sign for a reaction or a – sign for no reaction; C is recorded if the eyes are closed due to trauma. Also record if the pupils respond briskly or sluggishly to light, and the size of the pupils (Davies & Hassell 2007). These should be between two and four millimetres in diameter (Williams 2000).

Motor response (GCS top score is 6)
This is to assess the level of consciousness, how deep a coma the patient is in, and if simple commands can be obeyed (Waterhouse 2005). Check if Leah obeys simple commands, for example squeezing the nurse's finger (6/6); if she does not respond then central painful stimulus is used to assess the level of consciousness and a response will score 5/6. This can either be by pressing the supraorbital ridge or by using the trapezius squeeze (Waterhouse 2005). The experienced intensive care nurse will be observing Leah for normal or abnormal movements. The lowest score is (1/6) if there is no movement.

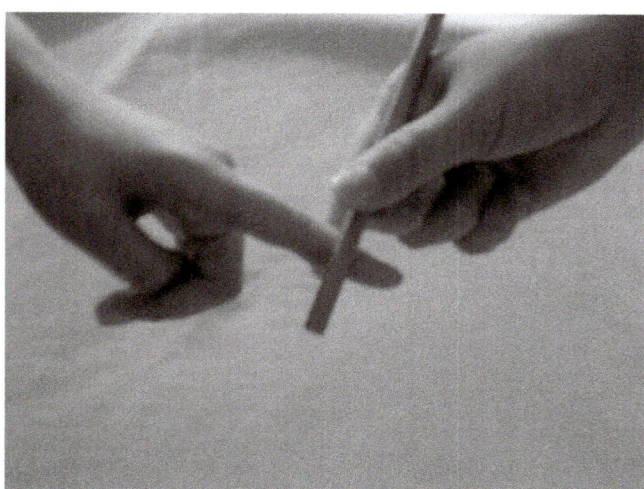

FIGURE 17.3 Assessing response.

Please note: the hand rests on the patient's head and the flat part of the thumb is placed on the supraorbital ridge gradually increasing the pressure for a maximum of 20 seconds. *This is not to be used if there are facial or skull fractures.*

Please note: apply gradual degrees of pressure until the patient attempts to localise pain for a maximum of 20 seconds (not suitable for children under five).

Verbal response (GCS top score is 5)

This provides the children's nurse with information about the patient's speech, ability to understand and functioning areas of the higher, cognitive centres of the brain (Waterhouse 2005).

As Leah is ventilated and sedated she will have an ET tube *in situ*-, therefore she can only score (1/5).

COUGH

ET suction is an important part of the care in intensive care but this suctioning needs to be kept to a minimal as coughing increases ICP (Tume & Jinks 2008). The nurse can assess the cough reflex during ET suction.

GAG

The gag reflex can be assessed when performing oral suction using a yankauer gently at the back of the throat (Davies & Hassell 2007).

SPONTANEOUS BREATHING

Breathing indicates that the brain stem is intact. Leah is ventilated, but an experienced intensive care nurse will be able to assess if she has spontaneous breathing.

Question 4(b). What other observations would you carry out?

The following observations are closely monitored to prevent any deterioration in Leah's condition. The heart rate, B/P and respiratory rate are recorded at least hourly. A falling heart rate (bradycardia) and a rising B/P (hypertension) combined with an irregular respiratory rate or apnoea (Cushing's triad) is an indication of a rising ICP. There will also be a decrease in the level of consciousness.

> BRAIN STEM

Heart rate range for a 10-year-old

Awake 60–140 (beats/minute) asleep 60–90 (beats/minute)

Systolic blood pressure (mmHg)

Range for a 10-year-old

Normal 90 + 2 × age in years

Lower limit 70 + 2 × age in years

Respiratory rate range for a 10-year-old

Breaths per minute 20–24

As Leah is in intensive care she will have ICP monitoring. Observe closely for any sustained rise in ICP.
Normal range of ICP in a 10-year-old

10–15 mmHg

Cerebral perfusion pressure (CPP)
Cerebral perfusion pressure (CPP) is mean arterial blood pressure (MAP) minus intracranial pressure (ICP). If the ICP is rising, the CPP will fall; it is therefore important to maintain a good blood pressure at all times. If the CPP falls, the blood supply to the brain is significantly reduced.
 An adequate CPP for a 10-year-old is >60 mmHg
 The hypothalamus is responsible for controlling body temperature. The importance of recording the body temperature cannot be underestimated; a rise in temperature increases the metabolic rate and therefore increases oxygen consumption. The children's nurse must be able to distinguish between pyrexia caused by infection or caused by a rise in ICP (Suadoni 2009).
 Plan: to minimise any further deterioration in the GCS:

- Nurse midline.
- Thirty degree head-up tilt (Feldman et al. 1992).
- Ensure good pain relief and sedation.
- Maintain $PaCO_2$ at lower end of normal (4.5–5.5 kPa); mild hyperventilation may be required.
- Maintain a blood pressure and a good CPP. To achieve this inotropes may be required, for example dopamine (further reading is required on inotropes – source BNF_C 2023).

A neuromuscular blockade, for example vecuronium bromide, may be considered but it does have complications including pneumonia and increasing the stay in intensive care (Tume et al. 2008) (further reading required on neuromuscular blockade: source BNF_C 2023).
 Medical staff will assess fluid requirements and may restrict fluids, but this will depend on blood pressure, perfusion, need for inotropes, and if a fluid bolus has been required.
 Maintain a normal body temperature. Further brain damage can be associated with hyperthermia (Davies & Hassell 2007).
 Consider the use of hyperosmolar therapy if there is a rise in the ICP, for example mannitol (further reading required source: BNF_C 2023).
 If cervical spine immobilisation is required using a spinal collar, ensure that this is not too tight, obstructing the jugular vein.
 If there is a sudden rise in ICP a computed tomography (CT) imaging of the head may be ordered by the neurosurgeons (NICE 2007).
 *Cerebral Function Analysing Monitoring (CFAM) is a monitoring device which records integrated encephalograms (EEG) which allows continuous observations of cerebral activity for prolonged periods. This is a useful tool to consider when children are being administered muscle relaxants in order to monitor seizure activity (Murdoch-Eton et al. 2001).
 Implicate and evaluate: using the Mead model now ensure all of the above has been effective and then write your evaluation.

Question 5. How would the children's nurse ensure adequate fluid balance?

Nutrition/hydration and elimination

Assess: all children admitted to hospital should have an accurate weight recorded to enable calculation of medications and fluids (NMC 2008). As Leah is critically ill and being admitted to an intensive care unit, it is appropriate to estimate her weight using the following formula.

Child aged 1–10 years

Weight (kg) = (age in years + 4) × 2 (Davies & Hassell 2007)

Ideally, Leah would be nursed on a weighing bed and when she has been stabilised, a more accurate weight can be obtained; this would also facilitate a daily weight to be recorded. Maintaining fluid balance is essential to health (Scales & Pilsworth 2008).

Normal fluid requirements for a child weighing 28 kg

Body weight	Fluid requirement per day (ml/kg)
First 10 kg	100 = 1000
Second 10 kg	50 = 500
Subsequent kilograms	20 = 160
Total	1660

Daily fluid requirement will be assessed by the medical staff; however, maintenance fluids will be calculated as per formulae above. Keeping an accurate fluid balance chart is an important part of hydration monitoring. The nurse must take into account all fluid administration when assessing how much fluid is to be administered on an hourly basis (intravenous fluids, enteral feeds, intravenous drugs). If a fluid bolus has been required, this is usually over and above the total 24-hour intake. All fluid administration is regulated by either infusion pumps or drivers and administrated as prescribed. Low intravascular volume is usually indicated by a rising heart rate and falling blood pressure (Cook 2005). In the critically ill it is also assessed by measuring the CVP.

Electrolytes require close monitoring, in particular sodium and potassium. Urea and electrolyte results dictate what type of intravenous fluids are prescribed by the medical staff.

CONSIDER RISK MANAGEMENT

It is important to avoid hyponatraemia (an electrolyte disturbance) in the acutely ill hospitalised child as this can occur during inappropriate rehydration or with maintenance fluids and may have serious advert effects, such as neurological impairment, and cause death (Jenkins et al. 2003). Therefore, it is vital that nursing and medical staff work effectively and efficiently to ensure care planning documentation is consistent, coherent, and standardised.

A nasogastric tube will be *in situ*, as enteral feeding is introduced as soon as possible following a traumatic injury, because the body requires an increased amount of calories. Early referral to the dietician is recommended and a high calorie feed commenced; prior to commencing feeds it is necessary to rule out any abdominal injury.

Check regular blood sugars; an insulin intravenous infusion may be required if the blood sugar level is persistently high.

Plan: record the fluid balance chart hourly as accurate intake and output is essential. Calculate the overall balance (intake minus output) at least six hourly. This is to ensure that Leah is neither in a large negative or positive balance. Check regular blood biochemistry (U&E). A urinary catheter will be *in situ*; record output hourly and note how many ml/kg/hour.

Normal urinary output for a 10-year-old: 1 ml/kg/hr

Regular urinalysis should be checked; the specific gravity (SG) will show if a patient s urine is dilute or concentrated (Scales & Pilsworth 2008). Following a head injury there can be a decreased production of the antidiuretic hormone (ADH) resulting in neurogenic diabetes insipidus (Davies & Hassell 2007). Avoid constipation as this can cause a rise in ICP due to straining (Suadoni 2009). A high fibre feed may be required.

Implicate and evaluate: whilst utilising the Mead model ensure all of the above planned care has been effective and then write your evaluation.

REFERENCES

British National Formulary for Children (2023) *British National Formulary for Children*. London: BNFc.

Cook, N.F. (2005) Fundamentals of fluids and hydration in the nursing of the neuroscience patient. *British Journal of Neuroscience Nursing*, **1**(2), 61–66.

Davies, J.H. & Hassell, L.L. (2007) *Children in Intensive Care. A Survival Guide*, 2nd edn. Edinburgh: Churchill Livingstone.

Feldman, Z., Kanter, M. & Robinson, C. (1992) Effects of head elevation on intracranial pressure and cerebral blood flow in head injury patients. *Journal of Neurosurgery*, **76**, 207–211.

Jenkins, J.G., Taylor, B. & McCarthy, M. (2003) Prevention of hyponatraemia in children receiving fluid therapy. *The Ulster Medical Journal*, **72**(2), 69–72. Note: this article incorporates the DHSSPS guidelines.

Martin, L.D., Bratton, S.L. & O'Rourke, P. (1999) Issues and controversies of neuromuscular blocking agents in infants and children. *Critical Care Medicine*, **27**(7), 1358–1368.

McClune, B. & Franklin, K. (1987) The Mead model for nursing-adapted from the Roper/Logan/Tierney model for nursing. *Intensive Care Nursing*, **3**(3), 97–105. cited in Viney, C. (1996) *Nursing the Critically Ill*. Edinburgh: Baillière Tindall.

Moppett, I.K. (2007) Traumatic brain injury: assessment, resuscitation and early management. *British Journal Anaesthesia*, **99**(1), 18–31.

Murdoch-Eton, D., Darowski, M. & Livingston, J. (2001) Cerebral function monitoring in paediatric intensive care: useful features for predicting outcome. *Developmental Medicine & Child Neurology*, **43**(2), 91–96. [Online]. Available at https://pubmed.ncbi.nlm.nih.gov/11221910 [Accessed 31st October 2022].

National Institute for Health and Clinical Excellence (2007) *Head Injury: Triage, Assessment, Investigation and Early Management of Head Injury in Infants, Children and Adults*, NICE clinical guideline 56. London: NHS.

Nursing and Midwifery Council (2008) *Standards for Medicines Management*. London: NMC.

One of the best clinical decision support tools for health professionals worldwide. www.bestpractice.bmj.com [Accessed 31st October 2022].

Pigula, F.A., Wald, S.L., Shackford, S.R. & Vane, D.W. (1993) The effect of hypotension and hypoxia on children with severe head injuries. *Journal of Pediatric Surgery*, **28**(3), 310–316.

Scales, K. & Pilsworth, J. (2008) The importance of fluid balance in clinical practise. *Nursing Standard*, **22**(47), 50–57.

Steffen-Albert, K.A. (2010) Management of patients with neurologic trauma, Chapter 63. In: Smeltzer, S.C., Bare, B.G., Hinkle, J.L. & Cheever, K.H. (eds). *Brunner & Suddarth's Textbook of Medical-Surgical Nursing*, 12th edn. Philadelphia: Wolters Kluwer/Lippincott Williams & Wilkins.

Suadoni, M.T. (2009) Raised intracranial pressure: nursing observations and interventions. *Nursing Standard*, **23**(43), 35–40.

Tume, L. & Jinks, A. (2008) Endotracheal suctioning in children with severe traumatic brain injury: a literature review. *Nursing in Critical Care*, **13**(5), 232–240.

Tume, L., Thorburn, K. & Sinha, A. (2008) A review of the intensive care management of severe paediatric traumatic brain injury. *British Journal of Neuroscience Nursing*, **4**(9), 424–431.

Waterhouse, C. (2005) The Glasgow coma scale and other neurological observations. *Nursing Standard*, **19**(33), 56–64.

Weinstein, S. (2006) Controversies in the care of children with acute brain injury. *Current Neurology and Neuroscience Reports*, **6**(2), 127–135.

Williams, A. (2000) Severe head injury in children: A case study. *Emergency Nurse*, **8**(1), 16–19.

BIBLIOGRAPHY

Bansal, S., Blalock, D., Kebede, T., Dean, N.P. & Carpenter, J.L. (2014) Levetiracetam versus (fos)phenytoin for seizure prophylaxis in pediatric patients with intracranial hemorrhage. *Journal of Neurosurgery Pediatrics*, **13**(2), 209–215. [Online]. Available at: https://pubmed.ncbi.nlm.nih.gov/24286154 [Accessed 31st October 2022].

Levin, H.S. & Diaz-Arrastia, R.R. (2015) Diagnosis, prognosis, and clinical management of mild traumatic brain injury. *The Lancet Neurology*, **14**(5), 506–517. [Online]. Available at: https://www.sciencedirect.com/science/article/abs/pii/S1474442215000022 [Accessed 31st October 2022].

Popernack, M.C., Gray, N. & Reuter-Rice, K. (2015) Moderate-to-severe traumatic brain injury in children: Complications and rehabilitation strategies. *Journal of Pediatric Health Care*, **29**(3), 1–7. [Online]. Available at https://pubmed.ncbi.nlm.nih.gov/25449002 [Accessed 31st October 2022].

PROFESSIONAL UPDATES

PANSTAR Course – Paediatric and Neonatal Safe Transfer and Retrieval.

Obesity

Janice Christie

CHAPTER 18

> **SCENARIO**

Treewood Primary School is located in a deprived inner-city location. Most of the parents with children attending the school have low incomes or are unemployed; many pupils live in single parent households. The surrounding community members often have negative stereotypes of the pupils and the school has a poor local image. Many of the Treewood students do not attain their full academic potential and under-achieve in performance tests.

The school is situated in a large public housing development known as Treeland. There are ten-storey flats and terraced housing in the development. Over the past few years, the area has become increasingly run down; there are many vacant dwellings that have been vandalised. Groups of young people, who have little else to do, break into empty houses or flats to take drugs and alcohol. Many older people, who are fearful of becoming victims of the rising crime rate within the estate, will not leave their homes in the evenings. Parents are reluctant to let their younger children play outside the home due to concerns about harm to their offspring arising from antisocial behaviour. Most people in the estate express hopelessness in their situation; they aim to live for today as they say that they have nothing to aspire to.

Treeland has few local amenities. There is a fast-food outlet that mostly offers fried foods, a small general store that sells staple foods (mainly processed foods) and an off-licence that sells alcohol. A youth club, for teenagers closed several months ago due to poor attendance and repeated vandalism of the premises. There are several green spaces within Treeland that could be used for play, but these are fouled with dog excrement and broken glass, often children end up playing in the small back gardens of terrace homes or in the corridors of flats. Few people living in Treeland have cars, most are dependent on public transport or private taxi hire for journeys. There is a local bus service that runs every 45 minutes in the evening. The nearest large food store is about a 30-minute walk (ten minutes by bus) away and the nearest leisure centre is about a 45-minute walk (or two ten-minute bus journeys).

The local housing authority is aware of problems in the estate and has helped residents form a neighbourhood committee in order to decide how to best tackle locality difficulties. This committee includes local residents and professionals (school, police, housing officers, health, and social care, etc.) working in the locality. A new headmaster (Mr. Jones) was appointed to Treewood school several months ago and he is determined to improve the school's image and increase life chances and academic standards within the school. The teachers in the school are supporting this new school vision.

Jane is a school nurse employed by a primary care trust and is attached (provides care) to Treewood primary school. Through the National Child Measurement Programme (NCMP) (NHS Choices 2021), she undertakes measurement of children's height and weight in the reception year (when children are aged 4–5 years) and in year 6 (children aged 10–11). Jane has identified that 20% of reception year students and 25% of year 6 pupils are obese. She knows that many children perform poorly at school. Jane has had to counsel some children who have low self-esteem and who have experienced bullying. The school has a canteen that provides healthy meals, but it is not used by all pupils, some parents give their children money to buy lunch and often these pupils buy chips (fried potatoes) from a local fast-food outlet that is near the school. Many children walk to school and all are offered 30 minutes per week of physical education/sporting activity.

Jane has been approached by Jake and his mother. Jake is ten-year-old boy who is obese, and both Jake and his mother are concerned and willing to take action about his recent accelerating weight gain. His two older brothers are both overweight and his mother, who is a single parent, is obese. Jake's mother has a part-time job in a local bakery. She starts work at 4 am, and finds she is too tired to cook for her family when she returns home after the end of her shift at 1 pm. All her children have different food preferences and she finds it hard to cater for all their needs, so she buys each a different ready meal. Jake says he never eats fruit or vegetables; his preferred meal is an adult-sized portion of macaroni cheese.

Jake has been showing attention difficulties in school, has poor academic performance and has low self-esteem. His mother asks his older brothers to help get him ready for school in the morning. Jake usually stays in bed for as long as possible most mornings, as he is later than his brothers there usually is no milk left for his breakfast cereal and often he leaves home without breakfast. His eldest brother leaves him at school before catching the bus to a local training programme. When Jake gets to school he finds it difficult to concentrate, especially during morning lessons.

Sometimes Jake's mother has time to make him lunch (usually white bread ham sandwiches, a packet of crisps and a sugary fizzy drink); at other times she gives him money to buy some food at the fast food shop. She does not want Jake to take free school dinners because of the stigma associated with free meals. Jake lives in a top-floor flat, often the lifts do not work and he uses the stairs to go home. Once at home, there is little to do other than to than to play his video games (his mother worries about the possible negative influence of his friends in the local neighbourhood).

Care Planning in Children and Young People's Nursing, Second Edition. Edited by Sonya Clarke and Doris Corkin.
© 2024 John Wiley & Sons Ltd. Published 2024 by John Wiley & Sons Ltd.

SOME HELPFUL ADDITIONAL INFORMATION

School nurses are responsible for health promotion and health maintenance of school-aged children, they support the wellbeing of individual children and attend to the public health of the school population; for further information of the public health role see Christie et al. (2009). In this section you will be asked to consider Jane's intervention for one child (Jake) and in addition, interventions for the school population. The Neuman system model (Neuman & Fawcett 2002) can be applied to one person, a group or population of people and therefore, it can be used as a model to develop a one-child and a public health school care plan.

You may find that some of your answers (particularly for questions 5 and 6) differ from the ones suggested. There are many possible acceptable responses for some questions, a good answer is based on evidence, so ensure that you use contemporary research and/or relevant local or national evidence-based guidelines when formulating your answers.

QUESTIONS

1. What is obesity and how is it usually defined?
   Resources:
   NICE (2013). *1 Recommendations | Weight management: lifestyle services for overweight or obese children and young people | Guidance | NICE*. [online] Available at: https://www.nice.org.uk/guidance/PH47/chapter/recommendations#recommendation-4-developing-a-tailored-plan-to-meet-individual-needs [Accessed 26 May 2021].

   World Health Organisation (2000) *Obesity: Preventing and Managing a Global Epidemic*. Report of a WHO consultation. Technical Report Series 894WHO

2. What are the risk factors for childhood obesity?
   Resource: Public Health England (2016). *Childhood obesity: applying All Our Health*. [online] GOV.UK. Available at: https://www.gov.uk/government/publications/childhood-obesity-applying-all-our-health/childhood-obesity-applying-all-our-health [Accessed 11 Aug. 2021].

3. Considering Neuman's system model/grand theory five variables; what are the possible consequences of childhood obesity for pupils, such as Jake?
   Resource: Public Health England (2016). *Childhood obesity: applying All Our Health*. [online] GOV.UK. Available at: https://www.gov.uk/government/publications/childhood-obesity-applying-all-our-health/childhood-obesity-applying-all-our-health [Accessed 26 May 2021].

4. Using Newman's model and the scenario at the start of this chapter, identify possible stressors and lines of defence or resistance for one pupil (Jake) by considering the five variables and their effect on his weight.
   Resource: Public Health England (2016). *Childhood obesity: applying All Our Health*. [online] GOV.UK. Available at: https://www.gov.uk/government/publications/childhood-obesity-applying-all-our-health/childhood-obesity-applying-all-our-health [Accessed 11 Aug. 2021].

5. Based on the information from questions 2–4, develop a healthy weight care plan for Jake.
   Resources: Department of Health and Social Care (2019). *UK Chief Medical Officers' Physical Activity Guidelines*. [online] *gov.uk*. Available at: https://assets.publishing.service.gov.uk/government/uploads/system/uploads/attachment_data/file/832868/uk-chief-medical-officers-physical-activity-guidelines.pdf.

   NHS Choices (2021). *The Eatwell Guide – Eat well*. [online] Available at: https://www.nhs.uk/live-well/eat-well/the-eatwell-guide [Accessed 26 May 2021].

6. Identify the possible stressors and lines of defence or resistance on healthy weight maintenance for the entire Treewood school population. Based on your assessment and the information from questions 2–3, can you develop a healthy weight care plan for the school?
   Resource: World Health Organisation (2008) *School Policy Framework Implementation of the WHO Global Strategy on Diet, Physical Activity and Health*. Geneva: WHO. [online]. Available at: https://apps.who.int/iris/handle/10665/43923.

PROPOSED ANSWERS TO QUESTIONS

Question 1. What is obesity and how is it usually defined?

Obesity is a condition that indicates risk to health, associated with excess body fat. It is usually defined according to body mass index (WHO 2020). Body mass index (BMI) is a ratio of a person's weight in kilograms divided by height in metres^2. For adults BMI can be classified as follows:

BMI <20 underweight

20–24.9 desirable/healthy

25–29.9 overweight

≥30 obese

BMI may be supplemented with waist measurements in adult with a BMI less than 35 kg/m² (NICE 2014); waist size has close link to morbidity (disease) and mortality (death) even in people who are not overweight (Harvard School of Public Health 2012).

It is more complicated to undertake an obesity assessment in children as BMI varies with age and gender. NICE (2014) suggests using the RCPCH *UK-WHO growth charts* (RCPCH, 2021). Children who are over the 91st centile on the BMI centile look up chart may be classified as overweight and those above the 98th centile, classified as obese. Children and young people who have excess weight are more likely to have an associated morbidity such as joint problems and pre-diabetes, they often have poor psychological wellbeing, be bullied and have more school absences (PHE, 2016). It is recommended that healthcare professionals should help identify children and families at risk (ASK), explain how to change to healthy behaviours (ADVISE) and refer for further support (ASSIST) (PHE, 2017). This discussion should be supportive, non-blame based, and factual. Refer to Figure 18.1 for boys growth charts.

Question 2. What are the risk factors for childhood obesity?

Obesity arises from an energy imbalance between energy intake (from food and drink) and energy expenditure (internal body processes and physical activity) (RCP et al. 2004). Weight gain occurs when energy intake (calories consumed) exceeds total daily energy expenditure for a prolonged period. Childhood obesity is associated with maternal and parental obesity, poor diet, and lower amounts of physical activity (PHE 2016). There is a complex mix of personal, social, and environmental factors that contribute to weight gain (PHE 2016), and Butland et al. 2007) suggests that genetics/biology loads the gun of obesity (makes people predisposed to obesity) and the environment factors pull the trigger (brings about the conditions in which obesity happens).

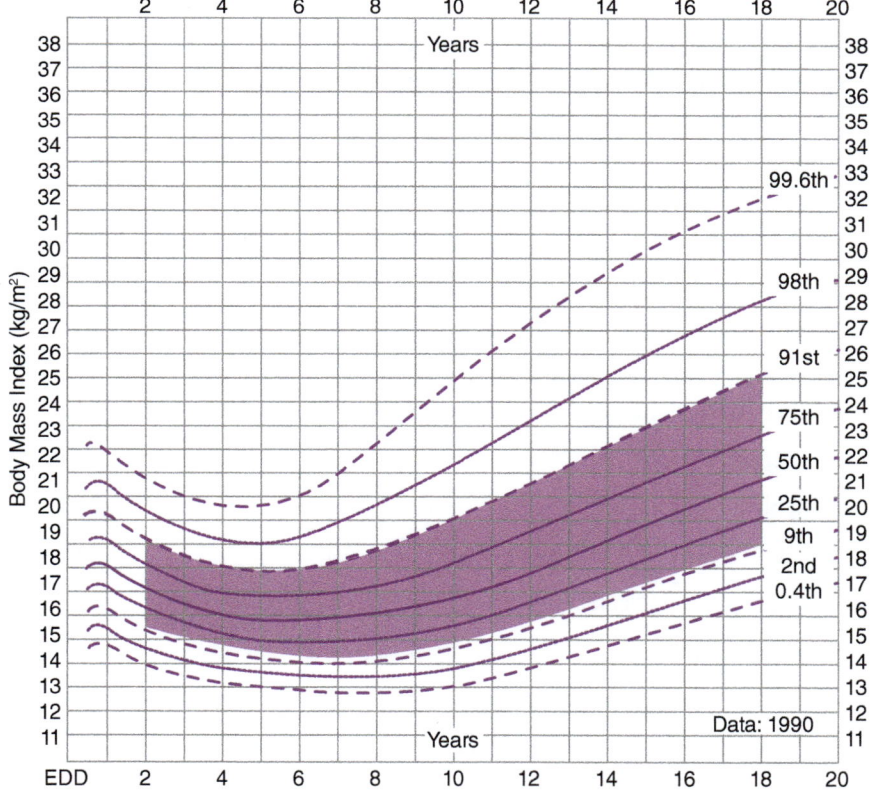

Notes: This chart is based on the UK population, not the IOTF populations.

FIGURE 18.1 RCPCH *UK-WHO growth charts for boys*.

Question 3. Considering Neuman's system model/grand theory five variables; what are the possible consequences of childhood obesity for pupils, such as Jake?

Neuman's system model (Neuman & Fawcett, 2002) identifies five client variables:

- Physiological = biochemical, physiological functioning of the body
- Psychological/cognitive = thought processes and emotions
- Socio-cultural = relationships, expectations, and activities
- Spiritual = human spirit and spiritual beliefs
- Developmental = lifespan growth

The consequences of obesity (drawn from PHE 2016) will be considered for each of these five client variables. Physiological consequences of obesity in childhood include:

- Breathing difficulties such as sleep apnoea and asthma, bone and joint problems such as ankle sprains, increased risk of fractures, knee problems
- Pre-diabetes
- High cholesterol and high blood pressure

Current evidence indicates that interventions that help improve diets and/or activity levels can promote more healthy weights in children up to 12 years of age (Brown et al. 2019).

Psychological/cognitive consequences of obesity in childhood include a lower self-esteem (PHE 2016). Socio-cultural consequences of obesity in childhood include stigmatisation, bullying and increased school absence (PHE 2016). There is currently little evidence about the spiritual consequences of obesity in childhood, however, adult studies with people with eating disorders suggest it may be associated with reduced hope and lower spiritual wellbeing (Boisvert and Harrell 2013a; 2013b). Developmental consequences of obesity in childhood may include a life course impact; obese children are more likely than their non-obese peers to become obese adults with an increased risk of ill health and premature mortality (PHE 2016).

Question 4. Using Newman's model and the scenario at the start of this chapter, identify possible stressors and lines of defence or resistance for one pupil (Jake) by considering the five variables and their effect on his weight.

Neuman's system model (Neuman and Fawcett, 2002) identifies three types of stressors that can act on individuals or groups of individuals' five variables. Stressors can be:

- Intrapersonal: within individuals or population
- Interpersonal: between individuals or populations and groups
- Extra-personal: these are factors outside the individual or population

Stressors can have actual (overt), potential (covert) or residual effects. The model also identifies that people have lines of defence or resistance that help protect the body from stressors.

Intrapersonal stressors include:

- Biological-genetic and physiological predisposition to weight gain (physiological, potential)
- Jake's erratic eating patterns (no breakfast) (physiological, actual)
- Large/adult food servings (physiological, actual)
- High fat and sugar, low in complex carbohydrate and fruit/vegetables diet (physiological, actual)
- Plays a lot of video games at home (socio-cultural, potential)
- Has low self-esteem (psychological, actual)

Interpersonal stressors include:

- Jake's other has difficulty finding time to prepare food and needs to cater for Jake's individual food preferences (physiological/psychological, potential)
- Bullying from other children (socio-cultural, residual)
- Jake has little physical activity and plays little with other children when at home (physiological/socio-cultural, potential)
- Other members of family are overweight (influence of family norms, socio-cultural, potential)

Extra-personal stressors include:

- Limited healthy eating resources outside school (physiological, potential)
- Limited exercise potential outside school (physiological, potential)
- Economic deprivation levels in the surrounding estate (socio-cultural, potential)
- Levels of crime and vandalism in the surrounding estate (socio-cultural, potential)
- Low hope in general community (spiritual, potential)

Jake's lines of defence and resistance could include:

- Walking to school and using stairs
- He says he wants to be a healthy weight
- Has some family support to make changes?

Question 5. Based on the information from questions 2–4, develop a healthy weight care plan for Jake

A Neuman system model assessment and intervention tool has been developed to help apply the model to the nursing process in practice settings, for more information about this tool please refer to Neuman and Fawcett (2002). Note, the author has adapted and modified the Neuman's system model care plan process to better support the learning aims of this book. When devising a care plan, please remember to identify the level of nursing intervention (as per Neuman's model) that you will use.

Neuman's system model identifies three levels of nursing interventions:

- *Primary prevention* occurs before a person or group of people react to a stressor. This can be by strengthening resistance to the stressor and/or by weakening the stressor.
- *Secondary prevention* occurs when a person or group of people have reacted to a stressor. This can be achieved through strengthening resistance to the stressor and/or removing the stressor.
- *Tertiary prevention* occurs after a person has had a secondary prevention intervention. It facilitates re-adaptation and prevention of future occurrences.

PHE (2016) recommends that health professionals should provide evidence-based advice about weight, diet and physical activity for children/young people and their families. In addition, NICE (2013) advises that healthcare professionals should assess the family for readiness and willingness to be referred to and attend a local effective lifestyle management service. If a child or young person is assessed as needing specialist support, they should also be referred to appropriate services (e.g. specialist obesity, paediatric of Child and Young People Mental Health Services (CYPMHS/CAMHS) services).

Jake's care plan

Assessed need	Plan	Type of intervention/implementation	Evaluation	Rationale
Jake has an imbalanced dietary intake contributing to unhealthy weight.	To increase Jake's consumption of healthy foods and drink within a month focusing on positive change.	Secondary prevention advice to Jake and his mother regarding: Food served on smaller plates to reduce food portion consumed. Regular meals to reduce binge eating. Increase in daily intake of water, complex carbohydrates, and fruit and vegetables consumption; to decrease sugary drink and fried food/processed intake. Ensure Jake and his mother are aware of local resources and services that support healthy eating and/or healthy weight.	Meet with Jake and his family weekly to discuss Jake's dietary intake and changes made.	Advice to follow the Eatwell guide (NHS choices, 2021).
Jake has low physical activity, contributing to unhealthy weight.	To increase Jake's level of physical activity to an average of at least 60 minutes of moderate to vigorous intensity physical activity (PA) per day across a week and minimise the duration of sedentary activity.	Secondary prevention: Reduce time of uninterrupted playing of video games (sedentary behaviour). Encourage walking to school. Encourage a range of different physical activities such as sport and climbing to build muscle and bone strength. Family activity at weekends. Ensure that Jake and his family are aware of local services and resources supporting physical activity e.g. sports clubs.	Meet with Jake and his family weekly to discuss physical activity undertaken and changes made.	Advice to follow UK Chief Medical Officers Physical Activity guidelines (2019).
Jake has low self-esteem and has few friends.	To improve self-esteem so that he believes in himself so that he can achieve a healthy weight within the next six months.	Secondary prevention: To repeatedly set realistic, easily achievable, short-term goals. To encourage and praise Jake for achieving goals. Encourage and support Jake in undertaking new activities. Conjointly work on coping strategies for situations and social interaction skills. Referral to school healthy club for peer support or other local support services or resources as appropriate e.g. Child and Young Peoples' Mental Health Services or YoungMinds.	Meet with Jake weekly and ask about his accomplishments, self-belief, and coping. Record monthly BMI readings for next six months with supportive feedback on progress.	Communicate supportively, using neutral and non-blaming language (PHE 2017).
Jake has previously been bullied and is at continued risk.	Within the next three months help Jake to deal with bullying behaviour effectively.	Tertiary prevention: Ensure that Jake and his mother are aware of school anti-bully policy procedures and empower and support the family in reporting incidents. Build Jake's self-esteem and teach assertive and communication skills strategies; offering support in line with school policy. Ensure that Jake and his family are aware of additional voluntary support services, such as Childline or ParentLine Plus.	During meetings with Jake and his family during the next three months, enquire about Jake's wellbeing and achievements, also his relationships with other children.	Adhere to DE (2017) and local guidelines on preventing and tackling bullying.

Question 6. Identify the possible stressors and lines of defence or resistance on healthy weight maintenance for the entire Treewood school population. Based on your assessment and the information from questions 2–3, can you develop a healthy weight care plan for the school?

Intra-school stressors:

- High levels of obesity (physiological, actual)
- Poor academic achievement, disruptive pupils, and bullying (socio-cultural, actual)
- Some pupils with low esteem and attention difficulties (psychological, actual)
- Low use of school canteen (physiological, potential)

Interschool stressors:

- Parents give students money for fatty fast foods (physiological, potential)
- Poor school image by local community (socio-cultural, potential)

Extra-school stressors:

- Limited healthy eating resources outside school (physiological, potential)
- Limited exercise potential outside school (physiological, potential)
- Economic deprivation levels in the surrounding estate (socio-cultural, potential)
- Levels of crime and vandalism in the surrounding estate (socio-cultural, potential)
- Low hope in general community (spiritual, potential)

School lines of defence and resistance:

- Weekly school sport activities
- School involvement with community neighbourhood group
- New headmaster with a vision for school improvement and motivated staff
- Existence of school canteen
- School nurse willing to tackle weight issues in school

School health plan

SUMMARY

Rates of obesity among children and young people are currently high in many countries and obesity has enduring impacts on health and wellbeing; due to these enduring impacts we now need across sector and community action to protect and improve child and young person health (Davies, 2019). There are many personal and environmental factors that impact attaining and maintain healthy weight (PHE 2016); therefore, it is appropriate supporting individuals and schools through pupil-specific and school-focused care plans. The Neuman grand theory/model (Neuman & Fawcett 2002) focuses on 'prevention' which makes this model relevant for nurses involved in promoting both public and personal health, as it supports nursing assessment and interventions for both individuals and populations. In addition, the model promotes assessment of psychosocial, physical, and developmental needs and this holistic focus means it can help address a wide range of factors that influence child and young person health. Thus, the Neuman model is a useful tool for care planning for children's and school nurses, engaged in individual child, young person, family, or community focused health promotion.

Assessed need Treewood	Plan	Type of intervention/implementation	Evaluation	Rationale
School has social, organisational, and environmental factors that are contributing to unhealthy food choices by pupils.	To help school pupils in making healthy food choices, thereby increasing the intake of fruit and vegetables and decreasing the amount of high sugar and high fatty foods eaten within the next six months.	Primary prevention Working with headmaster, pupils, and canteen staff regarding canteen image and marketing healthy foods on the menu. Working with teachers and pupils regarding classroom teaching about healthy foods, how to make food choices, and how to make basic healthy foods (resources for teachers are available via PHE 2021). Working with headmaster, school staff, parent committee, and pupils regarding holding family fun events to promote healthy eating and food preparation. Working with Treeland neighbourhood committee to improve local food amenities.	Evaluation of interventions put in place and monitor their effect on reception year and year 6 students by helping students complete a diary of foods eaten during school time and out of school time, in six months' time.	Work with school to support compliance with DE, (2019).
School has social, organisational, and environmental factors that are contributing to unhealthy physical activity levels in pupils.	To help school pupils to make healthy physical activity and thereby reduce sedentary behaviour and increase activity levels within the next six months.	Primary prevention: Working with teachers and pupils regarding increasing activity in classrooms, a range of active playground games, and additional PE/sports sessions in school week. Working with teachers regarding classroom teaching about healthy activity and increasing physical activity during class. (Resources for teachers are available via PHE 2021). Working with headmaster, school staff, parent committee, and pupils regarding holding family fun events to promote physical activities and improving school open spaces and playground to create active environments. Work with school and families to promote active travel to and from school. Working with Treeland neighbourhood committee to improve local play amenities.	Evaluation of interventions put in place and their effect on reception year and year 6. Monitor school physical activity rates and amount of sedentary behaviour by diary or using accelerometers* (during and outside school hours), in six months' time.	Ensure a multicomponent intervention and active environment in line with PHE (2020).
Some pupils are overweight or obese.	To decrease the percentage of overweight or obese pupils over a school year.	Primary prevention dietary and physical activity as above. Encourage school to register with Change4life School Zone (PHE, 2021) to access resources promoting health in the classroom. In addition: Secondary prevention. Healthy after school club set up for children who are overweight, offering professional advice/ support and peer support.	Evaluation of Healthy club outcomes and BMI recording at beginning and end of this school year.	Application of NICE (2013) guidelines for effective lifestyle programmes.
Some pupils who have been overweight or obese are now healthy weights.	To help previously overweight or obese pupils maintain healthier weights over their school career.	Tertiary prevention: Ongoing healthy club support for children who have regained normal weight, i.e. offering ongoing professional and peer support.	Evaluation of healthy club outcomes, BMI recording as required during their time at school.	There is a need for ongoing support to ensure long-term programme effects are sustained (Flynn et al. 2006).

*Accelerometers are recording devices that record body movement and distance moved.

ACTIVITY 18.1

Plot the following boys' heights and weight on the RCPCH Boys 2–9 years' growth chart (on final page of the leaflet). Then record their centiles for height and weight in the table below. Are any of these children's weight above the 75th centile or does any child have a height and weight on different centiles? If so, plot these children's centiles on the Body Mass Index (BMI)_centile look up chart. Based on this work, can you identify which child could be classified as 'very overweight' or obese?

Child's name	Gender And age	Weight	Height	Centile weight when plotted on the main chart	Centile Height when plotted on the main chart	Is the weight above 75th Centile or do weight and height centiles differ? Yes/no	If yes, plot your results on the BMI centile look up chart, what do you conclude?
Ahmed	Boy 6 years	16.5 kg	106 m	2nd	2nd	No	Not needed
Brendan	Boy 5 years	16 kg	97.5 cm	9th	0.4	Yes	50-75th okay
Christopher	Boy 7 years	21 kg	118.5 cm	25th	25th	No	Not needed
Dabir	Boy 8 years	26 kg	1.24 m	50th	25th	Yes	50-75th okay
Everton	Boy 9 years	36 kg	1.18 m	91st	0.4	Yes	Above 98

REFERENCES

Boisvert, J.A. & Harrell, W.A. (2013a) The impact of spirituality on eating disorder symptomatology in ethnically diverse Canadian women. *International Journal of Social Psychiatry*, **59**(8), 729–738.

Boisvert, J.A. & Harrell, W.A. (2013b) The effects of hope, body shame and body mass index on eating disorder symptomatology in women. *International Journal of Psychology*, **8**(3), 207–226.

Brown, T., Moore, T.H., Hooper, L., Gao, Y., Zayegh, A., Ijaz, S., Elwenspoek, M., Foxen, S.C., Magee, L., O'Malley, C., Waters, E. & Summerbell, C.D. (2019) Interventions for preventing obesity in children. *Cochrane Database of Systematic Reviews*, July 23; **7**(7), CD001871. doi: 10.1002/14651858.CD001871.pub4. PMID: 31332776; PMCID: PMC6646867.

Butland, B., Jebb, S., Kopelman, P. et al. (2007) *Foresight-tackling Obesities: Future Choices*. London: Government Office of Science.

Chief Medical Officers' Physical Activity guidelines (2019) https://www.gov.uk/government/publications/physical-activity-guidelines-uk-chief-medical-officers-report [Accessed 28 February 2023].

Christie, J., Parkes, J. & Price, J. (2009) Public health practitioner. In: Hughes, J. & Lyte, G. (eds). *Developing Nursing Practice with Children and Young People*. Chichester: J. Wiley and Sons, 87–101.

Davies, S. (2019) *Time to solve childhood obesity*. Department of Health and Social Care. Available at: https://assets.publishing.service.gov.uk/government/uploads/system/uploads/attachment_data/file/837907/cmo-special-report-childhood-obesity-october-2019.pdf [Accessed 28 February 2023].

Department of Health and Social Care (2019) *UK chief medical officers' physical activity guidelines*. [online] gov.uk. Available at: https://assets.publishing.service.gov.uk/government/uploads/system/uploads/attachment_data/file/832868/uk-chief-medical-officers-physical-activity-guidelines.pdf [Accessed 28 February 2023].

Flynn, M.A., McNeil, D.A., Maloff, B., Mutasingwa, D., Wu, M., Ford, C., & Tough, S.C. (2006). Reducing obesity and related chronic disease risk in children and youth: A synthesis of evidence with 'best practice' recommendations. *Obesity Reviews*, February; **7**(Suppl 1), 7–66. doi: 10.1111/j.1467-789X.2006.00242.x. PMID: 16371076.

Harvard School of Public Health (2012) *Waist size matters*. [online] Available at: https://www.hsph.harvard.edu/obesity-prevention-source/obesity-definition/abdominal-obesity [Accessed 28 February 2023].

Neuman, B. & Fawcett, J. (2002) *The Neuman Systems Model*, 4th edn. New Jersey: Prentice Hall.

NHS choices (2021) https://www.nhsinform.scot/healthy-living/food-and-nutrition/eating-well/eatwell-guide-how-to-eat-a-healthy-balanced-diet [Accessed 28 February 2023].

NICE (2013) *1 recommendations | weight management: lifestyle services for overweight or obese children and young people | guidance | NICE*. [online] Available at: https://www.nice.org.uk/guidance/PH47/chapter/recommendations#recommendation-4-developing-a-tailored-plan-to-meet-individual-needs [Accessed 26th May 2021].

NICE (2014) *Overview | obesity: identification, assessment and management | guidance | NICE*. [online] Available at: https://www.nice.org.uk/guidance/cg189 [Accessed 28 February 2023].

Public Health England (2016). *Childhood obesity: applying all our health.* [online] GOV.UK. Available at: https://www.gov.uk/government/publications/childhood-obesity-applying-all-our-health/childhood-obesity-applying-all-our-health [Accessed 26th May 2021].

Public Health England (2020) *What works in schools and colleges to increase physical activity?* [online]. Available at: https://assets.publishing.service.gov.uk/government/uploads/system/uploads/attachment_data/file/876242/Guidance_to_increase_physical_activity_among_children_and_young_people_in_schools_and_colleges.pdf [Accessed 28 February 2023].

Public Health England (PHE) (2021). *PHE school zone.* [online] Available at: https://campaignresources.phe.gov.uk/schools [Accessed 26th May 2021].

Public Heath England (PHE) (2017) *Let's talk about weight: a step-by-step guide to conversations about weight management with children and families for health and care professionals.* [online]. Available at: https://assets.publishing.service.gov.uk/government/uploads/system/uploads/attachment_data/file/649095/child_weight_management_lets_talk_about_weight.pdf [Accessed 26th May 2021].

Royal College of Physicians, Royal College of Paediatrics and Child Health, Faulty of Public Health (2004). *Storing up Problems: The Medical Case for a Slimmer Nation.* London: Royal College of Physicians.

RCPCH (2021) *UK-WHO growth charts – 2-18 years.* [online] Available at: https://www.rcpch.ac.uk/resources/uk-who-growth-charts-2-18-years [Accessed 27th Apr. 2021].

WHO (2020) *Obesity and overweight.* [online] Who.int. Available at: https://www.who.int/news-room/fact-sheets/detail/obesity-and-overweight [Accessed 27th Apr. 2021].

World Health Organisation (2000) *Obesity: preventing and Managing a Global Epidemic.* Report of a WHO Consultation. Technical Report Series 894WHO.

World Health Organisation (2008) *School policy framework implementation of the WHO global strategy on diet,* Physical Activity and Health. Geneva: WHO. [online]. Available at: https://apps.who.int/iris/handle/10665/43923.

Care of Neonates and Children with Respiratory Disorders

SECTION 4

Neonatal Respiratory Distress Syndrome

CHAPTER 19

Susanne Simmons

SCENARIO

Arthur is a 27-week gestation preterm infant born by lower segment Caesarean section (LSCS), following maternal pregnancy-induced hypertension. His Apgar score (Simon et al. 2021) was 3 at one minute and 7 at five minutes. Following delivery, Arthur was blue, floppy, made weak respiratory effort, and had a heart rate less than 100 beats per minute. Cord clamping was delayed, and Arthur was placed in a polythene bag at delivery and a hat was added to prevent heat loss (Resuscitation Council (UK) 2021). Infants less than 30 weeks' gestation are at risk of significant heat loss and trans epidermal water loss (TEWL). Placing these infants in a polythene bag at delivery, without drying, leaving the head free has been shown to limit/prevent both heat and water loss through the skin and maintain a core temperature between 36.5°C and 37.5°C (Sweet et al. 2019). He received five inflation breaths and was electively intubated and received positive pressure ventilation (Resuscitation Council 2021). Exogenous surfactant was administered via the endotracheal tube (ETT). Once stabilised, Arthur was transferred to the neonatal unit.

On admission to the unit, Arthur weighed 850 grams and was placed into a closed incubator with 80% humidity. An umbilical arterial catheter (UAC) and umbilical venous catheter (UVC) were sited. A chest X-ray verified the position of the ETT, UAC, and UVC and confirmed a diagnosis of respiratory distress syndrome (RDS). Volume-targeted ventilation (VTV) in combination with synchronised ventilation was provided and changes to Arthur's ventilator requirements were made in response to improving arterial blood gases (NICE 2019). Over the next few days, Arthur's respiratory function improved, and he was extubated onto nasal continuous positive airway pressure (nCPAP).

QUESTIONS

1. Assessment: How would you assess Arthur's respiratory needs?
2. Planning: What respiratory support will Arthur require?
3. Implementation: What care will Arthur require to optimise his respiratory function?
4. Evaluation: When will Arthur no longer require respiratory support?

This chapter will focus on the respiratory management of a preterm infant with RDS. Although the scenario is based on a premature infant, some of the principles of care outlined in the chapter are also relevant to the term neonate and infant. The neonatal mortality rate has declined significantly since 2000 (ONS 2019) with the demand for neonatal care increasing each year (RCPCH 2020). Approximately one in seven infants born each year will require admission to a neonatal unit, with preterm infants requiring specialist neonatal intensive care (BLISS 2021).

ANSWERS TO QUESTIONS

Activity of daily living: breathing.

Question 1. Assessment: How would you assess Arthur's respiratory needs?

The lungs *in utero* are filled with foetal lung fluid and the volume of this and amniotic fluid is crucial to normal lung development (Randall 2005). In addition, foetal breathing movements, seen *in utero* from as early as 12 weeks, are also thought to support the development of the diaphragm and chest

Care Planning in Children and Young People's Nursing, Second Edition. Edited by Sonya Clarke and Doris Corkin.
© 2024 John Wiley & Sons Ltd. Published 2024 by John Wiley & Sons Ltd.

Table 19.1 Overview of the stages of lung development.

Pseudo glandular stage (6–16 weeks)	The trachea, bronchi, and bronchioles are formed. Connective tissue, muscle, and blood vessels start to develop.
Canalicular stage (16–25 weeks)	The bronchioles continue to branch, and the vascular network develops alongside the airways. Type 2 cells begin to secrete small amounts of surfactant. The cells lining the alveolar are cuboidal, epithelial cells and are thick.
Terminal saccular stage (24 weeks to birth)	The alveoli develop and multiply. The alveolar epithelial lining thins (squamous epithelium) which allows closer contact with the capillaries. There is a surge of surfactant produced at 32–34 weeks' gestation.
Alveolar stage (32 weeks to childhood)	This stage continues after birth and into childhood. The alveoli develop further and mature. There are approximately 50 million alveoli present in the full-term infant and this reaches adult values of 300 million during childhood.

wall muscles. Lung development is characterised by stages (Moore, Persaud and Torchia 2019), which overlap and do not occur uniformly within each lung (see Table 19.1). The lungs need to be developed sufficiently to enable the alveoli to be involved in gaseous exchange and this is usually achieved by 32–34 weeks' gestation. At 27 weeks' gestation, Arthur's lungs will be immature in both structure and the amount of surfactant produced.

Respiratory distress syndrome is a pulmonary disorder caused by a lack of surfactant and is predominantly associated with prematurity. Surfactant is a complex mixture of proteins, lipids, and phospholipids and spreads across the liquid lined surface of the alveoli (Crawford & Davies 2020). It reduces surface tension and prevents the collapse (atelectasis) of the alveoli on expiration, therefore maintaining a positive pressure in the airways (functional residual capacity). The liquid lined surface of the alveoli facilitates normal gaseous exchange.

It is known that during a normal vaginal delivery the release of adrenaline promotes the switch of lung cells from producing foetal lung fluid to absorbing it. In addition, the pressure applied to the infant's ribcage during the delivery 'squeezes' the lung fluid out through the mouth and nose. As the infant takes its first breath a high intrathoracic pressure is generated which pushes the lung fluid into the pulmonary vascular and lymphatic system (Moore et al. 2019). As Arthur was delivered by an emergency LSCS, this process did not occur. Antenatal corticosteroids, given in time to have an effect, cross the placenta and appear to accelerate lung development (Sweet et al. 2019). However, antenatal steroids were not given prior to delivery. Arthur is therefore challenged at delivery in terms of his respiratory function.

Respiratory assessment of Arthur: airway and breathing

Airway
Neonates are predominantly nose breathers for the first few months of life. Arthur's airways are extremely narrow and his large tongue in relation to his small jaw can allow the tongue to fall back and obstruct his upper airway. In addition, the gag reflex is underdeveloped, and the large occiput of the neonate's head can push the chin downwards onto the chest when lying supine and cause airway obstruction. Due to surfactant deficiency his alveoli are collapsed (atelectasis) and a chest X-ray (Figure 19.1) reveals the lung fields have a ground glass appearance, with air bronchograms (the air-filled left and right main bronchi standing out black against the collapsed white lung fields).

Breathing
A normal respiratory rate for the neonate is below 60 breaths per minute. Without respiratory support, Arthur will demonstrate signs of respiratory distress due to surfactant deficiency. These signs include nasal flaring, subcostal (underneath ribcage) recession, intercostal (in-between ribs) recession, sternal recession, tracheal tug, and an expiratory grunt. Grunting occurs when an infant breathes out against a partially closed glottis in order to prevent alveoli collapse and preserve lung volume. Due to his compliant ribcage and small airways, Arthur also uses accessory abdominal muscles to ensure effective air entry. Therefore, a diaphragmatic breathing pattern is observed.

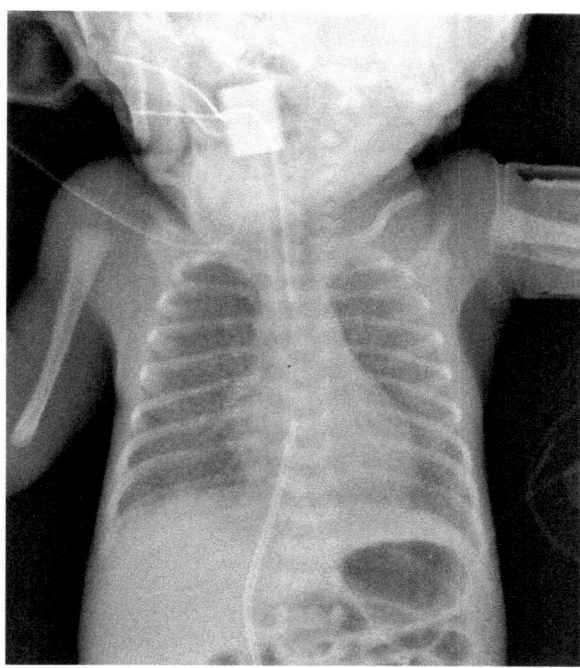

FIGURE 19.1 Chest X-ray.

Atelectasis results in ineffective gaseous exchange which means that Arthur would be hypoxic and hypercarbic (high carbon dioxide). Oxygen saturation monitoring and blood gas analysis is important in assessing respiratory function and metabolic parameters (Lynch 2009). Arthur's initial arterial blood gas on admission revealed a respiratory acidosis: pH 7.19, $PaCO_2$ 8.9, PaO_2 6.0, base excess − 2, standard bicarbonate 20.

Question 2. Planning: What respiratory support will Arthur require?

In RDS the lack of surfactant causes the alveoli to collapse and invasive ventilatory support may be needed to ensure the alveoli can participate in adequate gaseous exchange. Invasive ventilation can cause inflammatory changes and protein to leak onto the alveolar surface and form hyaline membranes. In uncomplicated RDS, surfactant production increases from approximately 36–48 hours and the infant's respiratory function then improves (Boyle 2020). The plan of care for Arthur is therefore to provide respiratory support until this occurs.

The primary cause of Arthur's respiratory distress is due to surfactant deficiency. Administration of exogenous surfactant has improved the outcome for neonates showing clinical signs of RDS. Currently, animal-based surfactants such as porcine derived Curosurf® are the treatment of choice as they reduce surface tension more effectively due to the presence of surfactant proteins (Sweet et al. 2019). In preterm infants, particularly below 30 weeks' gestation, improved outcomes have been achieved with the use of antenatal steroids and providing early nCPAP from birth. There has been a move away from prophylactic surfactant administration towards administering surfactant only if the infant is showing clinical signs of RDS. In the situation where the infant is not intubated and requires surfactant, the less-invasive surfactant administration (LISA) technique can be used (Bhayat & Shetty 2020). Trials with aerosolised surfactant administration have also been carried out (Jardine et al. 2021).

Arthur received surfactant at delivery in the labour ward. This was undertaken by an experienced practitioner skilled in neonatal resuscitation who was able to verify the correct position of the ETT without a chest X-ray. Following this initial dose of surfactant, Arthur required a further dose at 12 hours of age as he was still requiring ventilatory support and oxygen (NICE 2019).

The aim of ventilatory support is to maintain the pressures at which oxygen and carbon dioxide are dissolved in arterial blood within safe limits (Figure 19.2). This support should reduce the work of breathing for the infant and minimise the risk of lung injury. Advances in respiratory tech-

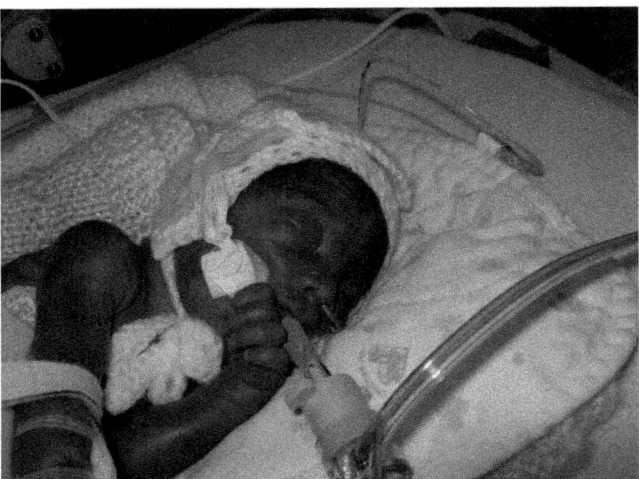

FIGURE 19.2 Ventilated neonate.

nology have resulted in the development of newer methods of volume targeted ventilation (Gupta & Janakiraman 2018). Modern neonatal ventilators have the facility to synchronise the ventilator breath with the respiratory pattern of the infant. Therefore, the infant does not receive a ventilator breath when they are breathing out.

Invasive ventilation can cause lung injury and contributes to the development of chronic lung disease (CLD) (oxygen requirement at 36 weeks). The plan of care is therefore to provide respiratory support until Arthur's lungs recover and to reduce the risk of CLD. Minimal ventilation is used to promote satisfactory lung inflations for gaseous exchange to occur, as high positive pressures are known to cause 'barotrauma' and high volumes of gas may cause 'volutrauma'. The amount of oxygen administered is carefully controlled as oxygen toxicity can cause lung damage (Sanoj et al. 2021). In infants less than 32 weeks' gestation, constant shifts in oxygenation are thought to be a contributing factor in the pathogenesis of retinopathy of prematurity (ROP) (Fleck 2013).

Ventilator requirements will be dependent on arterial or capillary blood gases. Blood gases may need to be taken frequently in the first 24–48 hours and this can contribute to iatrogenic blood loss, necessitating a replacement blood transfusion (Hellström et al. 2021). As invasive ventilation is known to cause lung injury the aim is to extubate Arthur as soon as possible onto nCPAP. This reduces the work of breathing for the infant and is a non-invasive method of respiratory support. The continuous pressure splints the infant's upper airway, reducing obstruction and apnoea, and providing a positive end expiratory pressure (PEEP) which promotes recruitment of alveoli and may also promote chest wall stability (Sweet et al. 2019).

There are a number of ways of delivering CPAP, but normally it is given via bi-nasal prongs. In bubble CPAP the CPAP pressure is generated by placing the distal limb of the CPAP circuit under a known depth of water, for example 6 cm H_2O (Gupta & Donn 2016). In variable flow CPAP there is an integrated nasal interface and pressure generator; the pressure is generated by the increased resistance as the gas leaves the nasal device and enters the infant's nasopharynx (Sweet et al. 2019).

Question 3. Implementation: What care will Arthur require to optimise his respiratory function?

Airway

It is important to ensure that Arthur has a patent and secure airway. There are a number of ways of securing the ETT, all with the aim of reducing the risk of accidental extubation. Whilst ventilated, the ETT provides an artificial airway, but its presence can cause problems. The size of the ETT should be big enough to allow effective amounts of gas to enter the lung but not so big that it causes pressure damage to the delicate epithelial lining of the pharynx, larynx, and trachea. A small tube will create resistance to the flow of gas and increase the amount of gas leak around the ETT, therefore compromising effective ventilation. The presence of the ETT reduces the normal mucocillary action within the respiratory tract.

Warming and humidifying ventilator gases are vital in loosening secretions and reducing the risk of drying and damage to the mucosa. Secretions will need to be suctioned to maintain an open airway. Suction should only be given if needed and not as a routine procedure and avoided, if possible, for at least 12 hours following administration of surfactant. Ideally it should be performed by two people and Arthur will need support throughout (see Chapter 13). The type and number of secretions obtained should be documented. The patency of the ETT can be assessed by observing Arthur's chest for equal movement on both sides, listening in to breath sounds with a stethoscope and ensuring that his oxygen saturations are within normal limits.

Once Arthur no longer requires ventilation, the ETT can be removed. Again, this procedure requires two people, one to carry out the procedure and one to support Arthur (see Chapter 13). The ETT may be suctioned prior to removal and any care that Arthur requires may be carried out beforehand. This means that once Arthur has been extubated, he can be left to settle after the procedure. The nasogastric tube should be aspirated and resuscitation equipment readily available. The CPAP device should be ready by the cot side so that Arthur can be placed onto nCPAP just before the ETT is removed, thereby minimising alveolar collapse. The tip of the ETT may be sent to the microbiology laboratory for microscopy, culture and sensitivity (M, C, and S).

The size of the nasal prongs and hat required by Arthur are measured using the manufacturer's template and adhering to the manufacturers and local unit guidelines. It is important to ensure that the bi-nasal prongs fit comfortably in the nares without causing pressure, as erosion of the nasal septum has been documented and is attributed to poor fixation (Haymes 2020). Observation of the nose is essential and is carried out when care is given. If redness is present, the use of a CPAP mask or appropriate hydrocolloid dressing may be indicated.

Ensuring patency of the airway is important. As CPAP may contribute to increased amounts of oral and nasal secretions, assessment of the need for nasal suctioning should be carried out regularly. Gentle suctioning of mouth and then the nares should be given. Loss of CPAP pressure may occur if the neonate's mouth is open. Use of a CPAP dummy (with parental consent) or a chin strap may help minimise this loss of pressure.

Breathing

Arthur's temperature, pulse, respirations, blood pressure, and oxygen saturations will be continuously monitored and recorded every hour. At the beginning of each shift the monitor alarm parameters will be set so that if there is an increase or a decrease in Arthur's vital signs the monitor will alarm. The position of the oxygen saturation probe is changed at least every four hours (or more often if instructed by the manufacturer) and documented to reduce the risk of thermal injury and tissue damage (MHRA 2001, 2021).

Arthur's respiratory function will be assessed by observing his respiratory pattern, auscultation of the chest and blood gas analysis. Improvements in blood gases mean that Arthur's respiratory function is improving and therefore the ventilation he is receiving can be reduced. The amount of oxygen administered to Arthur will depend on his oxygen saturations and can be increased or decreased according to his needs (Fallon 2012). In order to promote comfort and synchrony with the ventilation he is receiving, Arthur may require a continuous infusion of morphine (BNFC 2021) whilst ventilated (Kariholu et al. 2014). He also receives non-pharmacological pain relief throughout his stay on the neonatal unit (see Chapter 14).

The ribcage in the neonate is mostly cartilage rather than bone and so is very compliant. The ribs are horizontal rather than downward sloping and therefore the rigid 'bucket handle' action provided by the ribcage in the child and adult is missing (Randall 2005). It is known that the prone position can reduce the work of breathing for neonates and improve respiratory function. This effect is thought to be due to the mattress creating stability for the compliant ribcage. Arthur is nursed prone, and his parents are assured that this position is safe in the acute phase of his illness, as he is being continuously monitored. However, once monitoring is no longer needed, Arthur will be nursed supine (The Lullaby Trust 2021).

When extubated onto nCPAP the gastric tube can be left on free drainage and aspirated to reduce the gastric distension caused by air entering the stomach from CPAP. The neonate's abdominal muscles are immature and therefore the neonatal abdomen distends easily. Abdominal distension can cause respiratory compromise and assessment of the abdomen should be undertaken to ensure that it is soft, bowel sounds are present, and stools are being passed.

Apnoea of prematurity is common in neonates of less than 32 weeks' gestation (NICE 2019). It can be obstructive, central or mixed. It is demonstrated by frequent apnoeas and bradycardias, which may be reversed by gentle stimulation or, if life threatening, may require resuscitative measures, such as lung inflations. Caffeine is administered once daily either orally or intravenously as this medicine stimulates the respiratory centre of the brain (BNFC 2021). As Arthur's respiratory centre is immature, caffeine is prescribed to promote his respiratory drive. He is given a loading dose of caffeine and then receives a daily dose. Apnoeas and bradycardias can also be an indication of a blocked ETT, sepsis or gastro oesophageal reflux.

Question 4. Evaluation: When will Arthur no longer require respiratory support?

Once Arthur has been stable on nCPAP with good blood gases then he may be transferred to High Flow Nasal Cannula (HNFC) (Garg & Sinha 2014). During this time Arthur will be observed for signs of respiratory distress to assess if he needs more respiratory support or when HFNC can be discontinued. When HFNC is discontinued if Arthur still requires supplemental oxygen, then he can be changed to low flow nasal cannula which may be continued at home following discharge if needed.

It is likely that Arthur will remain on the neonatal unit until close to his expected date of delivery, that is, 13 weeks. Indications for discharge will depend on local unit guidelines. Discharge planning should commence on admission and Arthur's parents should be encouraged to participate in his care as soon as possible and throughout his stay on the unit (Bradford-Duarte & Gbinigie 2020). As a premature infant, Arthur is at increased risk of sudden unexpected death in infancy (SUDI) and therefore his parents will be taught infant cardiopulmonary resuscitation (CPR) prior to discharge (The Lullaby Trust 2021). Arthur will receive passive immunisation against respiratory syncytial virus (RSV) which causes lower respiratory tract infection and may cause severe illness in vulnerable infants such as those born preterm (NHS England & NHS Improvement 2021). Long-term studies of children born very prematurely suggest that prematurity can have wide-ranging physical and cognitive effects (Yanyan et al. 2021). Therefore, Arthur will be followed up closely over his first two years of life (NICE 2017) and may experience frequent readmissions to the children's ward with continuing respiratory needs.

REFERENCES

Bhayat, S. & Shetty, S. (2020) Less-invasive surfactant administration (LISA). *Paediatrics and Child Health*, **30**(4), 144–148.

BLISS 2021. *Neonatal care statistics*. Available from: https://www.bliss.org.uk/research-campaigns/neonatal-care-statistics [Accessed 27th October 2021].

BNFC (2021) *British National Formulary for Children*. London: BMJ Group.

Boyle, B. (2020) Management of respiratory disorders. In: Boxwell, G., Petty, J. and Kaiser, L. (eds). *Neonatal Intensive Care Nursing*, 3rd. London: Routledge.

Bradford-Duarte, R. & Gbinigie, H. (2020) Neonatal family integrated care: ensuring a positive parental experience. *Journal of Neonatal Nursing*, **26**, 284–290.

Crawford, D. & Davies, K. (2020) Biological basis of child health 5: development of the respiratory system and elements of respiratory assessment. *Nursing Children and Young People*, **32**(6), 33–42.

Fallon, A. (2012) Oxygen therapy in neonatal care. *Journal of Neonatal Nursing*, **18**(6), 198–200.

Fleck, B. (2013) Management of retinopathy of prematurity. *Arch Dis Child Fetal Neonatal Ed*, **98**, F454–F456. doi:10.1136/archdischild-2013-303933.

Garg, S. & Sinha, S. (2014) Non-invasive respiratory support in preterm infants: do we need more evidence? *Infant*, **10**(2), 44–48.

Gupta, S. & Donn, S. (2016) Continuous positive airway pressure: to bubble or not to bubble? *Clinics in Perinatology*, **43**(4), 647–659.

Gupta, S. & Janakiraman, S. (2018) Volume ventilation in neonates. *Paediatrics and Child Health*, **28**(1), 1–5.

Haymes, E. (2020) The effects of continuous positive airway pressure (CPAP) on nasal skin breakdown. *Journal of Neonatal Nursing*, **26**(1), 37–42.

Hellström, W., Martinsson, T., Hellstrom, A., Morsing, E. & Ley, D. (2021) Fetal haemoglobin and bronchopulmonary dysplasia in neonates: an observational study. *Arch Dis Child Fetal Neonatal Ed*, **106**, F88–F92. doi: 10.1136/archdischild-2020-319181.

Jardine, L., Lui, K., Liley, H., Schindler, T., Fink, J., Asselin, J. & Durand, D. (2021) Trial of aerosolised surfactant for preterm infants with respiratory distress syndrome. *Arch Dis Child Fetal Neonatal Ed*, 2022 Jan; **107**(1):51-55. doi: 10.1136/archdischild-2021-321645. Epub 2021 Jun 10. PMID: 34112722; PMCID: PMC8685619.

Kariholu, U., Banerjee, J., Selkirk, L., Warren, I., Chow, P. & Godambe, S. (2014) Managing neonatal pain while rationalising the use of morphine using a structured systematic approach. *Infant*, **10**(1), 30–34.

Lynch, F. (2009) Arterial blood gas analysis: implications for nursing. *Paediatric Nursing*, **21**(1), 41–44.

Medicines and Health Products Regulatory Agency (MHRA) (2001) *Tissue Necrosis Caused by Pulse Oximeter Probes*. SN 2001 (08). London: MHRA.

Moore, K.L., Persaud, T.V.N. & Torchia, M.G. (2019) *The Developing Human: Clinically Oriented Embryology*, 11th edn. Pennsylvania: Elsevier Science.

National Institute for Health and Care Excellence (NICE) (2017) *Developmental Follow-up of Children and Young People Born Preterm*. London: NICE.

National Institute for Health and Care Excellence (NICE) (2019) *Specialist Neonatal Respiratory Care for Babies Born Preterm*. London: NICE.

NHS England and NHS Improvement (2021) *Palivizumab Passive Immunisation against Respiratory Syncytial Virus (RSV) in at Risk Pre-term Infants*. London: HMSO.

Office for National Statistics (ONS) (2019) *Child and Infant Mortality in England and Wales: 2019*. London: HMSO.

Randall, D. (2005) Development of the respiratory system and respiration. In: Chamley Chamley, C., Carson, P. and Randall, D. (eds). *Developmental Anatomy and Physiology of Children*. UK: Elsevier Churchill Livingstone.

Resuscitation Council (UK) (2021) *Newborn Resuscitation and Support of Transition of Infants at Birth*. London: Resuscitation Council (UK).

Royal College of Paediatrics and Child Health (RCPCH) (2020) *National Neonatal Audit Programme Annual Report 2020*. London: RCPCH.

Sanoj, K.M., Ali, Mohammed, N., Qureshi, N. & Gupta, S. (2021) Oxygen therapy in preterm infants: recommendations for practice. *Paediatrics and Child Health*, **31**(1), 1–6.

Simon, L.V., Hasmi, M.F. & Bragg, B.N. (2021). Apgar score, national center for biotechnology information (NCBI): Statpearls publishing LLC. Bookshelf ID: NBK470569.

Sweet, D., Carnielli, V., Greisen, G. et al. (2019) European consensus guidelines on the management of neonatal respiratory distress syndrome – 2019 update. *Neonatology*, **115**, 432–450.

The Lullaby Trust (2021) Sudden unexpected infant death. Available from: https://www.lullabytrust.org.uk/safer-sleep-advice/what-is-sids [Accessed 27th October 2021].

Yanyan, N., Johnson, S., Marlow, N. & Wolke, D. (2021) Reduced health-related quality of life in children born extremely preterm in 2006 compared with 1995: the EPICure studies. *Arch Dis Child Fetal Neonatal Ed*, F1–F6. doi: 10.1136/archdischild-2021-322888.

CHAPTER 20

Cystic Fibrosis

Hazel Mills and Julie Hanna

SCENARIO

James is a five-year-old boy with cystic fibrosis (CF) admitted to hospital for intravenous antibiotics. He is an only child who lives at home with his parents Patrick and Sarah. James was diagnosed with CF at three weeks of age, by neonatal screening. At the time of diagnosis, James attended the hospital regularly, as an outpatient, for routine baseline investigations and parental education.

Cystic fibrosis is an inherited, multi-system disorder affecting infants, children, and adults as a result of a defect in the cystic fibrosis transmembrane conductance regulator (CFTR) gene. It results in dysfunction of the exocrine glands affecting particularly the respiratory tract, digestive tract, pancreas and sweat glands (Riordan et al. 1989).

The hallmark of cystic fibrosis is excessive mucus production, chronic respiratory infection, leading to airway inflammation and progressive lung disease, which is regarded as having the greatest role in morbidity. Other manifestations include pancreatic insufficiency, leading to fat malabsorption, failure to gain weight, and poor absorption of fat-soluble vitamins, high sweat chloride levels and later complications of liver disease and diabetes (Ratjen et al. 2015).

The clinical presentation may vary between individuals. Cystic fibrosis can present early, with meconium ileus on the first day of life, or later in life with infertility in otherwise healthy males.

The most common presentation of CF is with malabsorption, failure to thrive and chronic cough (Scott Bell et al.). The lower airways of patients with CF are typically infected with, initially, *Staphylococcus aureus*, later with *Haemophilus influenzae* and then often with *Pseudomonas aeruginosa* (PA) (Bhagirath et al. 2016).

Pseudomonas has been cultured from cough swabs since James was three years old. Initially this was successfully treated with a three-month course of oral ciprofloxacin and nebulised colistin. When James was four years old, PA grew again and this time the eradication therapy failed to clear the pseudomonas, resulting in admissions for intravenous antibiotics. James is reviewed 2–3 monthly at outpatient's clinic where, if required, admissions or a change of treatment is arranged. Intravenous antibiotics are usually required when James' cough and sputum production increases and appetite and energy levels decrease.

Peripheral venous access became difficult so James had a TIVAD (totally implantable venous access device) inserted when he was four years old. James finds accessing of the TIVAD frightening and uncomfortable despite much reassurance. Admissions are generally for 10 to 14 days during which time James is confined to his room.

QUESTIONS

1. How is CF diagnosed?
2. Discuss the medication prescribed to James, the newly diagnosed baby with CF.
3. What is a totally implantable venous access device (TIVAD)?
4. How would the children's nurse plan care to reduce James' anxiety during the accessing of the TIVAD?
5. Discuss how the children's nurse would devise a care plan to meet James' needs in relation to respiratory function.
6. What is the role of the community CF nurse specialist?

ANSWERS TO QUESTIONS

Question 1. How is CF diagnosed?

Based on the presence of clinical features, CF is confirmed by several different investigations. CF can present from birth through to adulthood and severity can vary from mild to severe. In the CF population 10–15% of babies will present with meconium ileus within 24–48 hours (failure to pass first stool). This may result in abdominal distension and vomiting. These babies should then be transferred to a regional

Care Planning in Children and Young People's Nursing, Second Edition. Edited by Sonya Clarke and Doris Corkin.
© 2024 John Wiley & Sons Ltd. Published 2024 by John Wiley & Sons Ltd.

paediatric surgical unit, for further treatment and investigations. Initially rectal gastrografin may be tried under radiological conditions. Gastrografin draws fluid into the bowel and helps to expel faecal matter. If unsuccessful, a surgical laparotomy will be required to relieve the obstruction. Bloods should be sent for genetic mutation analysis for CF (Farrelly et al. 2014).

What is immune reactive trypsin (IRT)?
Trypsinogen is a naturally occurring substance produced in the pancreas. In CF babies, the mucus they produce can prevent the trypsinogen from leaving the pancreas and reaching the small bowel. This then allows the trypsinogen level to build up in the blood.

When is the IRT test carried out?
A sample of blood is collected from the heel of a baby aged 5–8 days. This blood is placed on a special card which when dry is sent to biochemistry laboratory for analysis.

In August 2009, a national screening program was rolled out across the UK. Prior to this Northern Ireland had screened all babies born for CF on the routine heel prick test from 1983. The following route for screening is now been carried out:

1. Normal in full (IRT) → CF not suspected
2. Raised IRT → genetic analysis →no mutation → repeat IRT → normal limits → CF not suspected
3. Raised IRT → genetic analysis → two mutations identified → CF suspected → sweat test → confirmed diagnosis
4. Raised IRT → genetic analysis → one mutation identified → repeat IRT → raised IRT→ sweat test → confirmed diagnosis or carrier for CF gene

(Northern Ireland Bloodspot Screening Programme DHSSPSNI 2009)

Question 2. Discuss the medication prescribed to James, the newly diagnosed baby with CF

1. From time of diagnosis patients are usually commenced on an anti-staphylococcus prophylactic antibiotic for example, flucloxacillin. This will help to reduce staphylococcal infection and subsequent inflammation during the time of lung development when the lungs are most vulnerable. CF Trust, 2009.

2. Vitamin A, D, E supplementation is required daily. The rationale for giving these specific preparations is the malabsorption of fat-soluble vitamins due to pancreatic insufficiency in the CF person. Dosage varies according to age and plasma levels. Plasma levels should be checked annually to ensure an adequate dose is being prescribed and administered.

3. Pancreatic enzyme supplements are required by approximately 90% of the CF population. This is due to an inadequacy of their own pancreatic secretions. Pancreatic enzyme replacement should be started as soon as pancreatic insufficiency is established. Dosage should be adjusted according to weight gain, number and consistency of bowel movements. Enzyme replacement capsules, for example Creon 10,000, are administered immediately prior to all feeds (BNFC 2021–2022). They are opened and the small microspheres are placed on a spoon and delivered to the baby.

Question 3. What is a totally implantable venous access device (TIVAD)?

Totally implantable venous access devices were developed to overcome the problems associated with repeated venous access in patients needing long-term intravenous therapy. The implantable port is placed under the skin in the arm or chest by interventional radiologists or surgeons and usually under general anaesthetic.

It consists of two components (Figures 20.1 and 20.2):

1. A portal chamber made of titanium and a silicone septum (injection area).
2. A radio-opaque silicone catheter, which is introduced into the cephalic, jugular or subclavian veins.

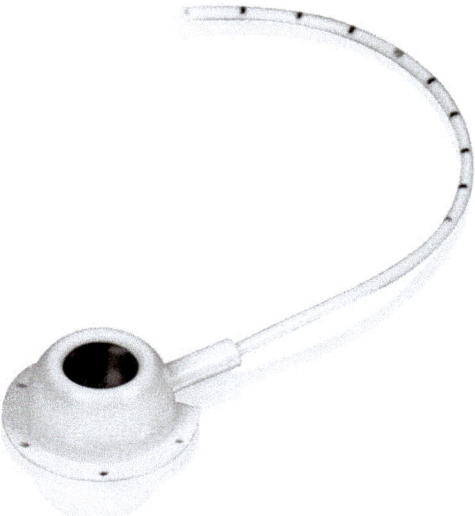

FIGURE 20.1 A totally implantable venous access device. Image provided by Vygon (UK) Ltd. and used with kind permission.

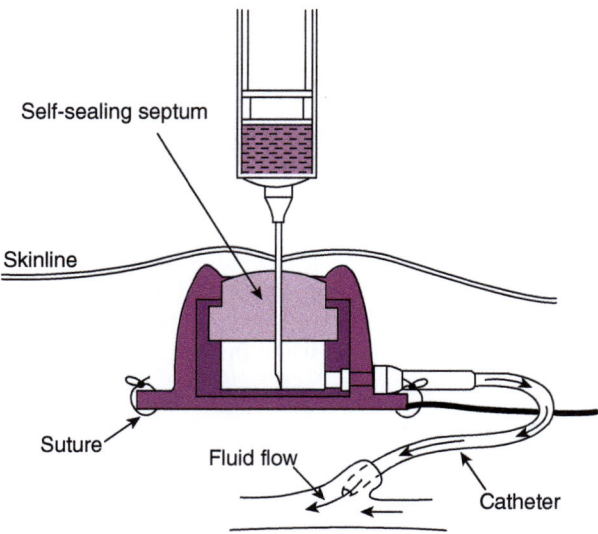

FIGURE 20.2 Diagram showing a needle inserted through the skin and silicone septum into the portal chamber. Image provided by Vygon (UK) Ltd. and used with kind permission.

Medication is given into the TIVAD by inserting a non-coring needle through the skin into the portal chamber and injecting or infusing the drugs, which will travel along the catheter into the veins (Vygon 2020). A sterile, transparent, semi-permeable adhesive dressing is used to secure the needle in place. The intravenous system must be flushed and a heparin lock established following each usage and at least every four weeks between uses according to hospital protocol. Refer to Table 20.1 for the advantages and disadvantages of TIVAD devices.

Question 4. How would the children's nurse plan care to reduce James' anxiety during the accessing of the TIVAD?

Problem: communication (Roper et al. 2000).

James is anxious about having his TIVAD accessed.

Goal: to minimize James' anxiety.

Table 20.1 Advantages and disadvantages of TIVAD devices.

Advantages of TIVAD device	Disadvantages of TIVAD device
Fully implantable and can be cosmetically placed	A special non coring needles required for accessing device
Reduced risk of displacement compared to a central line	Device is expensive
Less interference with everyday activities – child is able to bath/shower/swim	Surgery required for insertion
Low maintenance – requires infrequent flushing	Two people required for flushing
	Other possible complications – access difficulties, blockage, leakage, or infection.

Nursing action

- Assess level of anxiety.
- Plan strategies to help reduce anxiety. A procedural preparation programme which involves the use of the play therapist and clinical psychologist may be required (Gjaerde et al. 2021).
- James should be settled into a child and family friendly environment, made comfortable with his surroundings and introduced to his named nurse on admission.
- A family-centred approach should be adopted to include the family's participation in aspects of care.
- If possible, give James a choice of where the procedure is carried out, for example treatment room or own side ward.
- Ensure James is in a comfortable position on examination couch/bed.
- Consider James' privacy needs during the procedure.
- Facilitate questions James or his parents may have regarding the procedure.
- Following discussion with the play therapist regarding information already communicated to James and his parents the children's nurse should give a brief explanation of the procedure including:
  – The use of local anaesthetic cream, for example Emla™, Ametop™
  – Cleansing of the injection site with antiseptic solution as this is an aseptic procedure
  – The port will be held in place whilst the needle is inserted
  – A slight prick and some pressure may be felt as the needle passes through the skin
  – Saline and heparin flushes will be administered through the TIVAD
  – The needle will be taped in place with a suitable dressing material
- If possible, allow James to decide when he is ready for the procedure to begin.
- Reassure James during the procedure.
- Keep James and his parents informed of what is happening during the insertion of the TIVAD needle.
- At the end praise and reward James for completing the procedure.

Evaluation: document all care, recording the strategies which were most useful at reducing anxiety.

Question 5. Discuss how the children's nurse would devise a care plan to meet James' needs in relation to respiratory function

Problem: breathing (Roper et al. 2000).
  James has been admitted for treatment of a chest infection.

Goals:

1. To relieve symptoms of respiratory distress
2. To safely administer medication to treat infection

Nursing action

1. Record vital signs – temperature, pulse, respiratory rate, oxygen saturations and blood pressure.
2. Report any deviation from within normal limits to doctor or nurse in charge.
3. Observe rate, rhythm and depth of breathing.
4. Observe for coughing and note colour and consistency of sputum.
5. Ensure James has sputum cartons to allow expectoration of sputum.
6. Nurse sitting upright beside suction and oxygen.
7. Inform physiotherapists of admission to initiate chest physiotherapy and exercise.
8. Encourage oral fluids to maintain hydration and help reduce viscosity of sputum.
9. Administer medication as prescribed; observe for effects and side effects.
10. Following the administration of nebulised medication ensure equipment cleaned and disinfected (Bell et al. 2020).
11. Refer to respiratory physiologist for pulmonary function testing.

Evaluation: record and report to James and his parents, in suitable terms, changes in:

- Vital signs and lung functions
- Cough and mucus production
- Energy levels
- Appetite and weight

Problem: maintaining a safe environment (Roper et al. 2000).
  James has a TIVAD *in situ*.

Goal: to ensure safe administration of intravenous antibiotics and patency of line.

Nursing action

1. Access the device using aseptic technique.
2. Two registered nurses to check each antibiotic, name, dose, route of administration, expiry date.
3. Check patient details on drug Kardex® and patient armband – name, date of birth, and hospital number.
4. Inform James of administration and alleviate any anxieties.
5. Administer antibiotics using the protocol for TIVADS.
6. Observe site for redness, swelling, and pain – stop administration if James experiences any problems and report immediately to doctor or nurse in charge.

7. Record administration of medication.
8. Observe for any side effects and report immediately to doctor or nurse in charge and take appropriate action.
9. Nurse beside oxygen and suction in case of emergency.

Evaluation:

- Record and report changes in respiratory function.
- Observe port site for redness and swelling when needle removed at end of IV course.

Question 6. What is the role of the community CF nurse specialist?

In Northern Ireland, all children with CF attend the Regional Paediatric Centre in Belfast. Between the regular check-up visits or hospital stays, the community CF nurse visits the home to provide assessment of health, advice, and support to both children and their parents. Treatments can also be initiated at home, which reduces hospital attendance. Home visits can allow parents, who are often anxious, to ask appropriate questions that they may feel unable to do in a hospital environment. At time of diagnosis the CF nurse links closely to the child's other health providers, for example GP and health visitor, educating them on the individual treatment and management of the CF child. The community CF nurse will liaise with schools at time of starting, transferring or at other times when issues may arise, to ensure the child with CF is given every aid as required with their education. Indeed, throughout the child's years until they transfer to the adult services the CF nurse is there to provide all possible assistance that these families and children may need. The community CF nurse is fortunate to be part a dedicated team of professionals who look after these children and can contact colleagues for advice when required.

Since the first edition of this book was published, precision medicines have been developed to treat specific CF mutations. This group of drugs called modulators tackle the underlying causes of the disease by helping the CFTR protein work effectively. The newest, Kaftrio (elexacaftor, tezacaftor, ivacaftor) has been found to be highly effective in randomised controlled trials in patients aged 12 yrs and older. From baseline through to 24 weeks, there was a 14.3% mean improvement in lung function, 63% reduction in pulmonary exacerbations and significant increase in BMI compared to those on placebo (Middleton et al, 2019).

The use of Kaftrio is expected to result in significant reductions in requirements for IV antibiotics in people with CF. James will soon be eligible for these drugs when the license is extended to children his age.

REFERENCES

Bell, J., Alexander, L., Carson, J., Crossan, A., McCaughan, J. & Mills, H. (2020) on behalf of the Northern Ireland Working Group on Nebuliser Care and Hygiene in Cystic Fibrosis Review Nebuliser hygiene in cystic fibrosis: evidence-based recommendations. *Breathe*, Jun **16**(2).

Bhagirath, A.Y., Li, Y., Somayajula, D., Dadashi, M., Badr, S. & Duan, K. (2016) Cystic fibrosis lung environment and *Pseudomonas aeruginosa* infection. *BMC Pulmonary Medicine*, **16**(174), Published online 2016 Dec 5,, doi: 10.1186/s12890-016-0339-5.

BNFC (2021–2022) *British National Formulary for Children*. London: BMJ Group.

The Department of Health, Social Services and Public Safety Northern Ireland (DHSSPSNI) (2009) *Northern Ireland Bloodspot Screening Programme, MCADD and Revised CF Screening Implementation. April 2009*. Northern Ireland: DHSSPSNI.

Farrelly, P.J., Charlesworth, C., Lee, S., Southern, K. & Baillie, C. (2014) Antibiotic Treatment for cystic fibrosis Third edition. May 2009 Fighting for a Life Unlimited Antibiotic treatment for cystic fibrosis – 3rd edition Report of the UK Gastrointestinal surgery in cystic fibrosis: a 20 yr. *Journal of Paediatric Surgery*, Feb **49**(2), P280–283.

Gjærde, L.K., Hybschmann, J., Dybdal, D. et al. (2021) Play interventions for paediatric patients in hospital: a scoping review. *BMJ Open*, **11**, e051957. doi: 10.1136/bmjopen-2021-051957.

Middleton, P.G., Mall, M.A., Dřevínek, P., Lands, L.C., McKone, E.F., Polineni, D., Ramsey, B.W., Taylor-Cousar, J.L., Tullis, E., Vermeulen, F., Marigowda, G., McKee, C.M., Moskowitz, S.M., Nair, N., Savage, J., Simard, C., Tian, S., Waltz, D., Xuan, F., Rowe, S.M. & Jain, R., (2019) VX17-445-102 study group elexacaftor–tezacaftor–ivacaftor for cystic fibrosis with a single Phe508del allel.

Ratjen Felix, B., Scott, C., Rowe Steven, M., Goss Christopher, H., Quittner Alexandra, L. & Bush, A. (2015) Cystic fibrosis. *Nature Review Disease Primers*, 2015 May **14**(1), 15010.

Riordan, J.R., Rommes, J.M., Kerem, B., Alon, N., Rozmahel, R., Grzelczak, Z., Lok, S., Plavsic, N., Chou, J.L. et al (1989) Identification of the cystic fibrosis gene: cloning and characterization of complementary DNA. *Science*, 1989 Sep 8, **245**(4922), 1066–1073.

Roper, N., Logan, W.W. & Tierney, A.J. (2000) *The Roper-Logan Tierney Model of Nursing: Based on Activities of Living*. Edinburgh: Elsevier Health Sciences.

Vygon (UK) Ltd (2020) Ports product guide. The Pierre Simonet Building. V Park, Gateway North, Latham Road, Swindon, Wiltshire. Code: DXjB0004017V00194v1.

Asthma

CHAPTER 21

Barbara Maxwell, Gillian Gallagher, Katie McMullan, and Catherine Russell

SCENARIO

George is a six-year-old boy (weighing 19 kg), who lives at home with his eight-year-old sister and both parents (smokers). George's sister, Daisy, suffers from eczema and was diagnosed three years ago with exercise-induced asthma and often self-administers a dry powder bronchodilator prior to playing hockey.

George's previous history included bronchiolitis when he was a five months old, when he required hospital admission. Since then George has been susceptible to intermittent 'wheezy' episodes with viral illnesses. His mum administers a bronchodilator metered dose inhaler (MDI) to George as and when required. To date he has never needed inhalers at school. However, over the past two years George has generally needed his bronchodilators more frequently during the summer months.

Today, as part of his summer school trip, George went to visit a local farm where he and his friends met and stroked farmyard animals. When George's mum picked him up from school at 3 p.m. he was slightly breathless, complaining about tightness in his chest and unable to tell his mum about his school trip. George's mum brought him to be assessed by his GP.

On auscultation the GP observed George to have an expiratory wheeze accompanied by marked respiratory effort. He prescribed ten puffs of a bronchodilator (100 mcg per dose) via a yellow aero chamber. George's symptoms did not improve so he was referred to his local children's hospital.

In A&E, the triage nurse noted George to have an audible wheeze, nasal flaring and that he was unable to complete sentences. His respiratory rate was 56, heart rate 128 and oxygen saturations 88% in room air. Refer to Box Activity 21.1 to 21.4

ACTIVITY 21.1

Please read the SIGN,158 British guideline (2019) on the management of asthma.

QUESTIONS

1. What is asthma?
2. Discuss the importance of monitoring vital signs.
3. What are the risk and trigger factors of asthma?
4. Explain the importance of asthma medication and education.
5. Plan George's discharge from hospital.

ANSWERS TO QUESTIONS

Question 1. What is asthma?

Asthma is a common and chronic inflammatory disorder of the airways and it can affect both adults and children of all ages (Price et al. 2004).

During an exacerbation of asthma, bronchoconstriction causes obstruction in the airways and therefore limits airflow. The obstruction in the airway is partially or completely reversible and this

Care Planning in Children and Young People's Nursing, Second Edition. Edited by Sonya Clarke and Doris Corkin.
© 2024 John Wiley & Sons Ltd. Published 2024 by John Wiley & Sons Ltd.

occurs either spontaneously or due to therapeutic interventions. The smooth muscle goes into spasm; there is also increased mucus secretion and cellular infiltration of the airway walls mainly by eosinophils, which leads to epithelial damage (Scullion 2005).

The tightness George felt in his chest was as a direct result of his airways narrowing and spasm of the smooth muscle, probably as a result of the exposure to the farmyard animals.

ACTIVITY 21.2

Blow out a candle until you have expelled all the air in your lungs. Inhale approximately 50% of air back into your lungs. Fully exhale again and once more inhale 50% of what you've just exhaled back into your lungs. If you keep repeating this task for a few minutes, the sensation you feel should be one of a 'tight' chest.

Reflect upon the scenario: apply Roper et al. (2009) model of care.

Activity of living: breathing.

In A&E, due to low Sp02 88% the doctor prescribed nebulized 5 mg Salbutamol. It was administered by a member of the nursing team in accordance with Nursing and Midwifery Council guidelines (NMC 2018). Doses prescribed were based on the https://www.sign.ac.uk/our-guidelines/british-guideline-on-the-management-of-asthma/ (2003, revised July 2019). George's condition did not improve and he was beginning to feel agitated and frightened because of his breathing difficulties. He was reassured by the doctors and nurses. After 20 minutes he was reassessed by the medical team. The same prescribed dose of bronchodilator was administered again on two further occasions, unfortunately with no obvious improvement. George was also commenced on an oral steroid (prednisolone 30 mg). It was decided at this point that he needed to be admitted to the paediatric medical ward.

ACTIVITY 21.3

Write a care plan based on the Roper et al. (2009) model in relation to breathing, then compare with Appendix 7.

Question 2. Discuss the importance of monitoring vital signs

Activity of living: maintaining a safe environment.

On admission to the acute medical ward, George was tachypnoeic (respiratory rate: 52) and tachycardic (heart rate: 128). George was using his accessory muscles. Use of accessory muscles is indicated by nasal flaring, sternal recession and over-inflation of the chest wall. These symptoms are due to the respiratory system having to compensate for the narrowing of the airways.

George was pale, his oxygen saturations (SaO_2) were 88% in room air. Normal oxygen saturations are usually >95%, a reading of <93% will require oxygen (O_2) therapy.

SaO_2 is the percentage of Hb absorbed with the O_2 and measured in the arterial blood. SpO_2, meanwhile, is the process used for measuring pulse oximetry. Pulse oximetry, when performed correctly, is accurate to within plus or minus 3% of SpO_2 at higher ranges, but reflects SaO_2 less accurately when SpO_2 falls below 80% (Jubran 1999).

As part of good practice, paediatric nurses must assess the child holistically and not just rely on monitors, for example observing vital signs, monitoring patient's use of accessory muscles, shortness of breath and skin colour. Signs of pallor or cyanosis as well as low SpO_2 are all indicators that O_2 therapy may have to be prescribed and administered. In George's case two litres O_2 therapy was commenced via nasal specs, resulting in his SpO_2 rising from 88% to 95%.

When attaching the saturation probe to an infant's/child's thumb or toe, the light sensor needs to be attached directly opposite the probe to give a true reading (Booker 2008). It is also worth noting that nail varnish can interfere with SpO_2 readings and therefore needs to be removed where applicable (Booker 2007a).

Peak expiratory flow is generally used in the over five years age bracket not however used in acute exacerbations. More commonly air flow limitation is assessed using spirometry in an outpatient setting. Spirometry testing in children >5 years assesses airway obstruction. It is rarely useful during exacerbations of asthma, except where air leaks are suspected. However, it is useful when a diagnosis other than asthma is suspected (Townshend et al. 2007a).

Question 3. What are the risk and trigger factors of asthma?

It is important for medical and nursing staff to take a detailed history of symptoms during any consultation in a hospital ward/outpatients or a GP surgery.

In George's case he had a higher probability of developing asthma compared to his peers. Family history included George's sister, Daisy, who was known to suffer from asthma and eczema. Both parents were smokers and George had had a previous history of bronchiolitis and recurrent episodic viral induced wheeze episodes.

A risk factor increases the probability of a person developing asthma, whereas a trigger factor may be the instigating factor during an exacerbation of asthma.

Risks: family history of asthma, atopy/allergy, gender (more common in males than females), birth history, passive smoking, certain foods, and recurrent respiratory infections.

Triggers: Non allergic – viruses, cold air, menarche, emotion, smoking, chemical odours, pollution, exercise, certain drugs. Allergic triggers – house dust mites, animal dander, pollens, moulds, food (Scullion 2005).

Both of George's parents were smokers. Smoking during pregnancy increases the child's risk of respiratory conditions by 35%. Also, children whose parents smoke face a 50% increased risk of developing asthma (Asthma UK 2005).

George's sister Daisy also had a history of eczema. Atopic conditions such as eczema and rhinitis increase the probability of asthma (British Guideline on Management of Asthma 2019).

Daisy's asthmatic symptoms became worse when playing outdoor sports. In George's case his symptoms became worse once he was exposed to farmyard animals. Skin prick testing could confirm George's allergens. If positive, George would then avoid known trigger factors. This would be completed at a future outpatient appointment. Bloods for specific IgE to aeroallergens and Eosinophil count can be requested during admission but it is not a routine test.

One reason why atopic asthma patients wheeze with viruses is due to the fact that they are born with smaller airway dimensions than those who do not wheeze (Townshend et al. 2007b).

Question 4. Explain the importance of asthma medication and education

George's symptoms improved with the assistance of various medications:

1. Bronchodilators: open up the airways
2. Steroids (inhaled and oral): reduce airway inflammation
3. Montelukast: leukotriene receptor antagonist – non steroidal anti-inflammatory effect plus mild bronchodilation.

George's respiratory symptoms initially did not improve with the aid of an MDI via spacer device. He was prescribed and administered bronchodilators via a nebuliser device which was attached to the O_2 mains by his bedside. Nebulisers are instruments designed to atomise liquid drugs into fine mists for inhalation into the lungs (Booker 2007a). Booker (2007a) also states that nebulisers require a driving gas flow rate of 6–8 litres. Nebulisation of normal volume of drug (2–4 ml) should be complete in about ten minutes. Realistically it may be necessary to reduce the time to around five minutes when administering nebulisers to infants. Toddlers often find the mist from nebulisers quite scary and generally do not like to be held for long periods.

The mist of the drug can only be delivered to the lungs once the patient has inhaled. Therefore the nebulised drug is wasted during exhalation (Booker 2007a). Since so much of the drug is wasted it is important to keep the nebuliser mask sealed to the child's face and not wafting from a short distance from the face to ensure that maximum dose is administered.

Nebulised salbutamol 5 mg was prescribed hourly and reassessed thereafter. Due to poor response to the beta2 agonist, ipratropium bromide 0.25 mg (a B2 agonist) was added in. As George's symptoms improved, the interval between bronchodilator nebuliser therapy was gradually stretched from one to four hourly. His mum noticed that George's hands had started to shake.

Side effects of bronchodilators include fine tremor of the hands, tachycardia, and hypocalcaemia (BNF$_C$ 2021–2022). Around 12% of the nebulised drug which leaves the chamber enters the lungs, but the majority of the drug stays in the apparatus (Rees 2005).

Once George's symptoms improved and vital signs settled to within normal limits, that is, heart rate 98, respiratory rate 28, and SpO$_2$ 95% in room air he was changed to an MDI via a yellow spacer device. Aero chamber Plus generally fit all forms of MDIs. They are available in five different sizes:

- **Orange**: has mask attached, suitable for children <1 year.
- **Yellow**: has mask attached, suitable for children aged 1–5 years.
- **Green**: has mouthpiece attached, suitable for children aged 5+ years
- **Purple**: facemask attached, suitable for 5+ years children unable to use mouthpiece.
- **Blue**: has mouthpiece attached, suitable for children 12+ years and adults, also available with facemask.

Other medium to large spacers are available.

ACTIVITY 21.4

Describe how you would demonstrate to a child the most effective way to administer inhalers. See photos of children using an MDI with aero chambers (Figures 21.1 and 21.2).

When an MDI is used correctly, approximately 10% of the drug reaches the airways below the larynx. The rest of the drug is deposited no further than the oropharynx and is ultimately swallowed (Rees 2005). When using a spacer, tidal breathing (normal breathing rate) is not inferior to single breath and hold. Please note: MDI with spacer requires a slow, steady, deep inhalation(s), whereas dry-powdered devices require a sharp intake of inspiration. If used with a spacer device, Metered Dose Inhaler's (MDIs) are easier and more effective to use. Indeed it is recommended that all children should use an MDI with a spacer (Vincken et al. 2018).

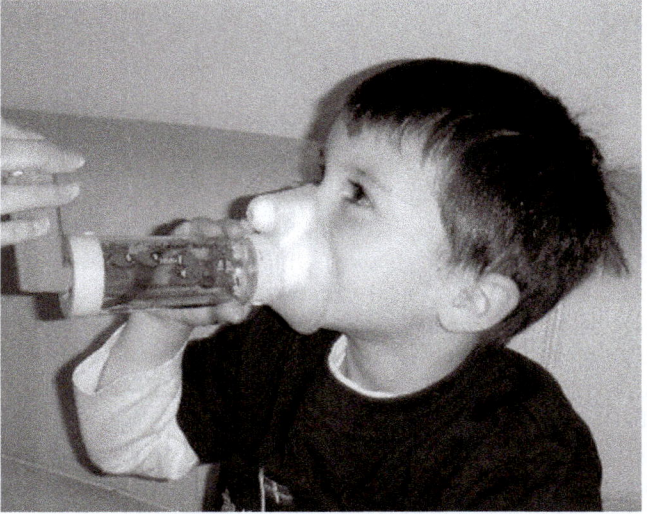

FIGURE 21.1 Child using an aero chamber with mask.

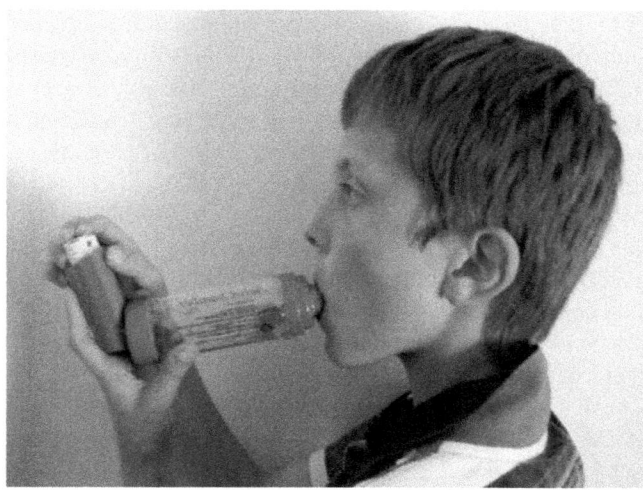

FIGURE 21.2   Medication via aero chamber.

George's nurse taught him and his parents the correct way to administer his MDI via his **green** spacer and correct breathing technique. When administering each dose George should be sitting or standing upright, with chin tilt slightly upwards. The MDI should be shaken, attached to the aero chamber and the mouthpiece should be inserted between the teeth and lips creating a good seal.

George was encouraged to take 5–6 slow steady deep breaths. If further doses are required, then wait 30–60 seconds, the MDI should be removed from the aero chamber and shaken in between each use. George's mum was also taught to rinse out the aero chamber every 1–2 weeks in warm soapy water and to leave it to air dry. Aero chambers should be replaced every 6–12 months (Rees 2005).

Older patients have the option of using dry powdered inhalers such as turbohalers and accuhalers. Inspiratory flow rate must be assessed using placebo devices prior to prescribing to ensure adequate inspiratory flow. Ideally the preventer and reliever inhalers should be the same type of device in order to ensure breathing techniques are not confused. Patients who are prescribed inhaled steroids should be encouraged to rinse their mouths after each use to prevent the common side effect of oral thrush and/or dysphonia (hoarse voice) (BNF_C 2021–2022).

Once George was stable on four-hourly bronchodilator MDI therapy, the doctor felt George was fit for discharge and was to go home on a regular ICS preventer inhaler. He was also to complete a three-day course in total of oral steroids (1–2 mg/kg). Over the next 3–5 days George may require some bronchodilator reliever inhaler. George's parents were given safety netting advice, regarding reliever use requirement.

Question 5. Plan George's discharge from hospital

Activity of living: communication (Casey 1988; Roper et al. 2009).

According to the BTS/SIGN guidelines (2019) after an exacerbation/attack, adults should be seen within 2–7 days and children within 1–2 working days. Unfortunately, this is not feasible in most primary care settings. Many people are at risk of readmission post attack. Often Asthma attacks are treated as a series of acute events, rather than as a chronic condition, that requires self-management skills. Education relating to ongoing day to day self-management skills for patients is often overlooked. According to the National Review of Asthma Deaths report (NRAD 2014), to this day, basic asthma care is poorly implemented throughout the UK, and implicated in the factors that lead to the preventable deaths examined and has therefore recommended improvement in this care provision.

Secondary care centres in Northern Ireland, have rolled out a regional pathway, offering a service of short term follow up for the patients admitted or attending Emergency Department with an asthma attack. In order to reduce readmission and prevent asthma deaths, but also reduce the burden on healthcare services. This pathway ensures patients receive verbal and written instruction on discharge, in order to be able to recognize failure to improve or any deterioration. Advice is provided on the appropriate action to take. It outlines their need for daily preventer treatment and ensures that a health professional has observed correct inhaler technique and checked understanding of safety netting advice. These patients are subsequently offered short-term outpatient follow up review, with an Asthma Nurse Specialist, initially within 2 weeks of attack and again on 2–3 occasions over an 8-week period total. The objective of this service is for asthma education to enable self-management of a chronic condition. This is known as the Safe Asthma Discharge Care pathway (SADCP); this was proven to improve patient outcomes and reduce re-attendance (Kennedy et al. 2022).

*For Safe Home Checklists (See Appendix 8).

Planning the discharge for any child from a paediatric ward should begin from admission. The BTS guidelines (2019) recommend that all patients with asthma should have a written, individualised asthma management plan (Townsend et al. 2007b).

Appendix 8 shows an example of written asthma plan and information leaflet used at a regional children's hospital. The details include name of patient, GP, hospital consultant, as well as emergency contact telephone numbers in the event of an asthma attack. Each treatment card should be personalised to each individual patient including clear, concise information and advice in regards to treatment and known trigger factors. The plans should include prescribed medication on a day-to-day basis as well as increased dosages required during an exacerbation of asthma. Parents and children should be aware that 'blue' inhalers are relievers (bronchodilators) and 'brown' inhalers are preventers (steroids which aim to prevent exacerbations of asthma). Please refer to the BNFc (2021–2022) to increase knowledge of short and long-acting inhaled bronchodilators and inhaled steroids.

Austin et al. (2005) has stated that children with asthma miss more days off school than their peers. Since George was only six years old, he still enjoyed school especially his school trips and was not keen to miss playing with his friends.

As part of discharge planning, the multidisciplinary team need to educate children as well as parents. Health professionals often talk to the carers instead of children, which can make children feel intimidated. Parents tend to see their role as carer and advocator (Iley 2007). Children need to take a certain amount of responsibility for their condition so that they recognise the warning signs because their parents will not always be with them. Parents also need to inform other people, for example relatives, teachers and other caregivers, about medication and action required during asthma attacks. Educating the family unit will benefit the whole family (Casey 1988). Children with asthma frequently tend to have a nocturnal cough. A child's cough can be distressing and also have a significant impact on their sleep, school performance and play (Shields et al. 2008). Therefore, effective therapeutic treatments will contribute to the whole family having undisturbed sleep.

While in the hospital ward, George and his mum were advised to avoid trigger factors such as farmyard animals. George was to be referred back to the hospital for skin prick testing to confirm potential allergens (Whaley & Wong 1999). George's mum and dad were also advised to stop smoking. Many parents are under the illusion that if they smoke 'out the back' they are not exposing their children to nicotine; this is not the case as cigarette smoke lingers on clothing for many hours.

George was discharged from hospital and was to be reviewed by his GP within two weeks. At each further consultation, whether at a GP centre or asthma clinic. Each asthmatic patient should have their inhaler technique reviewed to ensure good drug delivery and ongoing adherence to preventer treatment to maintain asthma control (BTS & SIGN 2019). By ensuring timely intervention with follow up review, this should reduce risk of future attack and help parents and children self manage their condition and in turn they should lead a relatively normal lifestyle.

REFERENCES

Asthma UK (2005) *A Moving Picture, Asthma in Northern Ireland Today*. 1–11. Belfast: Asthma UK.

Austin, J.B., Selvaraj, S., Godden, D. & Russell, G. (2005) Deprivation, smoking and quality of life in asthma. *Archives of Disease in Childhood*, **90**(3), 253–257.

BNF for Children (2021–2022) *BNF for Children*. London: BMJ Publishing group.

Booker, R. (2007a) Correct use of nebulisers. *Nursing Standard*, **22**(8), 39–41.

Booker, R. (2008) Pulse oximetry. *Nursing Standard*, **22**(30), 39–41.

British Thoracic Society (2019) *Asthma | British thoracic society | Better lung health for all*. Available at https://www.brit-thoracic.org.uk/quality-improvement/guidelines/asthma [Accessed 14 November 2022].

Casey, A. (1988) A partnership with child and family. *Senior Nurse*, **8**(4), 8–9.

Iley, K. (2007) The impact of asthma on childrens lives: A social perspective. *Primary Health Care*, **17**(8), 25–29.

Jubran, A. (1999) Pulse oximetry. *Critical Care*, **3**(2), 11–17.

Kennedy, L., Gallagher, G., Maxwell, B. et al. (2022) Implementation of a children's safe asthma discharge care pathway reduces the risk of future asthma attacks in children-a retrospective quality improvement report, Frontiers in Pediatrics. https://www.frontiersin.org/articles/10.3389/fped.2022.865476/full?&utm_source=Email_to_authors_&utm_medium=Email&utm_content=T1_11.5e1_author&utm_campaign=Email_publication&field=&journalName=Frontiers_in_Pediatrics&id=865476 [Accessed 14 November 2022].

(2014) *The National Review - Asthma + Lung UK*. Available at https://www.asthma.org.uk/293597ee/globalassets/campaigns/nrad-full-report.pdf [Accessed 14 November 2022].

National Review of Asthma Deaths report (NRAD) (2014) Why asthma still kills. London: RCP.

Nursing and Midwifery Council (2018) *The Code – Professional Standards of Practice, and Behaviour for Nurses and Midwives*. London: NMC.

Price, D., Foster, J., Scullion, J. & Freeman, D. (2004) *Asthma and COPD*. London: Churchill Livingstone.

Rees, J. (2005) ABC of asthma, methods of delivering drugs. *British Medical Journal*, **331**, 504–506.

Roper, N., Logan, W.W. & Tierney, A.J. (2009) *The Roper-Logan-Tierney Model of Nursing: Based on Activities of Living*. Edinburgh: Churchill Livingstone.

Scullion, J. (2005) A proactive approach to asthma. *Nursing Standard*, **20**(9), 57–65.

Shields, M.D., Bush, A., Everard, M.L., McKenzie, S. & Primhak, R. and on behalf of the British Thoracic Society Cough Guideline Group (2008) Recommendations for the assessment and management of cough in children. *Thorax*, **63**, 1–15.

Townshend, J., Hails, S. & McKean, M. (2007a) Management of asthma in children. *British Medical Journal*, **335**, 253–257.

Townshend, J., Hails, S. & McKean, M. (2007b) Diagnosis of asthma in children. *British Medical Journal*, **335**, 198–202.

Vincken, W. *et al.* (2018) *Spacer devices for inhaled therapy: Why use them, and how?* ERJ Open Research. U.S. National Library of Medicine. Available at https://www.ncbi.nlm.nih.gov/pmc/articles/PMC6004521/#__ffn_sectitle (Accessed 14 November 2022).

Whaley, L.F. & Wong, D.L. (1999) *Nursing Care of Infants and Children*, 6th edn. St Louis: Mosby.

Care of Infants and Young Persons with Cardiac Conditions

SECTION 5

Cardiac Catheterisation

CHAPTER 22

Pauline Carson

SCENARIO

David is 13 years old and has a history of pulmonary valve stenosis and asthma. When he was three years old David underwent a balloon pulmonary valvuloplasty to relieve the stenosis, and has had routine yearly cardiac follow up since then. During his last clinic visit some restenosis of his pulmonary valve was identified, and it was decided that a second balloon pulmonary valvuloplasty was required to relieve the stenosis and he has now been admitted for cardiac catheterisation and a balloon pulmonary valvuloplasty. David's asthma was diagnosed when he was six; it is well controlled with inhalers and he has not required hospitalisation since his initial diagnosis. He administers his own inhalers but often has to be reminded to do so by his parents.

David is in his second year at senior school, where he has lots of friends who he enjoys spending time with. He enjoys playing football and cricket, swimming, and playing on his Xbox with friends and is a sociable and active teenager. Apart from becoming wheezy when he plays football neither of his conditions has restricted his education or his involvement in sports. On admission to the ward David is very quiet, his parents answer most of the questions and also tell you that David has recently started to argue with them all the time. On talking to David afterwards he tells you that his parents think he should not play football and they do not allow him to stay over with friends or go on overnight trips with school because of his heart and asthma problems and that's what causes the arguments. He says his older brothers tend to protect him although he does not want to be different from his friends and wants to do all the things they do. David also says he is worried about being in hospital and having an 'operation' as he does not remember the first one and he is also concerned that his friends will not be allowed in to visit.

QUESTIONS

1. What is congenital heart disease and how are defects classified?
2. What is pulmonary stenosis and how is it treated?
3. What is a cardiac catheterisation?
4. What is transitional care?
5. Using the nursing process and Orem's self-care model, how would the nurse assess and plan care to alleviate David's anxiety?
6. David has reached an age where he now needs not only to begin taking control of his medical conditions, but also to start the transition process which will lead to transfer to the adult service in a few years' time. Using Orem's model and the nursing process, how can David and his parents be supported in this?

ANSWERS TO QUESTIONS

Question 1. What is congenital heart disease?

Congenital heart disease (CHD) is a term used to describe a problem with the heart that is present from birth. This includes structural defects, arrhythmia's, and some types of cardiomyopathies and range from problems that can be managed with medicine to complex structural problems requiring either heart surgery or a transcatheter intervention (key hole technique) sometimes just hours after birth (National Institute for Cardiovascular Outcomes Research, NICOR 2022). Structural defects are often

Care Planning in Children and Young People's Nursing, Second Edition. Edited by Sonya Clarke and Doris Corkin.
© 2024 John Wiley & Sons Ltd. Published 2024 by John Wiley & Sons Ltd.

classified as either cyanotic or acyanotic defects (Gaskin & Daniels 2021), but they can also be classified in terms of the blood flow through the heart, i.e. defects with increased or decreased pulmonary blood flow, obstructions to blood flow, or mixed blood flow (Schroeder et al. 2019).

Question 2. What is pulmonary stenosis and how is it treated?

Pulmonary stenosis is one of the most common obstructive defects, where there is narrowing or stenosis above (supravalvular), below (subvalvular), or at the site of the pulmonary valve itself (valvular). The degree of stenosis can vary from mild to severe, with treatment either non-surgical or balloon valvuloplasty, or surgical, such as pulmonary valvotomy, depending on the severity and degree of stenosis present (Jones et al. 2009). In the scenario above David is scheduled to have a balloon valvuloplasty in the catheter laboratory.

Question 3. What is cardiac catheterisation?

Cardiac catheterisation is an invasive procedure used for therapeutic interventions, electrophysiological evaluation, and treatment and diagnostic purposes. However, as echocardiography and other non-invasive diagnostic imaging methods advance the latter is decreasing, although it is still a necessary procedure if pressure measurement is required (Dhillon et al. 2009). Procedures performed during interventional catheterisation include creation and device closure of atrial and septal defects, device closure of ventricular septal defects, coil occlusion of a patent ductus arteriosus, and balloon valvuloplasty for pulmonary and aortic valvular stenosis. The procedure itself is carried out in the cardiac catheterisation laboratory and in children and young people usually under general anaesthetic; therefore they will not be allowed to eat or drink prior to the procedure.

During the procedure a radio-opaque catheter is inserted through a peripheral blood vessel, usually a femoral vessel, allowing pressures in the heart chambers to be recorded, angiography contrast material to be delivered, and defects to be corrected using occlusive devices and balloons. After the procedure the catheter is removed and pressure is applied to the site. Close observation is required for 24 hours for any side effects or adverse reaction to the contrast medium or for complications such as bleeding, haematoma, arrhythmias, thrombosis, cardiovascular accident, perforation, cardiac tamponade, and/or cardiac arrest. Refer to Box Activity 22.1.

ACTIVITY 22.1

Review the pathophysiology of congenital heart disease and related nursing care in the following textbooks:

Cook, K. & Langton, H. (2009) *Cardio-thoracic Care for Children and Young People*. Chichester: Wiley-Blackwell.
Glasper, A; Richardson, J and Randall, D (2021) A textbook of children's and young people's nursing 3rd edition London Elsevier.
Gormley-Fleming, E and Peate I. (2019) Fundamentals of children's applied pathophysiology an essential guide for nursing and health care students: Chichester: Wiley-Blackwell.
Hockenberry, MJ; Wilson, D and Rodgers, CC. (2019) *Wong's Nursing Care of Infants and Children*, 11th edition. St. Louis: Mosby.

Question 4. What is transitional care?

The National Institute for Clinical Excellence guidelines, Transition from children's to adults' services for young people using health or social care services (NICE 2016) provides guidance for those caring for young people moving from children's to adult services around the period before, during, and after a young person moves with the aim of improving the experience for both the young person and their carers.

> **ACTIVITY 22.2**
>
> Access and read the following document.
> What key principles of transition can you identify?
> National Institute for Health and Care Excellence (2016) Transition from children's to adults' services.

Question 5. Using the nursing process and Orem's self-care model, how would the nurse assess and plan care to alleviate David's anxiety?

ASSESSMENT

> **BOX 22.1 ASSESSMENT: OREM'S SELF-CARE MODEL**
>
> | | Normal self-care/dependent care ability | Current self-care | Self-care deficit |
> |---|---|---|---|
> | **Universal self-care requisite** | | | |
> | Maintenance of a balance between solitude and social interaction.

Promotion of normalcy. | David has lots of friends. He plays football and cricket, swims, and enjoys playing on his Xbox by himself and with his friends.

Usually very happy and doesn't worry about anything.

David's parents do not allow him to stay over with friends or go on overnight trips with school and restrict the amount of time they allow him to play football. | In hospital and away from his social network of friends.

Very quiet, anxious, and apprehensive about procedure.

David is in the early phase of adolescent development, peer group connections are becoming very important to him, and he will not want to be seen to be different. | Feelings of isolation in an unfamiliar environment and unable to maintain normal contact with his friends and peer group.

Lacks knowledge about procedure and is very anxious and apprehensive about undergoing cardiac catheterisation and having a general anaesthetic.

David feels that he is different from his friends and is beginning to resent his parents for restricting the activities he can do with his friends. |
> | **Developmental self-care requisite** | | | |
> | David is 13 years old | Parents have been responsible for meeting all of David's needs, including his healthcare needs, since his birth. | David has now entered adolescence and will be starting to move towards achieving independence from his parents. | David's knowledge and understanding of his asthma and pulmonary stenosis needs to be developed.

Parental input into meeting David's healthcare needs will begin to decrease as he gains independence. |

PLANNING

Maintenance of a balance between solitude and social interaction.
   Problem: David is feeling isolated in an unfamiliar environment and is unable to maintain normal contact with his friends and peer group.
   Goal/aim: David will become familiar with the ward environment and also be able to maintain contact with his friends and peer group. Nursing interventions will include:

- Allocate David a bed space with other adolescents, preferably in a designated adolescent bay if available.
- Familiarise David with the ward environment and ensure he knows where the bathroom facilities and kitchen facilities are; where he can use his mobile phone and where the adolescent activity/games room is, if available.
- Introduce David to the ward/hospital youth worker if one is available.
- Inform David and his parents of the visiting times and reassure him that his friends are able to come and visit him while he is in hospital.

- Make David aware that there are PlayStations, Xboxes, and DVD players available for him to use and that he can bring in his own games and DVDs for them.

Nursing action: educative/supportive (Orem 1995; Pearson et al. 2005).

Promotion of normalcy
Problem: David lacks knowledge about procedure and is therefore very anxious and apprehensive about undergoing cardiac catheterisation and having a general anaesthetic.

Goal/aim: David will know and understand what the procedure entails will feel less anxious about it.

Nursing interventions:

- Encourage David to express his concerns and take time to listen to what he has to say.
- Explain the cardiac catheterisation procedure to David in terms he will understand.
- Provide literature and use online resources aimed at adolescents which explain cardiac catheterisation.
- Arrange a preliminary visit to the cardiac catheterisation laboratory.
- Arrange for David to meet with the adolescent cardiac liaison nurse.
- Reassure David that the medical and nursing staff will explain any procedures to him before they carry them out and that it is all right for him to ask questions if he is unsure about what they are going to do.
- Explain the preoperative procedure and ensure David understands what it entails.
- Explain the postoperative procedure, i.e. the observations that will be carried out and the length of time he will have to remain in bed and ensure he understands why this is necessary.
- Reassure David that his parents can accompany him to the catheterisation laboratory, stay with him until he goes to sleep, and be with him when he wakes up.

Nursing action: educative/supportive (Orem 1995; Pearson et al. 2005).

Problem: David feels that he is different from his friends and is beginning to resent his parents for restricting the activities he does with his friends.

Goal/aim: David will equate himself with his peers and will not feel he is different to them just because he has asthma and pulmonary stenosis.

Nursing interventions:

- Talk to David's parents to establish what their understanding is with regard to asthma and pulmonary stenosis and the activities David can participate in.
- Explain to David's parents that while it is normal for them to want to protect David with regard to his asthma and pulmonary stenosis he is at an age and stage of development where it is important for him to be able to spend time with his friends.
- Encourage David and his parents to identify activities that he and his friends can do together which his parents will be less apprehensive about him doing.
- Arrange for David and his parents to meet with the cardiac liaison nurse and asthma specialist nurse to discuss how best to manage David's activities when he goes home so that he does not feel he is any different to his friends.
- Provide David's parents with information on parent support groups.
- Provide David with information about the adolescent support group within the GUCH (grown up congenital heart) support group and adolescent asthma support groups and asthma camp.

Nursing action: educative/supportive (Orem 1995; Pearson et al. 2005).

Question 6. David has reached an age where he now needs not only to begin taking control of his medical conditions, but also to start the transition process which will lead to transfer to the adult service in a few years' time. Using Orem's self-care model and the nursing process, how can David and his parents be supported in this?

DEVELOPMENTAL SELF-CARE REQUISITE

Problem: David needs to become more independent in managing his asthma and pulmonary stenosis but his knowledge and understanding of both is very limited.

Goal/aim: David will become more independent in meeting his own healthcare needs as he begins the process of transition which will eventually lead to the transfer over to adult services when he is older.

Nursing interventions:

- Explain to David and his parents what the term transition means and what it will involve for both David and his parents.
- Allow both David and his parents the opportunity to ask questions and express any fear; anxiety or apprehensiveness they may have regarding this process, i.e. why it starts at such an early age.
- Arrange for David and his parents to meet with the asthma transition nurse and the cardiology transition nurse to begin to plan David's transition to adult respiratory and cardiology services.

Nursing action: educative/supportive.

REFERENCES

Dhillon, R., Sharland, G., Robinson, A.M., Clay, C. & Bearne, C. (2009) Presentation and diagnosis. In: Cook, K. and Langton, H. (eds). *Cardio-thoracic Care for Children and Young People*. Chichester: Wiley-Blackwell.

Gaskin, K.L. & Daniels, A. (2021) Caring for children and young people with cardiovascular problems. In: Glasper, A., Richardson, J. & Randall, D. (eds). *A Textbook of Children's and Young People's Nursing*, 3rd edn. London: Elsevier.

Glasper, A., Richardson, J. & Randall, D. (2021) *A Textbook of Children's and Young People's Nursing*, 3rd edn. London: Elsevier.

Gormley-Fleming, E. & Peate, I. (2019) *Fundamentals of Children's Applied Pathophysiology an Essential Guide for Nursing and Health Care Students*. Chichester: Wiley-Blackwell

Hockenberry, M.J., Wilson, D. & Rodgers, C.C. (2019) *Wong's Nursing Care of Infants and Children*, 11th edn. St Louis: Mosby.

Jones, T., Cook, K., Dhillon, R. et al. (2009) Treatment options/management. In: Cook, K. & Langton, H. (eds). *Cardio-thoracic Care for Children and Young People*. Chichester: Wiley-Blackwell.

National Institute for Cardiovascular Outcomes Research (2022) Congenital heart disease in children and adults (Congenital audit)Accessed

NICE (National Institute for Health and Care Excellence) (2016) Transition from children's to adults' services for young people using health or social care services. NICE guideline [NG43].[Available at https://www.nice.org.uk/guidance/ng43 Accessed 6 march 2023]

Orem, D.E. (1995) *Nursing: Concepts of Practice*, 5th edn. St Louis.: Mosby.

Pearson, A., Vaughan, B. & FitzGerald, M. (2005) *Nursing Models for Practice*, 3rd edn. Edinburgh: Elsevier

Schroeder, L.M., Baker, A.L., Bastardi, H. & O'Brien, P. (2019) The child with cardiovascular dysfunction. In: Hockenberry, M.J., Wilson, D. & Rodgers, C.C. 2019 (eds). *Wong's Nursing Care of Infants and Children*, 11th edn. St Louis: Mosby Elsevier

CHAPTER 23

Infant with Cardiac Failure

Pauline Carson

SCENARIO

Dora (seven months old) is being admitted to the ward via the walk-in centre accompanied by her parents, Jane and Paul. Her older sister, Lily, is at nursery school. The referral letter gives a provisional diagnosis of congestive cardiac failure, stating that Dora's respirations are 45 per minute, heart rate 184 beats per minute, temperature 37.4°C, and oxygen saturations 92%.

Dora's parents took her to the walk-in centre because she has been restless and irritable during the night. They were unable to see the GP today but have been consulting the doctor frequently about their worries over Dora's faltering growth. Her birth weight was 3.2 kg, and she is now 4.5 kg. Jane stopped breastfeeding when Dora was 12 weeks, and Dora now has formula feeds, however, she can take 45 minutes to finish a bottle, sometimes falling asleep during the feed, she has also started a weaning diet four weeks ago, which she has twice a day.

Dora is a restless sleeper, waking frequently, often seems distressed and does not settle when offered a night feed. She was a full-term baby delivered vaginally and did not require admission to special baby care. On admission Dora is awake but lethargic and looks pale. She has good head control but cannot sit unaided. Movement in all four limbs is noted but they are mottled and cool to touch. Eye contact is present, and Dora turns to locate the source of any sound. She smiled when offered a toy, grasped it with both hands, moving it from one hand to another.

Jane works as a hotel manager, so she is worried about missing work whilst Dora is in hospital. Dad, Paul, is a transport manager at a local firm. Dora's grandmother provides childcare. Dora is being admitted for further investigation of congestive cardiac failure (CCF).

QUESTIONS

1. Using Roper, Logan, and Tierney's model of nursing (Holland & Jenkins, 2019):
   (a) Review the scenario and highlight any information which is relevant to Dora's holistic assessment.
   (b) Note the additional assessment information needed about Dora to ensure safe and effective nursing care during her first 24 hours in hospital. Think about family history, observation, interviewing, and measurement during this process.
2. Cardiac failure is a symptom and always has an underlying cause. List some probable causes of Dora's cardiac failure.
3. Some children with CCF are cyanosed. Explain why cyanosis occurs in heart disease.
4. Write a holistic care plan for Dora's first 24 hours in hospital, giving a rationale for the prescribed nursing actions.
5. Explain the immediate investigations that Dora may need to establish the possible cause of her cardiac failure.

Dora's initial assessment should provide sufficient information to highlight her immediate problems, establish a plan of care, and commence treatment. It is a challenging activity because Dora lacks the verbal skills to guide the nurse, and her physical immaturity may mean that rapid and serious deterioration is possible. Her parents may be distressed, anxious, and unable to answer some initial enquiries.

A calm and sympathetic environment will benefit Dora, with an initial visual assessment providing further useful information about Dora's physical condition, level of consciousness, and behaviour. It should be performed prior to physical contact and the use of medical devices because the use of equipment may upset Dora, causing her to cry and thereby changing baseline measurements.

A systematic approach should help to prevent omissions from the assessment.

Care Planning in Children and Young People's Nursing, Second Edition. Edited by Sonya Clarke and Doris Corkin.
© 2024 John Wiley & Sons Ltd. Published 2024 by John Wiley & Sons Ltd.

ANSWERS TO QUESTIONS

Question 1. Using Roper, Logan, and Tierney's model of nursing (Holland et al. 2019)

Using Roper, Logan, and Tierney's model of nursing (Holland et al. 2019)

(a) Review the scenario and highlight any information which is relevant to Dora's holistic assessment.

Breathing

At the walk-in centre, Dora's respiratory rate and apex heart rate exceeded the normal range for her age group (Kelsey 2021), and her oxygen saturation rate was below the usual rate of 95–98% (Kelsey & Rylatt 2021). These rates need to be re-assessed to provide baseline measurements and should be performed whilst Dora is relaxed and calm.

Dora's respiratory rate and oxygenation saturations should be recorded, and a visual assessment of her respiratory effort should be made to observe for any evidence of cyanosis, peripheral or central. Whilst Dora is calm her respirations should be counted for a full minute, these are likely to be high as tachypnoea is a common feature of CCF. The pattern and effort of her breathing should also be assessed for any signs of respiratory distress, such as head bobbing, nasal flaring, sternal or intercostal recession (Royal College of Nursing (RCN) 2017). Her oxygen saturations should be monitored as a saturation of 92% in air is low (Kelsey & Rylatt 2021) and a stethoscope should be used to auscultate Dora's chest to assess for any abnormal breath sounds, as fluid will interfere with the conduction of normal breath sounds (Kelsey & Rylatt 2021).

Dora's heart rate and capillary refill time (perfusion) should also be assessed and recorded. In children under 2 years of age an appropriately sized stethoscope should be used to count Dora's apex heart rate for a full minute (Kelsey & Rylatt 2021); it will also be necessary to palpate a peripheral pulse to ensure consistency with the apex rate and to assess the depth, volume, and rhythm (RCN 2017). In children with CCF, tachycardia will be present as the cardiovascular system has the capacity to initiate compensatory mechanisms to sustain and increase cardiac output. However, any changes in these compensatory mechanisms, such as a weak and thready pulse may indicate that the compensatory mechanisms within Dora's heart and circulatory system are weakening, and her condition is deteriorating (Gaskin & Daniels 2021).

Capillary refill time should be measured centrally on the chest as Dora's limbs are cool to the touch and this would affect the result. Normal capillary refill should be within two seconds, a slower capillary refill alongside pallor and mottling of the skin would indicate low cardiac output and poor systemic perfusion (Veal & Bailey 2018)

Measurement of blood pressure may provide additional information and if attempted it is essential to use the correct cuff size, as a cuff that is too large or too small will give an incorrect reading (Gormley-Fleming 2022). However, changes to blood pressure are a late indicator of problems in young children (Kelsey & Rylatt 2021) and it is also likely that Dora will move around during this procedure, also affecting the result and limiting the value of any reading.

Temperature control

Dora's temperature of 37.4°C is within the normal range for her age group but she may feel clammy and sweaty. This happens because of sympathetic nervous system stimulation as the heart tries to compensate for falling cardiac output (Schroeder et al. 2019) and additionally, may have caused Dora to have cradle cap.

Sleep

Dora wakes during the night and is difficult to settle, indicating that orthopnoea/dyspnoea may be a problem, whilst falling asleep during feeds indicates fatigue, poor exercise tolerance and might be contributing to her poor weight gain. Dora's sleep pattern may also affect her parents' ability to get enough sleep, impacting upon their ability to recognise Dora's needs and respond appropriately.

Nutrition

Dora's history indicates that she is formula fed and has commenced a weaning diet but has not been gaining weight so it will be important to assess and monitor her weight and intake. Enquire about Dora's normal feeding pattern, the amount of formula offered, and the foodstuffs offered as a weaning diet. Her parents may want to continue to give her feeds, so discuss their preferences. Dora should also be weighed to establish a baseline measurement to monitor the effects of prescribed therapy and feeding regimes. Infants with CCF will have an increased metabolic rate due to their increased heart and respiratory rate and due to fatigue, their ability to take in sufficient calories to meet their needs is limited and hence they do not gain weight (Schroeder et al. 2019). In addition, the true extent of poor weight gain may not always be evident due to the presence of generalised oedema, caused by water and sodium retention, a common feature of CCF. (Schroeder et al. 2019).

Mobility
Dora might be expected to be sitting unaided by this age (Boyd & Bee 2014); however, children with cardiac failure lack energy and tire easily (Roberts 2019), so Dora may only be able to sit unaided for short periods. Her ability to transfer a toy from one hand to another however would indicate that fine motor skills are developmentally appropriate (Boyd & Bee 2014).

Safety
At seven months, Dora is dependent on her parents and carer's to maintain her safety both at home and in the hospital. Policies and guidelines should be followed to ensure Dora's safety whilst in hospital for example when administering medication. It is also important to find out if Dora has ever been given any medications, either prescribed, over the counter or herbal and if she has any known allergies. However, it should be remembered that Dora will still be encountering new substances and her reaction to them cannot be predicted. Finding out about her immunisation history to date from her parents will also be important as Dora's age increases her risk of infection.

Communication
Dora lacks the ability to verbalise her needs. However, she will be conscious of the visual and auditory information around her and play games such as 'peek a-boo' show displeasure when a toy is removed and reach out to be lifted (Kidd & Rodgers 2019). At 7 months she has also developed the muscle control needed to allow her to combine a vowel sound with a consonant sound and begin babbling (Boyd & Bee 2014). Dora has also developed a sense of object permanence and may begin to experience distress if separated from her parents (separation anxiety), or when encountering strangers so facial expressions and crying patterns should be observed for signs of anxiety or increasing distress (Kidd & Rodgers 2019).

Elimination
Ask about the number of wet and dirty nappies Dora normally has each day and find out if there have been any recent changes to frequency, consistency, or smell of urine or stools. It is advisable to test Dora's urine to exclude infection and to check the napkin area for any signs of irritation or nappy rash.

Cleansing and dressing
Ask the parents about bath times, and clothing preferences. Dora's parents may want to meet her hygiene needs, so note their choices.

Playing
Play is essential for a child's normal growth and development (Boyd & Bee 2014) and enables children to experience, connect, and interact with the world around them (Shapcott 2018). At 7 months Dora should be reaching out to grasp small toys, transfer them from hand to hand and shake rattles deliberately to make a sound (Kelsey 2021). Dora's abilities and her play preferences should be discussed with her parents and they should be encouraged to bring some of her favourite toys with them to the hospital, to provide an essential link with home, aid normality, and minimize her stress and anxiety. Quiet play activities should be explored with her parents to decrease Dora's oxygen requirements and mitigate against any potential regression that could come about because of hospitalisation.

Dora is too young to understand the biological differences between females and males, but her parents may have definite ideas about gender differences, so establish if Dora's parents have any specific preferences related to toys or clothing.

Death and dying
Dora will lack any concept of death, but her parents may have fears about the possibility of Dora dying, as many people associate heart problems with early death. Conversely, they may not have

considered this possibility, so limit discussion to any current fears or anxieties. Further discussion can be initiated by clinicians when more concrete information about the cause of Dora's problems is known.

Question 1. Using Roper, Logan, and Tierney's model of nursing (Holland et al. 2019):

Using Roper, Logan, and Tierney's model of nursing (Holland et al. 2019):

(b) Note the additional assessment information needed about Dora to ensure safe and effective nursing care during her first 24 hours in hospital. Think about family history, observation, interviewing, and measurement during this process.

Obtaining a detailed health history, such as concerns about poor feeding, and a family history is important when assessing an infant with a heart condition as it can provide further relevant information about Dora's diagnosis. Parents who have had a congenital heart malformation themselves or who already have had an affected child are at increased risk of having a child with cardiac problems (Schroeder et al. 2019).

Question 2. Cardiac failure is a symptom and always has an underlying cause. List some probable causes of Dora's cardiac failure

Congestive cardiac failure is caused by cardiac dysfunction and occurs when the heart is unable to pump sufficient blood around the body to meet its metabolic demands for nutrients, the transport of blood gases, and electrolytes (Schroeder et al. 2019). It is characterised by either pulmonary or systemic venous congestion or indeed both, which in turn leads to inadequate peripheral oxygen delivery (Roberts 2019). There is always an underlying cause of CCF with congenital heart malformation the most common cause in infants and children. Something happens during foetal life to disrupt the normal development of the heart structures and/or the vessels leading to or from the heart. This might be a missing heart valve or chamber, a hole between two chambers, or a narrowing in a valve, artery, or vein. Such problems can occur singly or in combination. Other acquired heart problems seen in older children (Table 23.1) can also cause CCF.

Question 3. Some children with CCF are cyanosed. Explain why cyanosis occurs in heart disease

Cyanosis is a bluish discolouration of the skin and mucous membranes when children are hypoxic (Mills et al. 2019); however, some children with congenital heart conditions will also present with cyanosis due to the structural malformation of their heart and the presence of deoxygenated blood in the arterial circulation. Blood enters the arterial system from the right side of the heart without going to the lungs to collect oxygen, due to the malformation or abnormal opening in the heart or its

Table 23.1 Causes of congestive cardiac failure.

Common congenital heart malformations		Other causes
Acyanotic	**Cyanotic**	
Patent ductus arteriosus	Tetralogy of Fallot	Infective endocarditis
Atrial septal defect	Tricuspid atresia	Myocarditis
Ventricular septal defect	Transposition of the great arteries	Rheumatic fever
Coarctation of the aorta		Kawasaki disease/syndrome
Aortic stenosis		Bacterial endocarditis
Pulmonary stenosis		Henoch-Schonlein purpura cardiomyopathy severe anaemia
		Hyperthyroidism
		Sepsis

Adapted from (Roberts 2019).

surrounding vessels, for example Tetralogy of Fallot or Transposition of the Great Arteries. For more detail on these and other cyanotic heart defects please read Chapter 9 Disorders of the Cardiac System in (Roberts 2019).

Question 4 Write a holistic care plan for Dora's first 24 hours in hospital, giving a rationale for the prescribed nursing action (see Chapter 10)

Write a holistic care plan for Dora's first 24 hours in hospital, giving a rationale for the prescribed nursing action (see Chapter 10)See Box 23.1.

BOX 23.1 CARE PLAN

Problem	Goal	Nursing action
Breathing		
Dora is breathless with tachycardia,	To ensure a respiratory rate between 20 and 45 breaths per minute (Kelsey & Rylatt 2021).	Ensure Dora is nursed in a sitting position using a baby chair when awake (45 degrees). Tilt cot when Dora is sleeping (45 degrees).
	To ensure a resting apex/pulse rate of 110 and 160 (Kelsey & Rylatt 2021).	Monitor and record apex and respiratory rate every four hours using auscultation/manual palpation techniques and an appropriately sized stethoscope.
		Use continuous bedside monitoring of oxygen saturations, using an appropriately sized and placed oxygen saturation probe and ECG trace.
		Observe and report any undue pallor or cyanosis.
		Administer humidified oxygen if prescribed.

This care plan is based on Dora's history given at the beginning of the chapter highlighting the activities of living which differ from normal and can be supported in the acute setting. The nursing actions described are often required by children with cardiac failure and will often form the basis of any initial care plan. However, children in cardiac failure will require further supportive therapy depending on the additional assessment information collected, the cause of the cardiac failure, the medical plan of care, and the wider needs of the family.

Rationale

Positioning Dora in a semi-upright position and administering prescribed oxygen can reduce respiratory distress (Schroeder et al. 2019).

Her heart rate and respiratory rate should be measured for a full minute to provide an accurate rate and assessment. In children under 2 the apical route provides the most accurate heart rate measurement (Veal & Bailey 2018); however, manual palpation of central pulses such as the brachial or femoral pulse should also be carried out to assess the rate, rhythm, and volume, and ensure the rate is consistent with the apex beat (RCN 2017). Dora's breathing pattern and effort should be assessed for any signs of respiratory distress, also her oxygen saturations should be monitored in order to provide a complete respiratory assessment and enable early identification of any changes/deterioration in Dora's condition. In some children with heart conditions, the level of oxygen circulating in the blood stream can be reduced. Therefore it is important to establish Dora's normal oxygen saturation level and if it is expected to fall outside the normal acceptable limits for oxygen saturations it should be documented to ensure the paediatric early warning score (PEW) is calculated correctly (Veal & Bailey 2018).

Children with cardiac conditions can require oxygen therapy to reduce heart and respiratory rates and decrease the effort of breathing (Schroeder et al. 2019).

	Temperature control	
Dora's temperature regulation is physiologically immature.	Dora's body temperature remains 36–37.5°C. Dora is free of the signs of fever or hypothermia.	Monitor temperature four hourly using the tympanic or axillary route and report any pyrexia. Investigate and treat pyrexia. Wrap warmly if cold.

Rationale
Pyrexia and low body temperature both increase the consumption of oxygen (Schroeder et al. 2019).

	Safety	
Dora is at risk of hospital-acquired infection.	Dora will remain free of infection throughout her stay in hospital.	Explain and demonstrate infection control measures to parents, including hand-washing technique, appropriate disposal of nappies, towels, and bedding.
Dora maybe commenced on medication to improve cardiac function.	To administer medication as prescribed.	Ensure name band *in situ* and checked prior to all administration episodes.
	Monitor and report any side effects of prescribed medications.	Calculate, check doses, and record administration according to local policy.
		Ensure no known allergy to administered substances.
		Note and report any side effects.

Rationale
The use of infection control measures reduces the risks of transmission via hands and clothing.

Dora could be prescribed a range of medications to improve the function of her heart and/or reduce the fluid retention associated with cardiac failure, it is therefore important that guidelines for medicine management (RCN 2020) are followed to diminish the chance of inaccurate calculation or administration.

Communication

Dora is pre-verbal and cannot make her needs known.	Dora will not be distressed by separation and stranger anxiety.	Explain all procedures and interventions to parents, negotiating their role. Encourage parents to hold and speak to Dora during nursing/medical interventions.
Dora's parents may be anxious about her hospital admission.	Dora will maintain developmental milestones during admission.	Replicate home routines where possible.
Dora's mother worried about missing work time.		Allocate nursing staff consistently and minimise number of practitioners working with her.
		Provide toys and play materials as discussed with parents.
		Explain parental residence and visiting policy to parents.
		Negotiate the parent's role in Dora's daily living activities.
		Negotiate parent's level of participation in nursing interventions.
		Establish which friends and family might visit Dora and whether they will be providing any daily care activities when parents cannot be present.

Rationale
The presence and support of parents and family members should be soothing for Dora, preventing separation anxiety. Her parents will be able to provide informed consent for any further investigations or treatments.

Negotiation related to visiting and care activities will help parents to prioritise activities and balance their other commitments.

Nutrition

Dora is having difficulty feeding with poor weight gain.	Dora will gain weight.	Offer feeds three hourly for a maximum of 30 minutes.
		Introduce top-up NG feeds if Dora remains unable to finish feeds.
		Consult dietician about feeding supplements and calorie dense weaning foods.
		Weigh daily at same time on same scale.
		Complete a daily fluid balance chart.

Rationale
Dora may find frequent, smaller feeds easier to finish which will facilitate weight gain. However, frequency of feeding should not be less than three hourly to allow sufficient rest and sleep (Schroeder et al. 2019). However, if feeds remain incomplete, NG feeding will increase the calorie intake associated with milk feeds.

A daily weight will provide information about the success of the feeding regime. The fluid balance chart will highlight any fluid retention. Combined scrutiny of this information will assist the medical practitioner's decisions about on-going treatment.

Sleep

Dora's sleep is disturbed. Parental tiredness	Dora will sleep soundly overnight and have a short nap(s) during the day.	Cluster daily activities and nursing care to ensure rest periods of 2–3 hours and an unbroken sleep pattern.
		Involve family members in comforting activities to try to minimise crying.
		Negotiate regular breaks with parents. Encourage adoption of routines which facilitate sleep.

Rationale
Clustering Dora's care to allow for periods of uninterrupted sleep and rest will help to reduce the workload placed on Dora's heart (Gaskin & Daniels 2021) and conserve her energy. Dora may be less tired and more able to feed if given frequent rest periods. Minimising Dora's stress and preventing episodes of crying will also help to conserve her energy.

Encouraging the parents to take adequate breaks should help them maintain their physical fitness and ability to recognise Dora's needs.

Cleansing and Dressing

Dora is at risk of skin breakdown due to possible oedema and sweating.	Dora's skin will remain intact throughout her hospital admission.	Daily bath.
		Change nappies prior to all feeds.
		Inspect pressure points for redness and abrasions during hygiene procedures and following daily weight.
		Change Dora's position following feeds.
		Use a skin assessment tool such as the Glamorgan scale to assess Dora's skin.

Rationale
Cleansing Dora's skin, assessing her skin regularly, using a skin assessment tool, and changing her position will reduce the chances of redness and pressure ulcers caused by tissue compression developing (Schroeder et al. 2019).

Question 5. Explain the immediate investigations that Dora may need to establish the possible cause of her cardiac failure

Initially Dora will be assessed by the medical staff who will take a detailed history about Jane's pregnancy and Dora's birth.

A chest X-ray will provide information about the size and shape of the heart, demonstrating any enlargement and any congenital problem, which has changed the silhouette (Gaskin & Daniels 2021).

An ECG will provide a record of the electrical activity of Dora's heart, including the rate, rhythm, and spread of the electrical impulse, conduction problems, and age-related changes in children (Gaskin & Daniels 2021).

Echocardiography uses high-frequency sound waves to provide visual images of the structure of the heart and surrounding vessels allowing any structural defects or abnormalities to be identified before and after birth and for on-going assessment (Schroeder et al. 2019).

Cardiac catheterisation is an invasive diagnostic procedure, usually combined with angiography, that child may undergo to obtain further diagnostic information from within their heart and involves the insertion of a radio-opaque catheter through a peripheral blood vessel into the heart (Gaskin & Daniels 2021; Schroeder et al. 2019).

Blood tests carried out include haematocrit, haemoglobin, and red cell count, giving further information related to oxygenation. Sodium, potassium, and calcium levels may be assessed.

Follow-up action plan

Dora's case history has introduced the problems of an infant with cardiac failure, but the practitioner will need to broaden their knowledge. Further study is recommended related to:

1. The anatomy and physiology of the normal heart.
2. Signs and symptoms associated with the disorders listed in Table 23.1.
3. The pathophysiology of congestive cardiac failure in all age groups.
4. Medications which are used to support children with cardiac problems, including cardiac glycosides, angiotensin-converting inhibitors, and diuretics.

REFERENCES

Boyd, D.G. & Bee, H.L. (2014) *The Developing Child*, 13th edn. Harlow: Pearson.

Gaskin, K.L. & Daniels, A. (2021) Caring for children and young people with cardiovascular problems. In: Glasper, A., Richardson, J. and Randall, D. (eds). *A Textbook of Children's and Young People's Nursing*, 3rd edn. London: Elsevier.

Gormley-Fleming, E. (2022) *Children and Young People's Nursing Skills at a Glance*. Chichester: Wiley-Blackwell.

Holland, K., Jenkins, J. & Solomon, J. (2019) *Applying the Roper, Logan & Tierney Model in Practice*, 3rd edn. Edinburgh: Churchill Livingstone.

Kelsey, J. (2021) Physical growth and development in children. In: Glasper, A., Richardson, J. and Randall, D. (eds). *A Textbook of Children's and Young People's Nursing*, 3rd edn. London: Elsevier.

Kelsey, J. & Rylatt, L.A. (2021) Respiratory illness in children. In: Glasper, A., Richardson, J. and Randall, D. (eds). *A Textbook of Children's and Young People's Nursing*, 3rd edn. London: Elsevier.

Kidd, M. & Rodgers, C.C. (2019) Health promotion of the infant and family. In: Hockenberry, M.J. & Wilson, D. (eds). *Wong's Nursing Care of Infants and Children*, 11th edn. St Louis: Mosby Elsevier.

Mills, E., Court, R. & Fidment, S. (2019) Disorders of the respiratory system. In: Gormley-Fleming, E. & Peate, I. (eds). *Fundamentals of Applied Pathophysiology, an Essential Guide for Nursing and Health Care Students*. Oxford: Wiley Blackwell.

Roberts, S. (2019) Disorders of the cardiac system. In: Gormley-Fleming, E. and Peate, I. (eds). *Fundamentals of Applied Pathophysiology an Essential Guide for Nursing and Health Care Students*. Oxford: Wiley Blackwell.

Royal College of Nursing (2017) *Standards for Assessing, Measuring and Monitoring Vital Signs in Infants Children and Young People*. London: RCN.

Royal College of Nursing (2020) *Medicines Management, an Overview for Nursing*. London: RCN.

Schroeder, L.M., Baker, A.L., Bastardi, H. & O'Brien, P. (2019) The child with cardiovascular dysfunction. In: Hockenberry, M.J., Wilson, D. & Rodgers, C.C. 2019 (eds). *Wong's Nursing Care of Infants and Children*, 11th edn. St Louis: Mosby Elsevier.

Shapcott, J. (2018) Effective communication with children and young people. In: Price, J. & McAlinden, O. (eds). *Essentials of Nursing Children and Young People*. London: Sage.

Veal, Z. & Bailey, J. (2018) Care of children and young people with cardiovascular problems. In: Price, J. & McAlinden, O. (eds). *Essentials of Nursing Children and Young People*. London: Sage.

Care Planning – Surgical Procedures

SECTION 6

CHAPTER 24

Tonsillectomy

Jodie Kenny and Doris Corkin

SCENARIO

Mark weighs 40 kg, is eleven years of age, and is in the concrete-operational stage of development (Bee & Boyd 2013). He is an only child and lives with his mum, Anna, and dad, Patrick. Mark has no known health problems, apart from mild asthma which is well controlled using Seretide® 50 mcg two puffs twice daily and Ventolin 100 mcg two puffs as required. He is allergic to ibuprofen which exacerbates his asthma. Other than that, Mark has no known allergies. He has never been in hospital and has never had a general anaesthetic.

For the past two years Mark has suffered from recurrent tonsillitis, requiring antibiotic treatment at least five or six times a year. As a result Mark has missed long periods off school and this is affecting his overall academic performance. His GP referred him for an ENT consultation. At this consultation the specialist advised that Mark should have his tonsils removed. The ENT surgeon explained to Mark and his parents what the surgical procedure would entail and possible complications. Mark's mum signed his consent form and Mark's name was placed on the waiting list for a tonsillectomy.

This surgical procedure requires a short admission to hospital and a general anaesthetic.

It can be very painful post-operatively and is occasionally complicated by bleeding.

Mark and his parents were invited to attend the pre-admission clinic, one week before his hospitalisation. At this clinic both parents and child are prepared for what is to happen both preoperatively and post-operatively and they are given the time to ask questions. Furthermore, it also gives them the opportunity to meet both the nurses and doctors who will be involved in their care. However, Mark's mum is very anxious about the surgery. Refer to Box Activity 24.1.

ACTIVITY 24.1

Please refer to British National Formulary for Children (BNFc 2020–2021).

1. As ibuprofen is a non-steroidal anti-inflammatory drug should Mark be prescribed this medication?

2. Using appropriate formula, what should the prescribed dose of paracetamol be for Mark, who weighs 40 kg? (see care planning in Chapter 28, for example of formula).

3. What should the prescribed dose of codeine be for Mark?

QUESTIONS

1. What is a tonsillectomy?

2. Having reflected upon the nursing process and models of care, how would the children's nurse prepare this young boy, Mark, and his family preoperatively?

3. Describe the nursing care of Mark on his return to the ward during the immediate post-operative period (first 24 hours).

4. What discharge advice will be given to Mark and his parents?

   Mark has been readmitted to ward with history of secondary post-operative bleeding. Blood results (Hb <7 g/dl; GAIN 2009) and history from his mum indicate a significant blood loss.

5. Discuss the nursing care of Mark when receiving a blood transfusion.

Care Planning in Children and Young People's Nursing, Second Edition. Edited by Sonya Clarke and Doris Corkin.
© 2024 John Wiley & Sons Ltd. Published 2024 by John Wiley & Sons Ltd.

ANSWERS TO QUESTIONS

Question 1. What is a tonsillectomy?

Tonsils are oval-shaped masses of lymphatic tissue located on either side of the back of the throat. Their function is to prevent the entry of bacteria and viruses into the body via the nose and throat, thus protecting the gastrointestinal system from infection (McConochie 2001).

A tonsillectomy is a surgical procedure carried out to remove the tonsils. Some of the indications for this can be: following recurrent throat infections, suspected malignancy, sleep apnoea, or peritonsillar abscess.

Each year in the UK thousands of children under fifteen years of age have their tonsils removed.

Question 2. Having reflected upon the nursing process and models of care how would you the children's nurse prepare this young boy Mark and his family preoperatively?

Assess/plan/preoperative implementation and evaluation.

Models of care (Casey 1995; Roper et al. 1996).

- On arrival at the ward Mark and his family are taken to his bed. He is shown where to put his belongings and how to activate his television. Mark is introduced to his 'named nurse'.

- A family-centred approach (Casey 1995) is adopted and Mark and his family are encouraged to participate in his care. They are shown around the ward, toilets, parent's facilities, theatres, and where the recovery ward is located.

- All available biographical details are confirmed with Mark's parents and when correct his patient identification armband is applied.

- Mark has baseline observations taken: temperature, pulse, respirations (TPR), oxygen saturation levels, and blood pressure (BP). These are recorded as per ward preoperative checklist.

- Mark's weight of 40 kg and height are recorded on his anaesthetic chart and medicine chart.

- A full medical history is taken and Mark's allergy to ibuprofen is highlighted on his medicine chart and anaesthetic chart. The nurse will establish if he has any current throat infections or head colds. If he does the anaesthetist must be informed and Mark's surgery would possibly be cancelled due to the higher risk of post-operative infection and bleeding.

- A family medical history is taken to establish any problems with general anaesthetic or bleeding.

- Mark and his family are introduced to the multidisciplinary team, consultant anaesthetist, consultant surgeon, ward doctor, nurses, and play therapist.

- Check that the consent form has been signed and dated by one of Mark's parents and they are fully aware what they have consented to.

- Check preoperative fasting times are adhered to: normally two hours for clear fluids and six hours for solids (RCN 2005).

    Note: Research has shown that drinking clear fluids one hour before surgery does not appear to increase the risk of aspiration (Kelly & Walker 2015). *However, it is advisable to adhere to anaesthetic instructions on fasting times.*

- Apply anaesthetic cream to venous accesssite as prescribed by doctor.

- Ensure Mark and his parents are given a full and clear explanation regarding what will happen in anaesthetic room. If it is hospital policy, a parent and 'named nurse' should be able to accompany the child until they are asleep.

- Preoperative checklist: confirm Mark's details are correct against his armband and both medical and nursing notes. Weight, baseline observations, allergies, any loose teeth (crowns or braces) should be noted. Confirm signed consent form, and pre-medication administered if ordered by anaesthetist. Also check fasting times have been adhered to and offer parents the opportunity to accompany Mark to theatre.

- Prepare Mark's bed space for his return. Ensure working oxygen and suction in case of emergency. Have cardiovascular monitoring ready (to be inclusive of SpO2, HR, and BP in the post-operative period) and nursing care documentation. Also a box of disposable tissues and emesis bowl should be available in case Mark feels nauseated post-operatively.

Question 3. Describe the nursing care of Mark in relation to the immediate post-operative period (first 24 hours), having returned to the ward

A tonsillectomy is considered one of the most painful procedures despite being recognised as a minimally invasive surgery thus optimal pain management is imperative in the post-operative period (Aldamluji et al. 2021).

Assess and plan post-operative intervention.

Activity of living: maintaining a safe environment (Roper et al. 1996).

- Family-centred care approach (Casey 1995), if hospital policy, parents will be brought into recovery to be with Mark as he starts to awaken. Mark and his parents will be involved in all aspects of his care. They will accompany him back to his bed space on the ward.

Implement post-operative intervention.

- If Mark is still asleep, attach him to monitor, explaining its purpose to his parents.
- Read medical and nursing notes and adhere to anaesthetist and surgeon's instructions.
- Document in nursing care plan medications and analgesia Mark has received in theatre and recovery.
- Monitor and record Mark's TPR, oxygen saturations, and BP on return to ward Post-operatively, Observations should be monitored at least half hourly for the first four hours and as often as the patient's condition dictate thereafter.
- Mark should be observed for any bleeding from his mouth or nose; dry and wet gauze can be weighed for blood loss accuracy and any findings should be reported to the surgeon immediately. Blood loss can sometimes be difficult to measure as the tonsil bed can ooze slowly over a long period of time however, staff must remain vigilant to potential post-operative blood loss. .
- Mark should also be observed for excessive swallowing and or pallor, as children will often swallow blood post-operatively.
- Person-centred care imperative – ask Mark how he is feeling as well as providing reassurance.
- Hospital policy must be adhered to regarding care of intravenous (IV) cannula, using a Visual Infusion Phlebitis (VIP) Scoring chart.
- If vomiting occurs, monitor and record amount, content and frequency, observing for any sign of fresh bleeding. Administer antiemetic as prescribed and monitor and record effect/side effects.
- Any fresh blood in vomit must be reported immediately to surgeon in case Mark needs to return to theatre.
- Administer analgesia as prescribed and monitor and record effect/side effects.
- When fully conscious and there are no obvious signs of bleeding, Mark can be given sips of water to drink initially. If tolerated then progress to free fluids and a light diet.
- It is important that Mark should drink and eat a normal diet post-operatively when considered appropriate. This aids healing by keeping the throat clean and moist.
- It is also important that Mark be given analgesia at least half an hour before meal times. If his throat is sore he will be reluctant to eat or drink, and there is then a greater risk of infection and post-operative bleeding.
- Ensure Mark's IV cannula is removed prior to discharge.

Question 4. What discharge advice will be given to Mark and his family?

Activity of living: communication (Roper et al. 1996).

Discharge advice

- Mark and his family will be advised of the importance of taking regular analgesia as prescribed. Try to take pain relief about half an hour before meals. The throat tends to be sorest first thing in the morning and at fifth day post-operatively.
- It is very important that Mark eats and drinks when he goes home so that he is well hydrated. This helps keep his throat moist and clean and aids healing.
- Some earache is normal; however, if pain is excessive see GP.
- At any sign of bleeding/haemorrhage either from the nose or throat Mark needs to be seen by an ENT doctor immediately. Parents are advised to contact the ward immediately, so that the doctor can be made aware of their impending arrival at A&E department.
- Mark is advised to stay off school for two weeks and stay indoors for the first two to three days, avoiding smoky atmospheres.
- Parents are given the ward contact number and told to phone at any time if they require advice.

Post-tonsillectomy haemorrhage is a common encounter/complication post surgery and can be categorised into two types:

There are two types of haemorrhage that may occur following a tonsillectomy:

- Primary
- Secondary

Primary haemorrhage occurs within the first 24 hours post-operative period while secondary haemorrhage occurs after the first 24 hours (Aldrees et al. 2022). Surgical intervention may be required for severe post-operative bleeding.

Secondary haemorrhage is usually associated with sloughing and/or infection at the operation site (Ikoma et al. 2014).

Question 5. Discuss the nursing care of Mark when receiving a blood transfusion

In relation to a blood transfusion, patient safety including minimising risk is crucial. Also ensure informed and valid consent (NICE Clinical Guideline NG24).

Activity of living: communication/maintaining a safe environment (Roper et al. 1996).
Refer to Box Activity 24.2.

Please note: it is very important that nurses adhere to hospital policy before, during, and after administering blood to patients, i.e. in exceptional circumstances, it may be recommended to send a 'group and save' to the laboratory pre-operatively.

ACTIVITY 24.2

Access and review the following resources:

Royal College of Nursing (2006) *Right Blood, Right Patient, Right Time: RCN Guidance for Improving Transfusion Practice.* London: RCN.
Thompson, C.L., Edwards, C. & Stout, L. (2008) Blood transfusions 2: signs and symptoms of acute reactions. *Nursing Times,* **14** (3), 28–9.
Serious Hazards of Transfusion (SHOT 2009) http://www.shotuk.org.
New, H.V., Beeryman, J., Bolton-Maggs, P.H. et al (2016) Guidelines on transfusion for foetuses, neonates and older children. *British Journal of Haematology,* **175** (5), 784-828.
http://www.learnbloodtransfusion.org.uk/e-learning for safe, effective and appropriate transfusion practice.

- Mark and his family should be fully informed by the doctor of his need for a blood transfusion, the likely duration of it and consent must be obtained and recorded in his medical records.
- Mark's pre-infusion observations should be taken and recorded: T, P, R, and BP.
- Ensure that Mark is wearing an identification armband, stating his name, date of birth, and hospital number.
- Blood must be prescribed by a doctor on the blood prescription sheet. This sheet must also have Mark's name, date of birth, and hospital number on it. The doctor must prescribe the blood product, infusion rate, start and finish times, and it must be transfused within four hours.
- Two registered nurses must complete **independent checks** to ensure Mark's details, blood group, expiry date and laboratory number correspond with his prescription sheet, blood bag and blood component form.
- Ensure two nurses bring all this documentation to Mark's bedside and then ask him to clarify his name and date of birth. This will be double checked by asking the child's parents the same details.
- Again, two nurses check Mark's name, date of birth, and hospital number against his wristband.
- Only when all checks are correct is blood administered.
- Sodium chloride 0.9% is first flushed through the blood infusion set, ensuring no air bubbles are present, before connecting blood transfusion.
- Mark and his parents are asked to inform the nurse should he experience any of the following symptoms:
  – Sweating
  – Mottled appearance
  – Dizziness
  – Rash
  – Flushed appearance pyrexia
  – Tachycardia
  – Nausea

Mark will be closely observed for any of these signs of an adverse reaction and will not be left unattended for the first 15 minutes of the blood transfusion or as policy dictates.

- Mark will also be observed for any major adverse reactions:
  – Rigors
  – Breathlessness/wheeze
  – Chest pain
  – Back or loin pain
  – Loss of consciousness
  – Collapse
- Should Mark experience any of these symptoms the blood transfusion should be stopped immediately and medical assistance called; the blood component should be retained.
- Marks observations T, P, R, and BP should be taken after the first 15 minutes of the blood transfusion commencing and again at the end of the transfusion or more frequently should his condition require.

- His infusion site should be checked at least hourly for any redness, swelling, tenderness, or leakage – using appropriate VIP scoring chart.
- When the blood transfusion is completed the children's nurse should ensure Mark's nursing notes are accurately recorded. Refer to Box Activity 24.3.

ACTIVITY 24.3

Answer these questions about blood transfusion.

1. When should a blood infusion be started following removal from refrigerator?
   a) 15 minutes
   b) 20 minutes
   c) 25 minutes
   d) 30 minutes

2. Which of the following do BCSH guidelines.com/(2009) recommend that the blood unit should be checked with:
   a) Doctor prescription
   b) Compatibility report
   c) Patient ID
   d) All of the above

3. Prior to administering blood, the giving set should be primed with:
   a) 0.5% dextrose
   b) 0.9% glucose
   c) 0.5% sterile water
   d) 0.9% sodium chloride

4. Current guidelines recommend that for every blood component transfused the following vital signs should be recorded *before* the start of each transfusion:
   a) Temperature, pulse, and respiration
   b) Temperature and pulse
   c) Temperature, pulse, respiration, and blood pressure
   d) Temperature, respiration, and blood pressure

5. Adverse reactions usually occur within
   a) First five minutes
   b) First 15–20 minutes
   c) First 60 minutes
   d) After transfusion complete

6. In prolonged transfusion of consecutive units the giving sets must be changed:
   a) After 2–6 hours
   b) After 8–12 hours
   c) After 12–16 hours
   d) No need to change giving set

7. A blood transfusion should be completed within
   a) 4 hours
   b) 3 hours
   c) 5 hours
   d) 8 hours

8. On completion of transfusion each/all packs must be kept at ward level for
   a) 12 hours
   b) 24 hours
   c) 48 hours
   d) 72 hours

ANSWERS TO ACTIVITIES

Answer to activity 24.1

1. Ibuprofen should not be prescribed as the patient is allergic to it.
2. Paracetamol 15–20 mg/kg 4–6 hourly per day. No more than four doses in 24 hours. Mark could be prescribed 800 mg per dose.
3. Codeine is prescribed 0.5–1 mg/kg 4–6 hourly. Mark could be prescribed 20 mg per dose.

Answers to activity 24.3

1. (d) 30 minutes.
2. (d) All of the above.
3. (d) 0.9% sodium chloride.
4. (c) Temperature, pulse, respiration, and blood pressure.
5. (b) First 15–20 minutes.
6. (b) After 8–12 hours.
7. (a) Four hours.
8. (c) 48 hours.

REFERENCES

Aldamluji, N., Burgess, A., Pogatzki-Zahn, E., Raeder, J. & Beloeil, H. (2021) PROSPECT guideline for tonsillectomy: systematic review and procedure-specific postoperative pain management recommendations. *Anaesthesia*, **76**, 947–961.

Aldrees, T., Alzuwayed, A., Majed, A., Alzamil, A., Almutairi, M. & Aloqaili, Y. (2022) Evaluation of Secondary Post-Tonsillectomy Bleeding among Children in Saudi Arabia: Risk Factor Analysis. *Ear, Nose & Throat Journal*, **101**(3), NP135-NP142. doi: 10.1177/0145561320944662.

Bee, H. & Boyd, D. (2013) *The Developing Child*, 13th edn. London: Pearson.

British Committee for Standards in Haematology (BCSH) (2009) *The Administration of Blood Components*. https://b-s-h.org.uk/guidelines/guidelines/administration-of-blood-components [Accessed 6 March 2023].

British National Formulary for Children (BNFc) (2020–2021) *British National Formulary for Children*. British Medical Journal. London: PS Publishing.

Casey, A. (1995) Partnership nursing: influences on involvement of informal carers. *Journal of Advanced Nursing*, **22**, 1058–1062.

Guidelines & Audit Implementation Network (GAIN) (2009) *Better Use of Blood in Northern Ireland: Guidelines for Blood Transfusion Practice*. Belfast: DHSSPS (GAIN, formerly known as CREST) https://nitransfusion.com/blood-20guidelines.pdf.

Ikoma, R., Sakane, S., Niwa, K. et al (2014) Risk factors for post-tonsillectomy hemorrhage. *Auris Nasus Larynx*, **41**(4), 376–379.

Kelly, C.J. & Walker, R.W. (2015) Perioperative pulmonary aspiration is infrequent and low risk in pediatric anesthetic practice. *Pediatric Anesthesia*, **25**, 36–43.

McConochie, J. (2001) Pathophysiology of tonsils, post – tonsillectomy bleed, treatment and nursing care. In: Sadik, R. & Campbell, G. (eds) *Client Profiles in Nursing: Child Health*. London: Greenwich Medical.

NICE 2015 Clinical Guideline NG24 – Blood Transfusion: assessment for and management of blood transfusions in adults, young people and children over 1 year old (health-ni.gov.uk).https://www.nice.org.uk/guidance/ng24 [Accessed 6 March 2023].

Roper, N., Logan, W. & Tierney, A.J. (1996) *The Elements of Nursing*, 4th edn. Edinburgh: Churchill Livingstone.

Royal College of Nursing (2005) *Perioperative Fasting in Adults and Children: An RCN Guideline for the Multidisciplinary Team*. London: RCN.

Royal College of Nursing (2006) *Right Blood, Right Patient, Right Time: RCN Guidance for Improving Transfusion Practice*. London: RCN.

CHAPTER 25

Appendicectomy

Fearghal Lewis
(acknowledge Lorna Liggett)

SCENARIO

Catarina, a seven-year-old girl, is admitted to the children's surgical ward with a history of vomiting and abdominal pain for the past six hours. Following an in-depth nursing assessment and medical examination Catarina is diagnosed as having appendicitis and has been prepared for theatre to have an appendicectomy.

Catarina and her parents have recently immigrated to the UK (United Kingdom) from Portugal. Catarina's father works in a local factory which involves 12-hour shifts, and her mother works part-time as a server in a local restaurant. Both can speak good English and do not need an interpreter for everyday situations.

Catarina attends the local primary school and is progressing well for her age.

The operation notes indicate that the appendix was slightly inflamed and therefore removed. The wound was sutured with six dissolvable sutures and a simple dressing was applied. Pain relief was given in the operating room. After a brief period in the recovery ward, Catarina was transferred to the ward where her mother was waiting for her.

Two aspects of care postoperatively will be addressed; these are wound care and communication.

QUESTIONS

1. Explain the pathophysiology of appendicitis.
2. What are the stages of wound healing and types of dressings?
3. How does the children's nurse plan the care for Catarina in relation to personal cleansing and dressing?
4. Discuss how the children's nurse would utilise a family-centred approach to Catarina and her mother to explain postoperative care in relation to wound care.

The proposed scenario incorporates two nursing models for planning care, i.e. Roper et al. (2000) and Casey (1988). The author recommends the student undertake the additional reading.

ANSWERS TO QUESTIONS

Question 1. Explain the pathophysiology of appendicitis

The appendix is located in the right iliac fossa region of the abdomen, where it is attached to the caecum. History would inform us, that the appendix has no function, although more recent studies have shown that the appendix provides a level of protection against invading pathogens in the gut (Smith 2022). In some circumstances, the appendix may become inflamed, and the patient can suffer acute appendicitis.

The exact cause of acute appendicitis remains unknown, but it is thought that half of all cases are caused by a blockage of the lumen due to hard impacted faeces, enlarged lymph nodes, foreign objects, or tumours (Rentea et al. 2017). As a result of the blockage, the intra-luminal pressure is raised and causes the wall of the appendix to become distended. Normal mucus secretions cause a further build-up of intra-luminal pressures and distension, which in turn cause compression and ischaemia of the mucosal walls.

Care Planning in Children and Young People's Nursing, Second Edition. Edited by Sonya Clarke and Doris Corkin.
© 2023 John Wiley & Sons Ltd. Published 2023 by John Wiley & Sons Ltd.

Because of a reduction in blood supply to the wall of the appendix, there will be little or no nutrition and oxygen reaching the appendix. As a consequence, a reduced supply of white blood cells and other natural fighters of infection found in the blood are being made available to the appendix. Eventually, if left untreated the appendix will become necrosed and the formation of pus, which increases the likelihood of perforation occurring. If perforation were to occur, the contents of the appendix and bowel can enter the abdomen causing peritonitis.

Pain in appendicitis is caused initially by the distension of the wall of the appendix, and later when the grossly inflamed appendix rubs on the overlying inner wall of the abdomen and then with the spillage of the content of the appendix into the general abdominal cavity (peritonitis). The pain is usually noted in the right iliac fossa region of the abdomen and is associated with abdominal tenderness, guarding, and vomiting.

Fever is brought about by the release of toxic materials following the necrosis of the wall of the appendix, and later by pus formation.

Question 2. What are the stages of wound healing and types of dressings?

Revise the stages of wound healing:

- Inflammatory stage
- Destructive stage
- Proliferative stage
- Maturation stage

For further reading please see National Institute for Health and Care Excellence Evidence Summary (2016).

When undertaking wound care, it is important to consider wound assessment, cleansing solutions, and type of dressing (see Table 25.1). Following an assessment of the wound, health professionals should consult with the multidisciplinary team as to which approach would be the most appropriate.

Table 25.1 Types of wound dressings.

Types of dressing	Examples	Use
Absorbent dressings	Primapore, Mepore	These can be applied directly to the wound or used as secondary absorbent layers in the management of heavily exuding wounds.
Low-adherence dressings and wound contact materials	Paraffin Gauze Dressing, Xeroform	These are usually cotton pads that are placed in direct contact with the wound. The addition of paraffin and similar substances is largely to stop the dressing from sticking to the wound.
Alginate dressings	Curasorb, Sea-Sorb, Sorbsan	These are highly absorbent and come in the form of calcium-alginate or calcium-sodium alginate, and they can be combined with collagen. The alginate forms a gel when in contact with the wound surface, which can be lifted off at dressing removal or rinsed away with sterile saline. Bonding to a secondary viscose pad increases absorbency.
Foam dressings	Allevyn, Biatain, Tegaderm Foam	These dressings normally contain hydrophilic polyurethane foam and are designed to absorb wound exudate and maintain a moist wound surface.
Hydrogel dressings	ActiformCool, Aquaflo	These consist of cross-linked insoluble polymers and up to 96% water. They are designed to absorb wound exudate or to rehydrate a wound, depending on wound moisture levels. They are supplied as flat sheets, as an amorphous hydrogel or as beads
Hydrocolloid dressings	GranuFLEX, NU DERM, Aquacel (Fibrous alternative)	These occlusive dressings are usually composed of a hydrocolloid matrix bonded onto a vapour-permeable film or foam backing. This matrix forms a gel that provides a moist environment when in contact with the wound surface
Antimicrobial dressings	Honey-, iodine-, and silver- impregnated dressings	Honey-impregnated dressings contain medical-grade honey, which is thought to have antimicrobial and anti-inflammatory properties and can be used for acute or chronic wounds.
		Iodine-impregnated dressings release free iodine, which is thought to act as a wound antiseptic when exposed to wound exudate.
		Silver-impregnated dressings are used to treat infected wounds, as silver ions are thought to have antimicrobial properties.

Adapted from Dumville et al. (2015).

Assessing the postoperative wound

It is important that the nurse checks the patient's wound before leaving the operating department, assessing the wound, the dressing, and if there are any drains in situ. The children's nurse should always read the operation notes to ascertain how the procedure went and any special instructions to be followed.

- Appearance: if a wound dressing is in place it is important not to disturb this, other than to inspect the wound dressing for signs of intermediary bleeding. If no dressing is in place the nurse must continue with the assessment of the wound.
- Size: the children's nurse must note the size of the wound and the location of any dehiscence.
- Drainage: the children's nurse must observe the location of the wound, colour, exudate, and odour.
- Exudate: fluid arising from the wound due to increased permeability of the capillaries; this will influence dressing type.
- Odour: an offensive odour is a sign of infection that needs to be assessed to identify an appropriate wound dressing.
- Inflammation: the children's nurse must observe for swelling and redness, though some slight swelling is normal in the early stages of wound healing.
- Infection: this needs to be addressed as it can affect wound healing. Swabs should be taken for microbiology to assess what is causing the infection.
- Pain: assess pain using an appropriate assessment tool (Wong et al. 2012).
- Drains/tubes: if any, which type of drain was used, the amount and colour of exudate in the reservoir.

Wound cleansing solutions

An aseptic non-touch technique is required for changing or removing surgical wound dressings. When cleaning the wound, it is advised that sterile saline water is used up to 48 hours after surgery; patients are advised that they may shower safely 48 hours after surgery. The use of tap water for wound cleansing is advised after 48 hours if the surgical wound has separated or has been surgically opened to drain pus (National Institute for Health and Care Excellence 2020).

Care planning for a child following an appendicectomy: in-depth focus

Question 3. How does the children's nurse plan the care for Catarina in relation to personal cleansing and dressing?

Activity of daily living: personal cleansing and dressing.
Potential problem: Catarina's wound is at risk of becoming infected.
Goal: to promote wound healing and prevent infection.
Nursing intervention:

- Explain to Catarina and her mother that the wound will be cleansed and redressed, to ensure they understand the intervention.
- Ensure strategies, such as pain assessment tools and distraction therapy, are in place to minimise wound pain before commencing, to ensure successful outcomes (Nilsson & Renning 2012).
- Educate Catarina and her mother regarding the importance of not removing the dressing until the wound has healed.
- Discuss the process of wound cleansing with Catarina and her mother.
- Prepare child, equipment, environment, and self to undertake aseptic technique.
- Carry out an aseptic technique using the non-touch technique (Bruce et al. 2022).
- Report and record on completion in order to promote continuity of care and collaboration between all professionals.

- Ensure Catarina is comfortable at all times.
- Encourage Catarina to ask questions and respond to these in an age-appropriate manner.
- Educate Catarina and her mother when it is appropriate to shower or have a bath.

Evaluation: the purpose of this stage of the nursing process is to evaluate the progress towards the set goal in the care plan. If progress is not being made or is slow then the nurse must report and document this. Then the care plan may require to be modified accordingly. If goals have been achieved then the care can stop. Any new problems which arise can be identified at any stage and measurable goals must be negotiated and agreed upon with Catarina and her family.

All documentation must be available to members of the multidisciplinary team to perform the agreed care and update if necessary. Examples of questions the nurse could ask herself:

- Is the wound healing?
- What is the status of the wound?
- What are the priorities for caring for Catarina?
- Is her condition stable?
- What are her clinical observations?
- Is she progressing, i.e. drinking, mobile, relatively pain-free?
- When will she be discharged, who will be at home with her?

The collection of data to determine the extent to which the set goals are achieved is crucial to the evaluation.

Question 4. Discuss how the children's nurse would utilise a family-centred approach to Catarina and her mother to explain postoperative care in relation to wound care. Refer to Box Activity 25.2

ACTIVITY 25.2

Review the key components of family-centred care: see Chapter 1.
Also references: Glasper et al. (2021) and Griffin and Celenza (2014).

Good communication is essential when working with children, young people, and their families since it assists in building up trust and encourages them to feel comfortable in seeking advice. Children, young people, and their families have the right to be fully informed and involved in all decisions about their treatment and plan of care (Bell & Condren 2016). The nurse must always communicate with children and young people in an age-appropriate manner and appreciate personal circumstances and the needs of the person. In order to build a good rapport, the nurse must show respect, understanding, and be honest throughout as this will have a positive impact on their lives (DfCSF 2010). Refer to Box Activity 25.3.

ACTIVITY 25.3

Reflect upon your practice using the Gibbs (1988) reflective cycle as seen in Figure 25.1.
Consider a recent experience in caring for a young person whilst in practice.
Explore your communication skills with the young person.

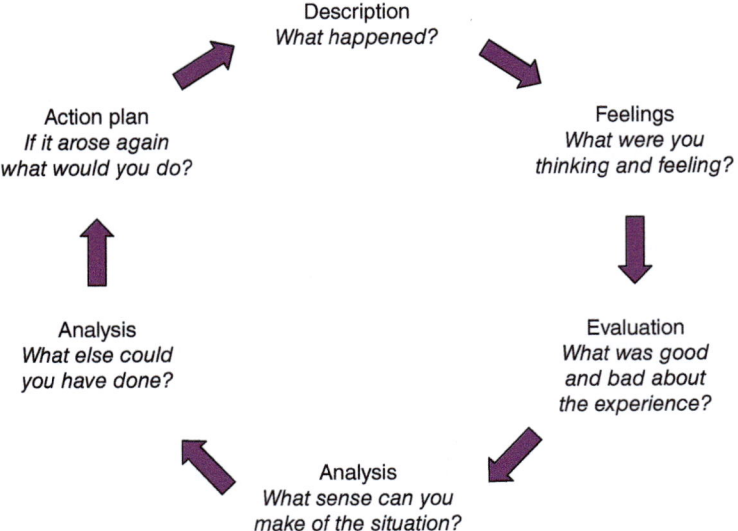

FIGURE 25.1 Activity of daily living – communication (adapted from Gibbs 1988).

Activity of daily living: communication (Gibbs 1988).
Potential problem: Catarina and her mother may not fully understand the information given to them and the medical terminology used. This could lead to misinterpretation and advice and guidance not being followed through.
Goal: to ensure Catarina and her mother fully understand the information given to them.
Nursing intervention: the children's nurse must:

- Take account of Catarina's cognitive ability (Crowley 2017).
- Use a family-centred approach throughout to promote collaboration and partnership (Glasper et al. 2021).
- Sit down with Catarina and her mother and speak slowly to ensure understanding.
- Appreciate the mother's ability to understand and contact a translator if necessary, so that the information is accurate.
- Determine Catarina and her parents' level of understanding regarding the surgery and subsequent care.
- Give time for them to ask questions, listen to them, and respond appropriately to ensure no misinterpretation.
- Reassess their understanding on a regular basis.
- Share all information with parent and child regarding progress, to promote understanding.
- Recognise the family's strengths and methods of coping.
- Encourage and facilitate parent-to-child support.
- Provide information leaflets to reinforce verbal information.
- Incorporate the developmental needs of Catarina to promote her independence.
- Provide play/distraction therapies.

Evaluation: this is an important aspect of nursing care which can be productive, satisfying, and rewarding. Evaluation of the care plan provides a tool to reflect on current practices, identify ways to improve care and services to patients, and also builds a solid foundation for continuous quality improvement initiative. Evaluation helps the nurse to learn how to meet the child and family's needs more efficiently and to follow progress over time. It also helps to identify things which are going well and provides positive feedback to the child and family.

- The nurse should select each point from the plan of care and report and record the outcome/progress.
- The children's nurse should explain the operation to Catarina's mother when Catarina returns to the ward.
- When Catarina awakes from the anaesthetic the nurse should explain that she has returned to the ward and her mother is there.
- Ensure Catarina is comfortable and relatively free from pain.
- The nurse will seek consent from Catarina to look at the wound site.
- The nurse should take time to explain the on-going care of Catarina to her mother: when she can have oral fluids, if she can sit up in bed or walk to the toilet and how long she may be in hospital for.
- Negotiate with Catarina's mother what aspects of care she wishes to be involved in.
- When Catarina is fully awake, relatively pain-free and clinical observation is within normal limits, the nurse should reassess her progress and report and record.
- Arrange for a play therapist to visit Catarina.
- Select appropriate leaflets for both to read.

REFERENCES

Bell, J. & Condren, M. (2016) Communication strategies for empowering and protecting children. *The Journal of Pediatric Pharmacology and Therapeutics*, **21**(2), 176–184.

Bruce, E., Williss, J. & Gibson, F. (2022) *The Great Ormond Street Hospital Manual of Children and Young People's Nursing Practices*. Chichester, UK: Wiley Blackwell.

Casey, A. (1988) The development and use of the partnership model of nursing care. In: Glasper, E.A. & Tucker, A. (eds). 1993. *Advances in Child Health Nursing*. London: Scutari Press.pp. 183–193.

Crowley, K. (2017) *Child Development: A Practical Introduction*. Los Angeles, CAL: SAGE.

Department for Children, Schools and Families (2010) *Effective Communication with Children, Young People and Families. Every Child Matters*. London: DfCSF. www.dcsf.gov.uk/everychildmatters/strategy/deliveringservices/commoncoreofskills.

Dumville, JC., Keogh, S.J., Liu, Z., Stubbs, N., Walker, R.M. & Fortnam, M. (2015) Alginate dressings for treating pressure ulcers. *Cochrane Database of Systematic Reviews 2015*. Issue 5. Art. No.: CD011277. DOI: 10.1002/14651858.CD011277.pub2.

Gibbs, G. (1988) *Learning by Doing: A Guide to Teaching and Learning Methods*. Oxford: Further Education Unit, Oxford Brookes University.

Glasper, E., Richardson, J. & Randall, D. (2021) *A Textbook of Children's and Young People's Nursing*. London, UK: Elsevier.

Griffin, T. & Celenza, J. (2014) *Family-centered Care for the Newborn: The Delivery Room and Beyond*. New York, NY: Springer Publishing Company, LLC.

National Institute for Health and Care Excellence (2016) *Chronic Wounds: Advanced Wound Dressings and Antimicrobial Dressings*. London: NICE.

National Institute for Health and Care Excellence (2020) *Surgical Site Infection: Prevention and Treatment of Surgical Site Infection*. London: NICE.

Nilsson, S. & Renning, A.-C. (2012) Pain management during wound dressing in children. *Nursing Standard*, **26**(32), 50–55.

Rentea, R., Peter, S. & Snyder, C. (2017) Pediatric appendicitis: state of the art review. *Pediatric Surgery International*, **33**(3), 269–283.

Roper, N., Logan, W.W. & Tierney, A.J. (2000) *The Roper-Logan-Tierney Model of Nursing: Based on the Activities of Living*. Edinburgh: Elsevier Health Sciences.

Smith, H. (2023) A review of the function and evolution of the cecal appendix. *The Anatomical Record*, **306**(5), 972–982.

Wong, C., Lau, E., Palozzi, L. & Campbell, F. (2012) Pain management in children: part 1 — pain assessment tools and a brief review of nonpharmacological and pharmacological treatment options. *Canadian Pharmacists Journal / Revue Des Pharmaciens du Canada*, **145**(5), 222–225.

Care of Infants and Young Persons with Orthopaedic Conditions

SECTION 7

Ilizarov Frame

CHAPTER 26

Sonya Clarke

SCENARIO

Patrick is 14 years old and lives in a two-storey town house with his parents and five-year-old-sister Annie. As an active seven-year-old Patrick regularly cycled in the local park. However, as he attempted to cross the busy road that leads to the park a car collided with him due to poor visibility. Patrick was taken to A&E, where his condition was stabilised and a diagnosis of a growth plate arrest injury confirmed; he was then transferred to the children's ward. Post-discharge Patrick's condition continued to be monitored long term under the care of an orthopaedic consultant. But over time the road traffic collision (RTC) resulted in a 6 cm leg length discrepancy (LLD), where one leg became shorter than the other due to the growth plate arrest.

A child with LLD walks on the toes of the short leg, with the heel never touching the ground, whereas the adult walks with a heel toe gait on short side and vaults over the long leg. The result is excessive up and down motion of the pelvis and trunk. Long-term effects include scoliosis, hip adduction, and flexion or recurvatum on the long side and equinus deformity on the short side. Patrick was subsequently monitored regarding his LLD.

Patrick now wears a 'shoe raise' which he hates as it makes him appear 'different', even though it equalises his leg length and aids mobility. During a consultation with his orthopaedic surgeon, it was agreed for Patrick to be admitted to hospital for elective surgery which involves application of an Ilizarov frame to his right tibia (see Figure 26.1) in order to correct the 6 cm leg length discrepancy. Limb lengthening will be achieved via osteogenesis distraction with the frame in situ for approximately six months (see Table 26.1 for principles of limb lengthening). Successful limb equalisation would mean Patrick would be able to wear normal shoes and trainers like his peer's following removal of the frame.

QUESTIONS

1. What is an Ilizarov frame/Ilizarov technique?
2. Reflecting upon the nursing process and a model of care how would the children's nurse prepare this young person and his family for application of an Ilizarov frame?
3. Discuss the nursing care of Patrick in relation to the immediate post-operative period (first 24 hours), having returned to the ward.
4. In an attempt to prevent pin site infection, how will Patrick (and his family) be educated and supported to undertake pin site care/management.
5. How would the children's nurse prepare Patrick and his family for discharge, following application of an Ilizarov frame?

The proposed answer plans offer 'lists of potential responses' with limited rationale. It is therefore recommended for the individual student/healthcare professional to explore the issues through further reading.

ANSWERS TO QUESTIONS

Question 1. What is an Ilizarov frame/Ilizarov technique?

Ilizarov frame/fixation is used for fracture fixation and stabilisation, limb reconstruction, deformity correction, and limb lengthening, using wires instead of pins and a circular frame instead of bars (Santy et al. 2009).

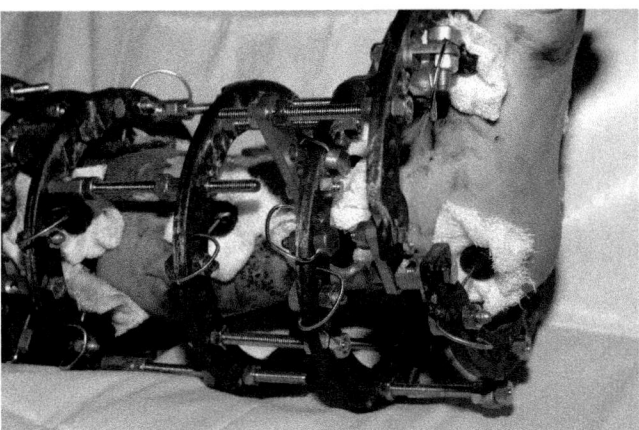

FIGURE 26.1 Ilizarov frame (Clarke and Richardson (2008), *reproduced with permission of Elsevier*).

Table 26.1 Principles of limb lengthening.

An established three-phase process was adopted (Zhang et al. 2019) – latency/delay, distract, and consolidate.
Minimal disturbance of the bone
Latency period/delay before distraction: this allows osteogenesis formation to begin
Rate of distraction: 1 mm a day (0.25 mm per 6 hours)
The duration of the consolidation phase depends on the amount of bone to be lengthened 6 cm = 6 months' consolidation

Ilizarov technique: a bone-fixation technique using an external fixator for lengthening limbs, correcting pseudarthroses and other deformities, and assisting the healing of otherwise hopeless traumatic or pathological fractures and infections, such as chronic osteomyelitis. The method was devised by the Russian orthopaedic surgeon Gavriil Abramovich Ilizarov (1921–1992) (G.A. Ilizarov – Ilizarov Centre).

Question 2. Reflecting upon the nursing process and a model of care how would the children's nurse prepare this young person and their family for application of an Ilizarov frame?

Activity of living: maintaining a safe environment.

Assess: determine the young person's and parents' level of knowledge in relation to all aspects of hospitalisation care.

Plan: the children's nurse must ensure Patrick and his parents are given appropriate preoperative preparation at ward level, which will involve physical and psychological care, the induction of a general anaesthetic (GA), pain management, the actual surgical procedure, and what to expect post-surgery regarding application of the Ilizarov frame (as shown in Table 26.2). All planned care should adopt an appropriate model of nursing, for example Casey (1988) and Roper et al. (1990). Please note, even though Roper et al. (1990) addresses 12 activities of daily living (ADL) (refer to Chapter 1) this chapter will only address the problems in preoperative and post-operative care in relation to the ADL – maintaining a safe environment.

Implement/preoperative interventions:

- Patrick should be settled into an allocated bed space appropriate for his age, be comfortable with the ward surroundings, and introduced to the nurse assigned to his care.

- Globally the needs of children and young people differ to those of adults and an increasing expectation is that children and young people should participate in health care decisions that affect them (Clarke 2021). Therefore, the care should have Patrick at the centre and be inclusive of the family, for example consideration given to their views, open visiting, and access to tea-making and overnight facilities for a parent if required. Explain what an Ilizarov

Table 26.2 Phases of treatment.

- Preoperative
- Latency period: initial post-operative period
- Distraction (approx. 1/3 of time in frame)
- Starts about 5–7 days post-operatively
- mm day divided into four increments or 0.25 cm every six hours
- Consolidation (approx. 2/3 of time in frame)
- Removal of frame (6–12 months approx.)
- Rehabilitation

frame is, show pictures, models and if possible, introduce Patrick and parents to another child with a frame *in situ*.

- Facilitate Patrick and his parents to raise any concerns they have regarding application of the frame, complications, returning to school, social activity, and the effects of altered body image for a 14-year-old boy.
- Complete and record base line vital signs on a paediatric early warning score (PEWS) chart, for example – temperature, pulse, pain score, respirations, SAO_2, and blood pressure (BP).
- Complete a ward urinalysis, if nothing abnormal detected (NAD) record and proceed, otherwise report and send mid-stream specimen of urine (MSSU) to laboratory for organism and sensitivity (O&S).
- Record weight and height accurately.
- Apply patient identification armband(s).
- Complete baseline venapuncture (may be undertaken by nurse or doctor) and send to laboratory as ordered by anaesthetist, full blood picture (FBP), and urea and electrolytes (U&E), plus 'group and hold' (blood for transfusion usually not ordered as operation carried out using tourniquet with minimal blood loss).
- Teach an appropriate pain assessment tool, a scale of 0–10 would be appropriate for a 14-year-old young person, where 0 is 'no pain' and 10 is the 'most imaginable pain' (Clarke 2003a).
- Discuss potential pain management options:
  – Patient controlled analgesia (PCA)
  – Continuous epidural infusion (Clarke 2003b; Wheetman 2006)
  – Intravenous paracetamol (Clarke & Richardson 2007) and step-down medication.
- Record full medical history, known allergies, establish if smoker/non-smoker, any family problems with a GA, etc.
- Facilitate informed consent (medical responsibility) through verbal, written, and visual display of an Ilizarov frame.
- Multidisciplinary approach and introduction to team: anaesthetist, consultant, named nurse, physiotherapist, occupational therapist (OT), and specialist Ilizarov nurse.
- Information on maintaining an Ilizarov frame, i.e. pin site care.
- Risk assessment using a dedicated tool, for example Waterlow (1998) score, and placed on appropriate pressure relieving device (bed and mattress).
- Plan discharge date.
- Preoperative fasting times as per anaesthetist's instructions (normally two hours for fluids and six hours for solids), patient shower, clean bed, gown *in situ*, and premedication administration if prescribed.

- Check out system; confirm patient details are correct, weight, allergies noted, notes, blood results and X-rays available, confirm signed consent form, and pre-medication administered if ordered. Gaining Patrick's verbal assent to the procedure, reinforces them as a service user and rights holder (UNCRC 1989). Also record if fasting times are adhered to and offer parents to accompany Patrick to theatre.

- Prepare Patrick's bed space to ensure a safe environment following his return from surgery – collect appropriate documentation, check oxygen and suction equipment is working, and gather any necessary monitoring or infusion devices.

- Evaluate all nursing interventions and complete all appropriate documentation as per hospital policy.

Question 3. Discuss the nursing care of Patrick in relation to the immediate post-operative period (first 24 hours), having returned to the ward

Activity of living: maintaining a safe environment.

Assess and plan post-operative interventions:

- Person-centred approach inclusive of parents, i.e. consider the parents when collecting Patrick from recovery and returning to the prepared bed space.

Implement post-operative interventions:

- Attach Patrick to appropriate monitoring and infusion equipment as per hospital policy.

- Read medical and nursing notes, adhering to anaesthetist and surgeon instructions.

- Ensure Patrick is comfortable, using appropriate tool, i.e. assess pain score (0–10), reposition Patrick, review risk assessment, for example Waterlow (1998).

- Observations to be completed and recorded on dedicated post-operative chart with appropriate action as per hospital protocol:
  – TPR, SAO_2 (oxygen saturations), and BP
  – Neurovascular observations of the operated lower limb are imperative, inclusive of pain intensity as he is at risk of developing acute compartment syndrome (RCN 2014)

- Check actual Ilizarov frame (as above), pin sites for ooze, bleeding, and signs of infection.

- Hospital protocol must be adhered to regarding care of cannula, i.e. patency and management of intravenous (IV) fluids

- Record all input and output on a fluid balance chart.

- Administer analgesia as ordered by anaesthetist. Patrick would most likely receive either a morphine based PCA, or an epidural infusion with a local anaesthetic. Both would be in conjunction with regular IV paracetamol. Nurse to observe for potential side effects of opioids. Analgesia can be used in conjunction with non-pharmacological methods, for example music.

- Monitor IV fluids and cannula site (as per hospital protocol). Patrick may also tolerate sips of water later in the day as directed by the anaesthetist. Also monitor output on fluid balance chart, reporting any concern to anaesthetist. Patrick may also have an indwelling urinary catheter – this often accompanies an epidural infusion (Wheetman 2006) which associated with orthopaedic surgery.

- Patrick to be reviewed by pain management team and physiotherapist.

- Occupational therapist to review Patrick to make foot splint which aims to prevent neurovascular complication, i.e. dropped foot.

- Consider Patrick's altered body image and privacy needs of a young person.

- Patrick to be reviewed by Ilizarov team: orthopaedic consultant, anaesthetist, physiotherapist and specialist nurse.

- Administer IV prophylactic antibiotics as per hospital protocol.
- Complete check X-ray as per consultant's instruction.

    Evaluate all nursing interventions and documents.

Question 4. In an attempt to prevent pin site infection, how will Patrick be educated and supported to undertake pin site care/management

A review by Georgiades in 2018:36 states, *'the goal of pin site care is to reduce, or where possible, prevent pin site infection'*. The author also reports on the care of external fixator pin sites to remain debated and researched among scholars, this has highlighted a number of variances and issues in pin site care. There is an absence of high-quality data and research to support any one particular type of dressing in reducing pin site infection, including the use of pin site crusts (Lethaby et al. 2013; Timms & Pugh 2012). The use of multiple pins has increased the risk of complications such as intractable pain, tethering and tenting of the surrounding skin, muscle spasm, swelling and soft tissue tension, and infection at the pin site, which is the main concern and can result in loosening of the pin, loss of fixation and osteomyelitis (Patterson 2005). In the UK the expert British nursing consensus group on pin site care (Lee-Smith et al. 2001) differentiate clearly between the term's 'reaction', 'colonisation', and 'infection' when discussing pin site care. Pin site care which is identified by Santy (2000) as requiring specialised nursing care is a psychomotor skill initially undertaken by the nurse and then executed by either the child or parent following appropriate education and a period of supervised practice. The most up-to-date Cochrane review on site care for preventing infections associated with external bone fixators and pins remains by Lethaby et al. in 2013 is presented in Table 26.3.

Like the first edition, Clarke and Richardson (2008) demonstrate the contemporary 'Russian' method (Table 26.4). Variations continue to be adopted by UK practitioners, for example figure of eight bandaging – recurring steps include weekly cleansing, use of pressure at pin sites, no showering of limb in-between showering and cleansing solution. This information should be used in conjunction with local guidelines for wound care, infection control and following discussion and agreement with other relevant members of the healthcare team and reviewed on an on-going basis.

ACTIVITY 26.1

Consider the impact on 'the family' when Patrick returns home with an Ilizarov frame on his leg for six months.

Table 26.3 Cochrane review by Lethaby et al. (2013) – current best level of evidence.

Summary
• A total of eleven trials (572 participants) were eligible for inclusion in the review but not all participants contributed data to each comparison.
• Three trials compared a cleansing regimen (saline, alcohol, hydrogen peroxide, or antibacterial soap) with no cleansing (application of a dry dressing), three trials compared alternative sterile cleansing solutions (saline, alcohol, peroxide, povidone iodine), three trials compared methods of cleansing (one trial compared identical pin site care performed daily or weekly and the two others compared sterile with non-sterile techniques), one trial compared daily pin site care with no care and six trials compared different dressings (using different solutions/ointments and dry and impregnated gauze or sponges).
• One small, blinded study of 38 patients found that the risk of pin site infection was significantly reduced with polyhexamethylene biguanide (PHMB) gauze when compared to plain gauze (RR 0.23, 95% CI 0.12 to 0.44) (infection rate of 1% in the PHMB group and 4.5% in the control group) but this study was at high risk of bias as the unit of analysis was observations rather than patients.
• There were no other statistically significant differences between groups in any of the other trials.

Table 26.4 'Russian pin site cleansing' (Clarke & Richardson 2007).

Points	Action	Rationale
1.	Prepare patient: seek verbal consent, check patient's position, and record pain score. Collect the required equipment: Dressing pack Sterile scissors Sterile gloves Bandages Non-sterile gloves Forceps (optional) Hydrex – pink chlorhexedine gluconate 0.5% w/v 70% v/v 'Non-woven' gauze squares	Potential pain during pin site dressings. Offer analgesia if appropriate. Day 2 post-surgery (approx.), reduce and renew dressings. Thereafter dressings will be changed at seven-day intervals (a shower can be taken prior to pin site care). No fibres to be left at pin site.
2.	Wash and dry hands, put on plastic apron.	Prevent cross infection.
3.	Pull back black rubber bungs (see below).	To provide access to existing dressings.
4.	Apply non-sterile gloves, remove existing bandages, dressings and discard in a clinical waste bag.	To expose pin sites.
5.	Inspect all pin sites.	Observe for signs of infection, etc.
6.	Wash hands.	Prevent cross infection.
7.	Open all sterile dressings and equipment to be used.	In preparation for aseptic technique.
8.	Apply sterile gloves.	To prevent cross infection.
9.	Prepare sterile gauze squares by making slit in the gauze (keyhole dressing; see below).	To allow gauze to fit over wire at the pin site.
10.	Using a separate piece of gauze (gloved finger or forceps), clean each individual pin site with Hydrex- 0.5% w/v 70% v/v alcohol solution using a sweeping action. Rubber bung	In an attempt to prevent infection at pin site.
11.	Do not remove crusts or scabs. Keep metal work socially clean.	In an attempt to prevent infection at pin site.
12.	Moisten all required gauze squares in Hydrex- 0.5% w/v 70% v/v alcohol solution and remove excess liquid from each gauze square.	In an attempt to prevent infection at pin site and reduce skin irritation.
13.	Apply the moistened keyhole gauze square dressing to each pin site. Keyhole dressing	Keyhole dressings of gauze, 2–3 layers thick moistened with Hydrex solution – alcoholic chlorohexidine. With excess liquid removed to prevent infection and skin irritation.
14.	Position the rubber bung onto each pre-soaked square gauze at each pin site (as demonstrated).	To secure gauze stays in position at pin site.
15.	Bandaging each pin site (optional) or alternative.	Bandaging in figure of eight to secure dressings and ensure that the bungs do not lift.
16.	Place solutions in a secure cupboard and discard all dressings, gloves, and apron in clinical waste bag/bin.	Health and safety. To prevent cross infection.
17.	Wash hands.	To prevent cross infection.

Table 26.4 (Continued)

Points	Action	Rationale
18.	Re-assess patient's pain score.	Review analgesia.
19.	Teach patient and family a similar regime.	Tampering with pin sites excessively can lead to infection.
	Keep regime simple and provide instruction.	Expect poor or non-compliance.
20.	Educate patient/family and community staff to look for signs of pin infection.	To identify problems early.
	In some cases, arrangements can be made to have the dressings completed by the Ilizarov nurse specialist.	
21.	Provide verbal and written information with contact numbers.	To reduce anxiety, increase compliance, and provide support.
	Provide opportunities to contact other patients and support groups.	
22.	Provide psychosocial support.	Pins/wires amount to a major insult to self-image.

Adapted from Davies et al. (2005) and Lee Smith et al. (2001).

Question 5. How would the children's nurse prepare Patrick and his family for discharge, following application of an Ilizarov frame?

Activity of living: maintaining a safe environment.

- Commence discharge planning on admission: reflect upon Patrick's stage of development and identify individual needs *(assess)*.
- Early *planning*: ensure Patrick is eating and drinking normally in conjunction with a normal urinary output and bowel function.
- *Implementation*: establish communication pathways with MDT and refer to community health care, i.e. children's community nurse.
- Physiotherapy input regarding mobilisation, check if Patrick can complete stairs and educate on elevation of limb with crutches to aid mobility.
- Educate Patrick on a healthy balanced diet and effects of smoking (it can interfere with bone healing).
- Occupational therapy referral (pre surgery) for potential housing aids, urinal, and wheelchair for distance, etc.
- Patrick to be taught and then demonstrate competence in undertaking the osteogenesis component of the distraction process.
- Promote good mental health – returning to school and socializing with friends.
- Also teach and observe Patrick's competence in cleaning his pin sites as per hospital protocol in conjunction with the signs of infection (Clarke & Richardson 2008).
- An adapted 'Russian method' of pin site cleaning is currently used across the UK (Davies et al. 2005; Santy 2006), practitioners await on an impending Cochrane Review to further guide practice in how to most effectively clean pin sites and reduce infection.
- Provide contact numbers to enable troubleshooting with specialist/ward nurse regarding potential problems, for example pin site infection, neurovascular compromise (e.g. swelling, discoloured toes, cool to touch), pain, or early consolidation (fracture of new bone growth – it goes 'pop'), etc.

- Outpatient date to be given to review Patrick's progress.
- Check X-ray to be completed and viewed – discharge to be confirmed by orthopaedic consultant *(evaluation)*.
- Doctor's letter for GP given to Patrick.
- Liaise with Patrick's school regarding returning to school or home tuition.
- Three-day supply of medication discussed, checked, and given to Patrick with his parents; may include paracetamol and short-term codeine for pain. Discuss possibility of constipation due to restricted mobility and medication, may also be prescribed a stool softener.
- Discuss future admission and procedure to remove Ilizarov frame.
- Allow Patrick and his parents to ask questions.
- Document all care and discharge interventions.

REFERENCES

Casey, A. (1988) A partnership with child and family. *Senior Nurse*, **8**(4), 8–9.

Clarke, S.E. (2003a) Orthopaedic paediatric practice: an impression pain assessment. *Journal of Orthopaedic Nursing*, **7**(3), 132–136.

Clarke, S.E. (2003b) Postoperative pain in children: a retrospective audit of continuous epidural analgesia in a paediatric orthopaedic ward. *Journal of Orthopaedic Nursing*, **7**(1), 4–9.

Clarke, S.E. (2021) An exploration of the child's experience of staying in hospital from the perspectives of children and children's nurses using child-centered methodology, comprehensive child and adolescent nursing, doi: 10.1080/24694193.2021.1876786

Clarke, S.E. & Richardson, O. (2007) Using intravenous paracetamol in children following surgery: a literature review. *Journal of Children's and Young People's Nursing*, **1**(6), 273–280.

Clarke, S.E. & Richardson, O. (2008) Skeletal pin site care, Chapter 42 In: Kelsey, J. and McEwing, G. (eds). *Clinical Skills in Child Health Practice*. London: Churchill Livingstone Elsevier, 379–387.

Davies, R., Holt, N. & Nayagam, S. (2005) The care of pin sites with external fixation. *Journal of Bone and Joint Surgery*, **87B**, 5, 716–719.

Lee-Smith, J., Santy, J., Davis, P., Jester, R. & Kneale, J. (2001) Pin site management. Towards a consensus: part 1. *Journal of Orthopaedic Nursing*, **5**, 37–42.

Lethaby, A., Temple, J. & Santy-Tomlinson, J. (2013). Pin site care for preventing infections associated with external bone fixators and pins. *Cochrane Database of Systematic Reviews*, (1): CD004551. doi:10.3109/02699206.2014.926994

Patterson, M. (2005) Multicenter pin site study. *Orthopaedic Nursing*, **24**(5), 349–359.

Roper, N., Logan, W. & Tierney, A. (1990) *The Elements of Nursing*, 3rd edn. London: Churchill Livingstone.

Royal College Nursing (RCN) (2014) Peripheral Neurovascular Observations for Acute Limb Compartment Syndrome. London : RCN

Santy, J. (2000) Nursing the patient with an external fixator. *Nursing Standard*, **14**(31), 47–52.

Santy, J. (2006) A survey of current practice in skeletal pin site management. *Journal of Orthopaedic Nursing*, **10**, 198–205.

Santy, J., Vincent, M. & Duffield, B. (2009) The principles of caring for patients with Ilazarov external fixation. *Nursing Standard*, **23**(6), 50–55.

Timms, A. & Pugh, H. (2012). Pin site care: guidance and key recommendations. *Nursing Standard*, **27**(1), 50–55.

UNICEF (1989) *A New Charter for Children 3/88*. UNICEF/UK Information Sheet No. 8. UNICEF, London.

Waterlow, J. (1998) Pressure sores in children: risk assessment. *Paediatric Nursing*, **10**(4), 22–23.

Wheetman, A. (2006) Use of epidural analgesia in postoperative pain management. *Nursing Standard*, **20**(44), 54–64.

Zhang, X., Zhang, T., Liu, T. et al (2019) Lengthening of free fibular grafts for reconstruction of the residual leg length discrepancy. *BMC Musculoskelet Disord*, **20**(2019), 66. https://doi.org/10.1186/s12891-019-2445-z.

Developmental Dysplasia of the Hip

CHAPTER 27

Sonya Clarke

SCENARIO

Wai-ki is a five-month-old baby girl who recently emigrated from China with her parents. During a routine visit to their GP (General Practitioner) concerns were raised regarding Wai-ki's lower limbs. A physical examination showed an uneven crease fold, leg length discrepancy, limited range of movement, with no evidence of pain. Both parents were present at the appointment with dad interpreting (mumum has limited English). Wai-ki was referred to a paediatric orthopaedic consultant following her clinical examination.

A second physical examination in conjunction with an X-ray of Wai-ki's hips confirms developmental dysplasia of the right hip (DDH). The parents agree to an elective admission to a children's orthopaedic ward following an informed discussion with the paediatric orthopaedic consultant. Wai-ki is scheduled for a closed reduction of her right hip, adductor tenotomy, and application of a hip spica cast (see Figures 27.1 and 27.2) under general anaesthetic.

Wai-ki undertakes the planned surgery (Dad was available to interpret) and returns to the ward in a double hip spica plaster with no complications.

The proposed case history incorporates two nursing models for planning care, i.e. Roper et al. (2000) and Casey (1988). The author recommends additional reading around the specialist area of orthopaedics, examples include the Royal College of Nursing (2019) Competency Framework for Orthopaedic and Trauma and relating publication on how the guidance was developed (Barnard et al. 2020).

QUESTIONS

1. What is developmental dysplasia of the hip (DDH)?
2. What is a hip spica, and what does it do for Wai-ki?
3. How does the children's nurse plan the care for Wai-ki in relation to *'controlling body temperature'*? (Use the commonly adopted model of care by Roper et al. (2000) and Casey's model of nursing (1988), which advocates working in partnership with children and their families.)

ANSWERS TO QUESTIONS

Question 1. What is developmental dysplasia of the hip (DDH)?

Vaquero-Picado et al. (2019, p. 548) suggest the term DDH *'includes a wide spectrum of hip alterations: neonatal instability; acetabular dysplasia; hip subluxation; and true dislocation of the hip'*. A change in terminology from congenital hip dysplasia (CDH) to DDH more accurately reflects the varying onset and types of hip abnormalities in which there is a shallow acetabulum, subluxation, or dislocation (Kneale & Davis 2005). Clinical screening (instability manoeuvres) should be carried out universally as a part of the physical examination of the new-born – after two or three months of life, limited hip abduction is the most important clinical sign (Vaquero-Picado et al. 2019). In a meta-analysis by Hundt et al. (2012) only familial aggregation, breech presentation, females and clicking

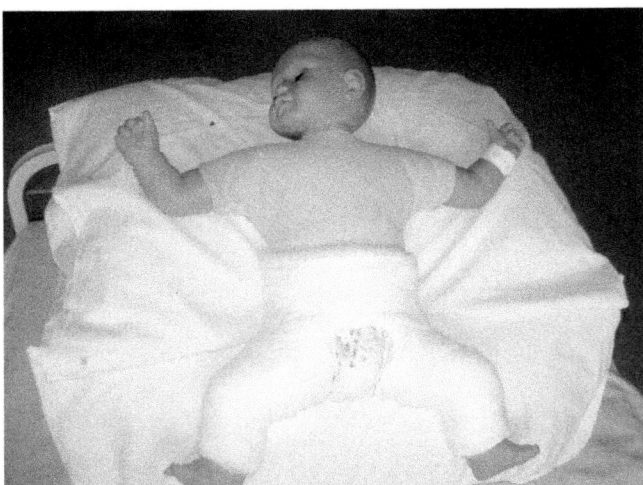

FIGURE 27.1   Child in hip spica cast. The nappy is effectively tucked into the hip spica.

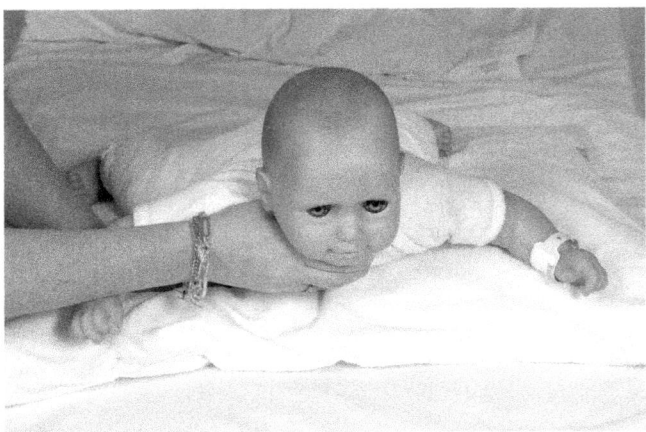

FIGURE 27.2   Child in hip spica cast, positioned prone with head supported.

hips in exploration demonstrated an increased risk for DDH. The higher the age at presentation, the worse the outcomes after intervention, it is also the main cause of a total hip replacement in young people – about 21–29% (Vaquero-Picado et al. 2019).

Question 2. What is a hip spica/spica cast and what does it do for Wai-ki?

Young children (under the age of five years) who present with the condition DDH or fractured femur continue to be managed using body casting (Apley & Soloman 2008; Clarke & Dowling 2003; Clarke & Drozd 2023; Vaquero-Picado et al. 2019). As no clear-cut term is used for body casting, confusion may arise for parents and health professionals (i.e. body cast/hip spica/frog plaster/spica cast). The hip spica is composed of plaster of Paris or synthetic material. Variations in spica cast position are influenced through child diagnosis, i.e. fracture versus DDH. The spica cast presents with the leg(s) +/– full extension, +/– hip(s) abduction, +/– knee flexion and either long or partial leg in plaster, i.e. double or one and a half spica cast. For the child in spica cast, a brief stay in hospital is necessary to dry the plaster and prepare for discharge. Table 27.1 includes general management information in relation to hip spica management. For additional information refer to Hip Dysplasia (DDH) via the 'STEPS Charity' (stepsworldwide.org).

The hip spica cast demonstrated in Figures 27.1 and 27.2 aim to maintain abduction of the femoral head within the acetabulum of the hip joint, as containment encourages normal femoral head development within the pelvis.

Care planning for child in hip spica: in-depth focus: see Figure 27.3.

Table 27.1 General hip spica information (adapted from Clarke & McKay 2006).

- Plaster of Paris is not waterproof.
- It will take at least 48 hours for the cast to dry.
- Special care must be taken to prevent damage to the cast during the first 48 hours.
- The child cannot bend at the waist! They should be nursed on pillows and turned every two hours during the day and every four hours at night until the cast is dry (*during hospitalisation as supervised by nurse as potential increased risk of 'sudden infant death' (SID) formally known as 'cot death'). Most deaths occur under 6 months old (Sudden infant death syndrome (SIDS) – NHS) (www.nhs.uk)
- Check circulation to the feet (neurovascular observations) (RCN 2021).
- The cast should be firm and fit snugly.
- The edges will be padded, a bar may be fitted to stabilise the cast and MUST NEVER BE USED TO LIFT WITH. When dry, a reinforcing layer can be added to strengthen the hip spica.
- When the cast is dry, the child can be positioned on a blanket either on the floor, or on a beanbag.
- Always put toys within reach of the child.
- The child may crawl in a safe environment.
- Do not allow your child to insert small toys or objects under the cast.
- Your child can be nursed, not carried, do not hip nurse, as the added weight is harmful to the carer's spine and posture.
- Standing in a cast is usually *not* advised.
- Care and attention need to be given to the child regarding temperature control, to avoid a febrile convulsion while in hip spica.

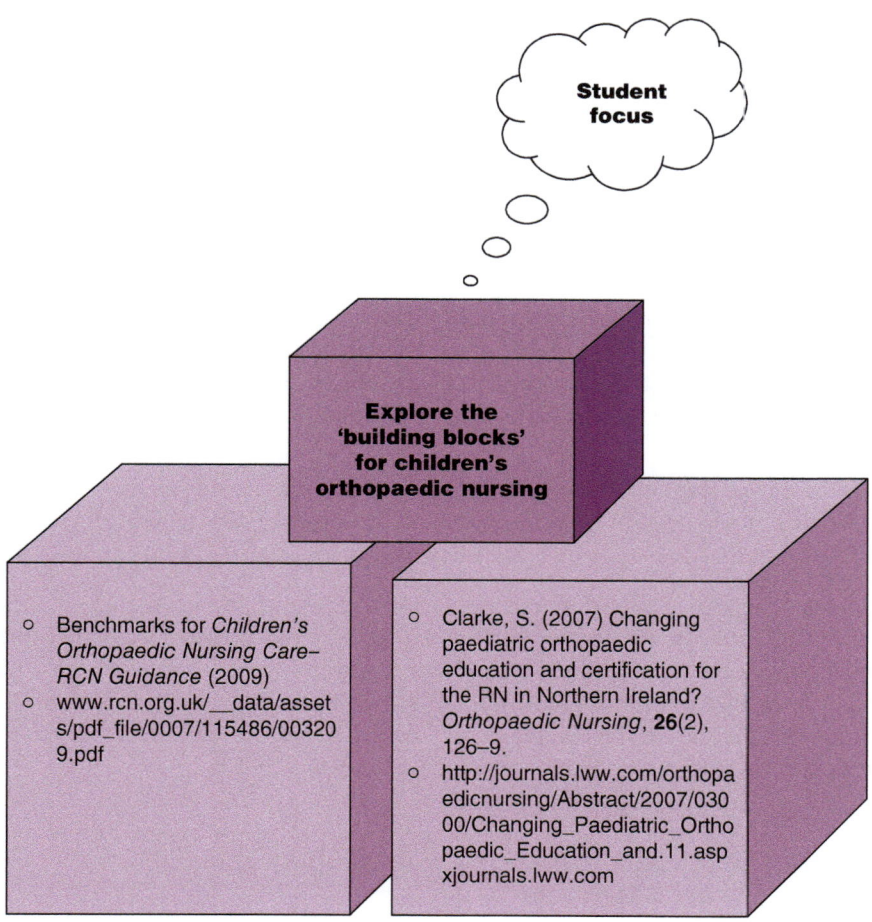

FIGURE 27.3 Student focus.

Question 3. How does the children's nurse plan the care for Wai-ki in relation to *'controlling body temperature'*? (Use the commonly adopted model of care by Roper et al. (2000) and Casey's model of nursing (1988), which advocates working in partnership with children and their families.)

Activity of daily living: controlling body temperature.

Potential problem:

Wai-ki is at risk of developing a pyrexia or febrile convulsion due to her age and application of a hip spica, i.e. legs, abdomen, and lower chest covered by plaster of Paris, stockinet, and padding.

Goal: to prevent or safely manage an elevated temperature, pyrexia, or febrile episode.

Nursing intervention:

- Educate parents on the implications of their daughter's underdeveloped hypothalamus in relation to controlling body temperature and the potential for 'regular assessment'.
- Inform parents on the normal temperature for their daughter at five months old, to be around 36.4°C but can vary slightly from child to child (NHS 2021).
- Educate parents on the 'basic signs' of fever, i.e. baby warm to touch, flushed, irritable, crying, sleepy, etc.
- Educate the parents on the relevant terms, i.e. fever/febrile (state of elevated temperature/fever), hyperthermia (elevated body temperature), and pyrexia (elevation of body temperature up to 38°C or more) (NICE 2018).
- Educate and determine parental competence in the application of a suitable tool that can evaluate their daughter's temperature; the ideal thermometer should be accurate, reliable, and safe. The National Institute for Clinical Excellence (NICE 2019) recommend using either an electronic or chemical dot thermometer in the axilla or infra-red tympanic thermometer to measure Wai-ki's body temperature.
- Position the child out of direct sunlight using safe moving and handling techniques.
- Educate the parents on how best to care for their child in a hip spica, washing, positioning, etc. (refer to Tables 27.1 and 27.2 plus Figures 27.1 and 27.2).
- Educate parents on the need for light bedding and clothing as a third of Wai-ki's body is covered in plaster of Paris and padding, which can act as an insulator.
- Educate on the effects/side effects and administration/dosage of antipyretics in the management of pyrexia. NICE (2018) guidance suggests guidance should include advice to parents/carers on the use of antipyretic treatment such as Paracetamol or Ibuprofen if the child is uncomfortable or distressed and not to routinely treat children who are well. They also report the non-use of Aspirin as an antipyretic.
- Educate the parents on the purpose of increasing fluids (with caution) and removal of upper clothing. NB. The child loses most of their heat through the head so care needs to be taken regarding the use of a hat.
- Educate on the safety/implications of older practice, i.e. tepid sponging, and fan therapy. A randomised controlled trial (RCT) by Thomas et al. (2009, p. 133) (N = 150) suggests 'apart from the initial rapid temperature reduction, addition of tepid sponging to antipyretic administration does not offer any more advantage in ultimate reduction of temperature; moreover, it may result in additional discomfort'. Refer to recent NICE guidance – Feverish illness in children: assessment and initial management in children younger than 5 years | Guidance | NICE.
- Discuss future admission and procedure to remove hip spica.
- Allow parents to ask questions.
- Document all care and discharge interventions.

Evaluation: Wai-ki's body temperature remained within normal limits post-surgery (remember to document).

Table 27.2 Care planning for the child in hip spica: quick general overview (adapted from Clarke & McKay 2006).

- **Washing and dressing**

    Problem: how do I wash my child's body and hair?

    Goal: to safely wash child's hair and body.

    Intervention:

    1. No baths. Wash with flannel or sponge using soap (if applicable) and moisturise skin.

    2. Wash hair over bath or basin: protect cast from water.

    Useful notes

    Wash child on bed turning from tummy to back.

    For hair washing the parent can sit on a chair or bed edge and support child's head on a plastic covered parent's knee over a basin or bath – use jug or shower.

    Rationale: to keep child clean and ensure good circulation.

    Use two people for carer and child safety.

    Check circulation – colour of skin should be pink and warm.

    Evaluate: outcome of care.

- **Mobilisation/positioning**

    Problem: can my child be comfortable?

    Goal: ensure child comfort.

    Intervention:

    1. Change position regularly (two hourly – on back/tummy/position at 30-degree tilt).

    2. Use pillows and wedge to change position.

    3. Older children can turn themselves. Encourage turning, as it will make the child more comfortable.

    4. Do not lift child by the arms but lift with hand supporting their bottom.

    Rationale: prevents pressure sores.

    Child at night should be on their back to reduce risk of SID.

    Younger children should sleep on their backs and in their parents' room (use pillows (with care) and wedge in cot so they not lying flat).

    Evaluate: outcome of care.

- **Elimination**

    Problem: how will my child go to the toilet?

    Goal: to attend to child's elimination needs effectively.

    Intervention:

    1. If your child uses a nappy continue to do so. If not, use a bedpan or urinal. Child may regress during time in hip spica, i.e. may need to use nappy if recently potty trained.

    2. Nappies, bedpan, and urinal may be available and free of charge from your health visitor/children's nurse.

    3. A child's nappy size may need to be reduced due to application of a hip spica (see Figure 27.1).

    Rationale: to ensure safe toileting/prevent skin breakdown/reduce cast smelling from unpleasant odours and structure breakdown.

    The ward nurse should address elimination needs prior to discharge.

    Evaluate: outcome of care.

- **Working and playing**

    Problem: how can I occupy my child?

    Goal: child is occupied, not bored or distressed.

    Intervention:

    1. Stimulating toys, TV, videos, reading, drawing, and computer (age appropriate).

    2. School-home tuition may be an option (age appropriate).

    3. Stimulation – good positioning of child so that they can see their surroundings, plus activities, will discourage bad behaviour.

(Continued)

Table 27.2 (Continued)

Rationale: to prevent boredom and encourage child development.

Evaluate: outcome of care.

- **Maintaining a safe environment**

    Problem: how will I take my child shopping and secure them safely in the car?

    Goal: always ensure child safety.

    Intervention:

    1. A suitable pram or special wheelchair may be available free or to rent prior to discharge.
    2. For a younger child suitable car seat should be bought and fitted prior to discharge (see www.safetyfirst.com).
    3. The ward staff can give full information on transport options. For the older child transport is problematic and an ambulance may be required.
    4. Parents are advised to contact their car insurance broker.

    Rationale: child safety, prevent prosecution – encourage social freedom.

    Evaluate: outcome of care.

- **Eating and drinking**

    Problem: do I feed my child a normal diet?

    Goal: ensure child receives age-appropriate diet/fluids and adequate intake.

    Intervention:

    1. Yes, but smaller amounts – the cast is restrictive; also monitor weight as potential weight gain due to reduced mobility.
    2. The child should be positioned at 45 degrees to aid digestion, comfort, and reduce the risk of aspiration or choking.

    Rationale: promote healing and prevent constipation. A balanced diet plus fluids.

    Evaluate: outcome of care.

ACTIVITY 27.1

What is the most recent evidence/effectiveness of tepid sponge and electric fan treatment for high fevers in children? Is there any harm in this treatment?

REFERENCES

Apley, A.G. & Solomon, L. (2008) *Concise System of Orthopaedics and Fractures*. Oxford: Butterworth Heinman.

Barnard, K., Judd, J., Clarke, S. et al. (2020) Updating the UK competence framework for orthopaedic and trauma nurses 2019. *International Journal of Orthopaedic and Trauma Nursing*. https://doi.org/10.1016/j.ijotn.2020.100780. [Accessed 6 March 2023]

Casey, A. (1988) The development and use of the partnership model of nursing care. In: Glasper, E.A. and Tucker, A. (eds). (1993). *Advances in Child Health Nursing*. London: Scutari Press, 83–93.

Clarke, S. & Drozd, M. (2023) *Orthopaedic and Trauma Nursing: An Evidence-based Approach to Musculoskeletal Care*, 2nd edition. London: Wiley Blackwell.

Clarke, S.E. & Dowling, M. (2003) Spica cast guidelines for parents and health professionals. *Journal of Orthopaedic Nursing*, **7**(4), 184–191.

Clarke, S.E. & McKay, M. (2006) Spica cast guidelines for parent and health professional: measure the effect of new evidenced based information using audit. *Journal of Orthopaedic Nursing*, **10**(3), 128–137.

de Hundt, M., Vlemmix, F., Bais, J.M.J. et al. (2012) Risk factors for developmental dysplasia of the hip: a meta-analysis. *Eur J Obstet Gynecol Reprod Biol*, **165**(1), 8–17.

Kneale, J. & Davis, P. (2005) *Orthopaedic and Trauma Nursing*, 2nd edition. Edinburgh: Churchill Livingstone.

National health Service (2021) NHS high temperature (fever) in children. Available at High Temperature (Fever) in Children – NHS. www.nhs.uk (accessed 4 June 2021).

NICE (2018) Feverish children- management summary. Available at Feverish children - management | Health topics A to Z | CKS | NICE (accessed 4 June 2021).

NICE (2019) Fever in under 5s: assessment and initial management. NICE Guideline [NG143]. Available at Recommendations | Fever in under 5s: Assessment and Initial Management | Guidance | NICE (accessed 4 June 2021).

Roper, N., Logan, W.W. & Tierney, A.J. (2000) *The Roper-Logan-Tierney Model of Nursing: Based on Activities of Living*. Edinburgh: Elsevier Health Sciences.

Royal College of Nursing (2019) *A Competence Framework for Orthopaedic and Trauma Practitioners*. London: RCN.

Royal College of Nursing (2021) *Peripheral Neurovascular Observations for Acute Limb Compartment Syndrome RCN Consensus Guidance*. London: RCN.

Thomas, S.V., Vijaykumar, C., Naik, R., Moses, P.D. & Antonisamy, B. (2009) Comparative effectiveness of tepid sponging and antipyretic drug versus only antipyretic drug in the management of fever among children: a randomised controlled trial. *Indian Pediatrics*, **46**(17), 133–136.

Vaquero-Picado, A., González-Morán, G., Gil Garay, E. & Moraleda, L. (2019) Development dysplasia of the hip:update of management. *EFORT Open Rev*, **4**(2019), 548–556. doi:10.1302/2058-5241.4.180019.

Care of the Gastro-intestinal Tract in Infants and Children

SECTION 8

Gastro-oesophageal Reflux

CHAPTER 28

Doris Corkin and Lynne Robinson

SCENARIO

Judith, now aged three months, was born at term weighing 3.7 kg and is in the sensorimotor stage of cognitive development (Bee & Boyd 2013). She was initially breastfed, but is currently bottle feeding on casein-based milk, demand fed every 3–4 hours, her weight is 5.0 kg, tongue-tie noted.

Judith has been admitted to hospital with a two-week history of vomiting following feeds and according to her mother appears to be in pain, as she is irritable, clenching her fists, and drawing up her knees. On admission to the ward the children's nurse advised Judith's mother to change Judith's casein-based milk back to whey, which is the preferred first choice.

Gastro-oesophageal reflux has been diagnosed after a few days, following a nursing and medical assessment and investigations. The doctor initially prescribed a trial period of infant Gaviscon and as it was unsuccessful then suggested thickening. Judith feeds with Carobel (Corkin 2008). However, Judith continues to vomit and is referred to the paediatric dietician who recommends an anti-reflux formula.

Judith is accompanied by her mother, a single mum, who is particularly anxious, and grandparents who are very supportive.

ACTIVITY 28.1

Plot Judith's weight on a centile chart. At birth Judith was assessed as within the 75th centile. At three months old Judith should now be between the 25th and 50th centile (see BMI chart in Chapter 18).

QUESTIONS

1. Discuss Judith's sensorimotor stage in cognitive development and possible characteristics.
2.a Explore the need for early identification of tongue-tie.
2.b Define gastro-oesophageal reflux.
3. What nursing and medical investigations are likely to have been undertaken?
4. How should gastro-oesophageal reflux be best treated and managed whilst being bottle fed?
5. Judith, three months old, weighing 5.0 kg has been prescribed oral omeprazole. When planning care what safety measures must the children's nurse consider prior to administration of medication?

ANSWERS TO QUESTIONS

Question 1. Discuss Judith's sensorimotor stage in cognitive development and possible characteristics.

Jean Piaget (1896–1980) has been the most influential child development theorist, extensively observing children, including his own (www.piaget.org). The sensorimotor stage represents the first major stage of cognitive development and has been identified as the period extending from birth to about 18 months of age, where the child is essentially engaged in their environment (Bee & Boyd

2013). During this time Judith will develop increased muscle control and should have a strong attachment to her mother. After Judith was born, she began to learn to use her senses and can understand the world through motor and sensory activities. She can focus and follow moving objects, distinguish between pitch and volume of sound, and see all colours. Now three months old, Judith can clearly recognise faces and respond to smiles and familiar sounds.

Question 2a. Early identification of tongue-tie.

There may be challenges for the mother who initially decides to breastfeed her infant with tongue-tie (also known as ankyloglossia), a congenital abnormality (Edmunds et al. 2011). Tongue-tie is characterized by an unusually thickened or shortened frenulum (membrane attaching tongue to floor of mouth), can be a barrier to breastfeeding, hindering the infant's ability to maintain an effective latch to breast (Hill & Pados 2020). Therefore needs to be explored as soon as possible by the primary healthcare professional, to prevent feeding difficulties and early cessation of breastfeeding. A Frenotomy consultation and procedure may significantly improve Judith's problematic feeding and articulation as she develops.

Question 2b. Define gastro-oesophageal reflux.

Gastro-oesophageal reflux is the passage of gastric contents into the oesophagus (Davies et al. 2015); it is a very common gastro-intestinal disorder in infants and tends to resolve following the weaning period. This is caused by the immaturity of the lower oesophageal sphincter which allows frequent reflux of gastric contents into the oesophagus. Vomiting (which is neither projectile nor bile-stained) can occur during or between feeds. Bleeding, however, may occur and appear as bright blood in the vomitus if oesophagitis is present. Commonly this may present as 'coffee ground' flecks of altered blood. Severe gastro-oesophageal reflux in some infants can lead to repeated episodes of aspiration and pneumonia and later present as faltering growth (National Institute for Health and Care Excellence (NICE), 2015). The diagnosis is established following a nursing assessment of the child's feeding pattern and a thorough physical examination by the medical team (Walls 2019).

Question 3. What nursing and medical investigations are likely to have been undertaken?

Assessment: on admission to hospital the children's nurse would undertake a detailed nursing assessment and establish Judith's weight and feeding pattern and this would include a test feed. In order to establish diagnosis the medical team investigations will involve:

- A health/family history
- Physical examination from head to toe
- Diagnostic tests, such as barium swallow or pH probe monitoring which measures the oesophageal pH and percentage of time the pH falls below 4 in 24 hours

Question 4. How should gastro-oesophageal reflux be best treated and managed whilst being bottle fed?

Activity of living: eating and drinking as per Roper, Logan, and Tierney model of care (Holland & Jenkins 2019); see Chapter 1 for further reading.

Plan: gastro-oesophageal reflux is a condition which nature will gradually resolve as Judith gets older. The children's nurse should aim to minimise the symptoms and keep Judith as comfortable as possible:

1. Thicken Judith's milk feed – following discussion with the medical team, this can be addressed by adding a thickener (Carobel) to the milk Judith is already receiving. The amount of Carobel can be increased, depending on the severity of the reflux. Alternatively, the paediatric dietician can be consulted and a formula tried, for example Enfamil AR or Staydown can be offered instead (Corkin & McDougall 2009).

2. It is important to highlight the need to calculate feeding requirements accurately based on Judith's weight and to educate her parent/grandparent regarding overfeeding, as it may be best to give Judith small frequent feeds initially until pain or discomfort eases. Breastfeeding more frequently is also encouraged to help ensure an adequate milk supply and to minimise symptoms in the breast-fed infant (Walls 2019).

3. Nurse Judith in a more upright position – infants benefit from being nursed in a suitable tilted bouncer/car chair or in buggy where their head is raised above the level of their feet. This allows gravity to help keep Judith's milk feed in her stomach. Furthermore, the head of Judith's cot can also be raised by placing some folded towels *under* the cot mattress at the head end. Also, it is important to make sure that the cot is stable and Judith is safe at all times. Make Judith's mother aware of cot death prevention advice, such as the 'feet to foot' position, so that Judith's feet are at the end of the cot, thus preventing her from wriggling under her covers (Public Health Agency 2021).

4. Encourage nappy changing prior to feeding and ensure accurate recording of intake and output on fluid balance chart while in hospital.

5. Paediatrician may prescribe Judith some medication – in some cases the doctor may prescribe an acid-reducing preparation such as infant Gaviscon (reduces oesophagitis) or omeprazole, which can be administered in liquid form (BNFc 2020–2021). However, these medications should not be used in combination with Enfamil AR or SMA Staydown as these milks need stomach acids present to be effective. Medications will allow Judith to tolerate her feeds by either promoting gastric emptying or reducing the acidity of Judith's stomach contents. This medication is similar to those used by adults with heartburn or ulcers. Medication can help reduce the pain which Judith is experiencing when reflux does occur.

6. Surgery such as a fundoplication (see Chapter 1, parents reflective account) may be performed in a minority of cases as a last resort (Walls 2019), especially those children with life-threatening conditions, for example a child with complex needs and a tracheostomy *in situ*.

7. Early weaning should be discouraged with Judith as the current government recommendation for starting weaning is six months (Public Health Agency 2021) or at the very earliest 17 weeks of age after careful consideration.

ACTIVITY 27.2

1. As Judith now weighs 5.0 kg, calculate her daily feeding requirements based on 150 ml per kg.
2. If Judith takes six bottle feeds in 24 hours how many millilitres would each one be?

Question 5. Judith, three months old, weighing 5.0 kg has been prescribed oral omeprazole. When planning care what safety measures must the children's nurse consider prior to administration of medication?

Administration of Oral Medication

Activity of living: maintaining a safe environment as per Roper, Logan, and Tierney model of care (Holland & Jenkins 2019).

Implementation: the administration of oral medicines is an important, complex aspect within the multifaceted role of the children's nurse (see Table 28.1). Standards for the profession are regulated by the Nursing and Midwifery Council (NMC 2015) and clearly highlight the nurse's responsibility to ensure safe practice when administrating medication. As medications can come in various forms for administration via multiple routes, it is essential for all nurses to have a working knowledge and understanding of these NMC standards as conventional drugs can have at least three names, for example:

Calpol – proprietary name
paracetamol – common (generic) name
acetaminophen – chemical name

Indeed, there are various omeprazole preparations available (British National Formulary for Children (BNFc) 2020–2021). Many generic companies manufacture omeprazole in capsule and tablet form. However,

Table 28.1 Administration of oral medication.

Action: administration of oral medication	Reason
1. The children's nurse should be aware of Judith's plan of care and incorporate a family-centred approach (Casey 1988) in order to gain consent and parental co-operation.	To ensure clear communication pathway is implemented.
2. The children's nurse should be able to correctly refer to a paediatric prescribing textbook, for example British National Formulary for Children (British National Formulary for Children (BNFc) 2020–2021).	To establish safe dose of medication, understand therapeutic effects and possible side effects.
3. Be aware of Judith's care plan, for example check for allergies, that prescription is valid, in keeping with Judith's age and weight and signed by doctor and dated.	To ensure safe practice and accurate calculation of dosage.
4. Children's nurses should wash their hands prior to and after procedure.	To prevent cross infection.
5. Safe administration of medication involves ten r's (Edwards & Axe 2015). Right dose • Right medicine (check expiry date) • Right infant/child (check unit number and details on hospital armband and records) • Right route (e.g. oral, nasogastric, etc.) • Right time • Right to refuse (patient/nurse) • Right knowledge • Right questions or challenges • Right advice • Right response or outcome Adhere to hospital policy, for example double checking by registered nurse/s involved at every stage of medicine administration process (NMC 2010).	Professional responsibility and accountability. To reduce risk.
6. The safe preparation, dispense, and storage of medication must be adhered to as per ward policy and pharmacist.	Patient safety.
7. The children's nurse should accurately and immediately record medication (RCN, 2020) after administration, or if refused by Judith, ensuring signatures of both nurses are clearly written with date and time. Ensure disposal of equipment used to administer medicine, disposal of unused medicine and monitoring of effectiveness of drug action.	Ensuring safe practice and continuity of care.

However, AstraZeneca manufacture Losec Mups® (omeprazole tablets dispersible in water) and Losec capsules® (e.g. contents can be sprinkled directly onto spoonful of food).

As the NMC (2010) supports the administration of medicines by a carer, the majority of parents should be encouraged by the children's nurse to take part in the administration of medicines to their child in the paediatric setting, thus advocating a partnership approach to care (Casey 1988). Although the responsibility to ensure the medication is given remains with the children's nurse, age-appropriate considerations should always be taken into account and there should be negotiation with the parent regarding mixing of medication with food to disguise any unpleasant taste. Please note this is different to 'covert administration of medicines', which is regarded as deception without informed consent (advice@nmc-uk.org).

Formula for calculating drug dosage: this is calculated as shown here (Watt 2003):

$$\frac{\text{what you require}}{\text{what you have}} \times \text{dilution} = \text{what you give}$$

A standardised formula can help reduce calculation/medicine errors, for example:

- 'What you require' is the prescribed dosage.

- 'What you have' is the concentration of drug in the medicine bottle.

- 'Dilution' is the amount of liquid in which the drug is dissolved.

CALCULATION OF DRUGS

The administration of prescribed medication to infants and children must be viewed by the children's nurse as a key aspect of nursing care that requires sound knowledge of pharmacology, numeracy skills, and the ability to communicate effectively with Judith and her family (Pentin et al. 2016b). To ensure accurate dosing, body weight is used more frequently for ease of paediatric calculations. In order to calculate drug doses accurately the children's nurse must be able to demonstrate an understanding of child development theory, the units of drugs in current use and approved abbreviations, for example:

- Gram = g
- Milligram = mg
- Millilitre = ml
- Microgram = must be written in full

Student nurses should be involved in the procedure of drug calculation and administration as a learning tool. However, in order to meet legal, local trust and professional guidelines student nurses should *NEVER* single check oral medication and administer unsupervised. As nurses administer medications on a regular basis there is the potential for errors to occur (Pentin et al. 2016a). According to Preston (2003) nurses' poor mathematical skills are an on-going problem and use of calculators is acknowledged as part of the dose checking process. Reports regarding medication incidents with children have included wrong drug, wrong strength, and wrong patient in 2008 (NPSA, 2009). A recent study (Simons 2010) has identified computerised prescription systems as having been shown to reduce medication errors.

STORAGE AND TRANSPORTATION OF DRUGS

Safe storage of drugs involves both environmental and security factors, such as medicines trolley and refrigerator. Children's nurses must ensure all medicines are stored in accordance with the patient/drug information leaflet. According to the Nursing and Midwifery Council (2010) registered nurses may transport medication to patients (including controlled drugs), where patients or their carers are unable to collect them, provided the registrant is conveying the medication to a patient for whom the drug product has been prescribed (e.g. from pharmacy to patient in community setting).

ANSWERS TO ACTIVITY 28.2

1. 50 × 5 = 750 ml in 24 hours
2. 750 ÷ 6 = 125 ml per feed

REFERENCES

Bee, H. & Boyd, D. (2013) *The Developing Child: Pearson New International Edition*, 13th edition. London: Pearson.

British National Formulary for Children (BNFc) (2020–2021) *British Medical Journal*. London: PS Publishing.

Casey, A. (1988) A partnership with child and family. *Senior Nurse*, **8**(4), 8–9.

Corkin, D. (2008) Artifical feeding, Chapter 14. In: Kelsey, J. and McEwing, G. (eds). *Clinical Skills in Child Health Practice*. Oxford: Churchill Livingstone, Elsevier.

Corkin, D. & McDougall, A. (2009) Preparation of infant feeds, Chapter 27. In: Glasper, A., McEwing, G. and Richardson, J. (eds). *Foundation Skills for Caring*. Hampshire: Palgrave Macmillan.

Davies, I., Burman-Roy, S. & Murphy, S. (2015) Gastro-oesophageal reflux disease in children: NICE guidance. *BMJ*, **350**, g7703.

Edmunds, J., Miles, S.C. & Fulbrook, P. (2011) Tongue-tie and breastfeeding: a review of the literature. *Breastfeeding Review*, **19**(1), 19–26.

Edwards, S. & Axe, S. (2015) The ten 'R's of safe multidisciplinary drug administration. *Nurse Prescribing*, **13**(8), 352–360.

Hill, R.R. & Pados, B.F. (2020) Symptoms of problematic feeding in infants under 1 year of age undergoing a frenotomy: a review article. *Acta Paediatrica*, **109**(12), 2502–2514.

Holland, K. & Jenkins, J. (2019) *Applying the Rope-Logan-Tierney Model in Practice*, 3rd edition. Edinburgh: Elsevier.

National Institute for Health and Care Excellence (2015) Gastro-oesophageal reflux disease: recognition, diagnosis and management in children and young people. (Clinical Guideline 193). www.nice.org.uk/guidance/NG1 (accessed on 5 October 2021).

National Patient Safety Agency (NPSA) (2009) *Review of Patient Safety for Children and Young People*. London: NSPA.

Nursing and Midwifery Council (2010) *Record Keeping – Guidance for Nurses and Midwives*. London: NMC.

Nursing and Midwifery Council (2015) *Guidelines on the Administration of Medicines*. London: NMC.

Pentin, J., Green, M. & Smith, J. (2016a) Undertaking safe medicine administration with children: part 1. *Nursing Children and Young People*, **28**(6), 35–41.

Pentin, J., Green, M. & Smith, J. (2016b) Undertaking safe medicine administration with children part 2: essential numeracy. *Nursing Children and Young People*, **28**(7), 37–43.

Preston, R.M. (2003) Drug errors and patient safety: the need for a change in practice. *British Journal of Nursing*, **13**(2), 72–78.

Public Health Agency (2021) *Birth to five*. http://www.publichealth.hscni.net

Royal College of Nursing (2020) *Medicines Mangement: An Overview for Nursing*. London: RCN.

Simons, J. (2010) Identifying medication errors in surgical prescription charts. *Paediatric Nursing*, **22**(5), 20–24.

Walls, E. (2019) Understanding reflux problems in infants, children and young people. *British Journal of Nursing*, **28**(14), 920–923.

Watt, S. (2003) Safe administration of medicines to children: part 1. *Paediatric Nursing*, **15**(4), 40–43.

Cerebral Palsy and Nasogastric Tube Feeding

CHAPTER 29

Susie Wilkie and Sonya Clarke

SCENARIO

Colin is an eight-year-old boy who was diagnosed as having cerebral palsy at the age of nine months, after his parents had concerns regarding his slow development. As he grew older Colin was able to learn to walk, first with a frame and then independently. He can competently carry out the activities of daily living, such as dressing and feeding himself. However, Colin has some difficulties with fine motor tasks; he has left-sided hemiparesis and has scoliosis.

Colin is cognitively intact, communicates verbally, and has a good social life with friends and family. He had been experiencing an upper respiratory tract infection for nearly a week; his condition then deteriorated and Colin was admitted to hospital with pneumonia. He was treated with antibiotics at first intravenously but then progressed to oral administration. Fluid intake was initially maintained intravenously. Although Colin's condition is improving he is still unable to maintain his fluid and nutritional needs orally and requires enteral feeding.

QUESTIONS

1. What is cerebral palsy?
2. Discuss the rationale for enteral feeding.
3. What is enteral feeding?
4. Using the nursing process and a model of care, how would the children's nurse prepare Colin and his family for the insertion of a nasogastric tube?
5. Describe the procedure for passing a nasogastric tube.

ANSWERS TO QUESTIONS

Question 1. What is cerebral palsy?

Cerebral palsy (CP) is an umbrella term used to describe a permanent non-progressive condition in which dysfunction of the brain affects movement, posture, and co-ordination.

The condition can arise before, during, or after birth. The severity and effects of the condition are wide ranging and less severe cases may not be detected until early childhood. Approximately 1 in every 400 children is diagnosed in the UK each year (SCOPE UK 2020) and the condition can affect individuals from any social background or ethnic group. There is a higher prevalence in children born prematurely (Sadowska et al. 2020).

The damage to the brain may occur prenatally between conception and birth, during birth or during early childhood. Prenatal causes include: inefficient placenta, genetic disorders, infections, maternal high blood pressure, or premature birth. Birth trauma may be due to prolonged labour, oxygen deficit or occasionally forceps delivery. Damage in the neonatal period may be caused by hypoglycaemia, respiratory problems, convulsions, blood group incompatibility, or infection (Sadowska et al. 2020).

Care Planning in Children and Young People's Nursing, Second Edition. Edited by Sonya Clarke and Doris Corkin.
© 2024 John Wiley & Sons Ltd. Published 2024 by John Wiley & Sons Ltd.

There are four main classifications of cerebral palsy: *spastic*, when the child's movement is difficult or stiff; *ataxic*, where there is loss of depth perception and balance; *athetoid or dyskinetic*, where movement is uncontrolled or involuntary; or the condition may be a mixture of any or all of these. Half of children born with cerebral palsy have an intelligence quotient within normal range; others will have some learning difficulties. Many children with cerebral palsy have swallowing problems due to poor tongue control.

Question 2. Discuss the rationale for enteral feeding

Poor nutrition is a complication of many childhood diseases which can affect the child's health by impairing immunity, delaying wound healing, reducing muscle strength, and impairing psychological drive (Kim et al. 2018). There are a number of reasons why illness may interfere with eating, digestion, and absorption. The desire to eat can be affected by many things such as: lack of appetite, nausea, vomiting, dysphasia, pain on swallowing, altered taste due to medications, and psychological factors. Ability to eat can be affected by impaired sucking, chewing, and swallowing mechanisms and respiratory or cardiac conditions leading to breathlessness when feeding (Nur et al. 2019). Digestion and absorption can be affected by altered pathophysiology of the gut, for example short-term conditions such as severe acute diarrhoea or long-term conditions including coeliac disease or short bowel syndrome.

When a child is at risk of suffering from under nutrition, enteral feeding can be considered, providing they have a functioning gastro-intestinal tract (Serjeant & Tighe 2021).

There are four main groups of children that may require enteral feeding. These include children with:

- Neurological disorders, such as cerebral palsy (Hopwood et al. 2021).
- Chronic conditions, such as cystic fibrosis, renal failure, and bowel disorders.
- Short-term feeding problems, including prematurity, cancer, and severe burns.
- Some miscellaneous conditions, such as anorexia nervosa (Falcoski et al. 2021). Refer to Box 29.1.

BOX 29.1 ASSESSMENT OF NEEDS

Colin is unable to meet his nutritional needs orally as he has no desire to eat. His increased respiratory effort makes it difficult for Colin to swallow and breathe at the same time. He feels thirsty and hungry but is unable to eat or drink normally. Colin is only able to manage sips of fluid to make his mouth more comfortable. Following discussion with the dietician, medical staff, Colin, and his parents, it has been decided that Colin will benefit from enteral feeding.

Question 3. What is enteral feeding?

Enteral feeding refers to the delivery of a nutritionally complete feed containing protein, carbohydrate, fat, water, minerals, and vitamins directly into the stomach, duodenum, or jejunum (NICE 2020).

Enteral feeding is an artificial method of providing nutrition to a child. There are three main routes for administration: orogastric, nasogastric, and gastrostomy.

- *Orogastric* feeding involves a tube passing through the mouth and oral cavity down the back of the throat, into the oesophagus and then into the stomach.
- *Nasogastric* feeding is when a tube is passed through the nostril, down the back of the throat, into the oesophagus and then into the stomach.
- *Gastrostomy* feeding is performed through a tube surgically placed through the skin of the abdomen into the stomach.

Nasogastric feeding is usually considered for the child requiring short-term nutritional support and can be used for anything between 6 weeks and 12 months depending on circumstances (Abdelhadi et al. 2020). Furthermore, it is suitable for those children unable to feed orally in acute or chronic illness. This is the most common method of enteral feeding, with nutrients being delivered directly into the gastrointestinal tract through a nasogastric tube. Although there is no direct guidance from NICE on enteral feeding specifically for children and young people, the Guidelines and Audit Implementation Network published guidelines in 2015 which recognised this deficit (GAIN 2015). Refer to Box 29.2.

> **BOX 29.2 PLANNING OF CARE**
>
> Colin has long-term needs resulting from his cerebral palsy and acute problems due to his respiratory infection. This has made it difficult for him to maintain his nutritional intake orally. With the use of antibiotics his condition should gradually improve and Colin will be able to eat and drink independently again. Therefore he only requires short-term assistance with meeting his nutritional needs and the nasogastric route would be the most suitable.

Question 4. Using the nursing process and a model of care, how would the children's nurse prepare Colin and his family for the insertion of a naso-gastric tube?

Activity of living: communication (Roper et al. 2000).

Best practice involves making sure Colin and his parents are fully informed regarding the benefits of inserting a nasogastric tube in order to meet Colin's nutritional needs. Information should be given verbally and when necessary supported by written information to meet the child and family's needs (National Institute of Clinical Excellence (NICE) 2021b). The individual's ability to understand must be considered when providing information with regard to language, culture, physical, sensory, or learning disabilities. Effective communication will need to take into consideration Colin's age, cognitive ability, personality, and coping skills. Misunderstandings can cause the child to become distressed; for a child there is no such thing as a minor procedure and often the severity of pain or discomfort does not correlate accurately with what the child feels they experience, as pain is personal, subjective, and complex (Pope et al. 2017). Children in hospital have described procedures as causing them fear and sadness (Clarke 2021) which is why effective communication is important.

The procedure should be explained to both the Colin and his parents and they should be encouraged to ask questions.

Goal: Colin and his parents will understand the need to commence enteral feeding. They will be fully informed regarding the procedure for passing a nasogastric tube.

Implement and evaluate:

- The need for Colin to be fed for a short period using the nasogastric route will be discussed with Colin's parents.
- Care will be planned with the parents on how best to proceed with the procedure causing the least distress possible to Colin.
- The procedure will be explained to Colin at his level of understanding using his own language, avoiding misinterpretations, and encouraging questions.
- Explore with Colin any fears he may have in relation to the procedure.

Activity of living: maintaining a safe environment (Roper et al. 2000).

Psychological preparation for an unpleasant procedure is essential (Rees et al. 2021). This will help the child and parents to manage the procedure effectively and help ensure the procedure is completed as efficiently and safely as possible (Hopwood et al. 2021). Passing a nasogastric tube is an invasive procedure and it could cause anticipatory anxiety in Colin and his parents. Past experiences of unpleasant procedures must be taken into account. Providing information to children about the experience, encouraging emotional expression of concerns, and establishing a trusting relationship with the healthcare professional will all help to reduce the stress of the procedure (Graham et al. 2019). Non-pharmacological interventions, such as parental presence, hugging and holding, distraction, deep breathing, and guided imagery and relaxation can all help reduce Colin's anxiety. Increasing parental participation can be achieved by providing them with a role such as active coaching to help the child through procedure.

Goal: Colin and his parents will have given consent for the procedure. Colin will be calm and compliant throughout the procedure and aware of the boundaries of behaviour and how to communicate distress. His parents will understand their role during the procedure. Management of the procedure will involve good organisation and planning ahead.

Implement and evaluate:

- If possible, both Colin and his parents should give verbal consent for the procedure to take place.
- Discuss with Colin what is expected of him and the limits of acceptable behaviour throughout the procedure.
- The procedure will be explained to Colin's parents, and their role during the procedure should be agreed.
- Age-appropriate books or other visual aids can be used.
- The procedure will be planned. Delays will be avoided that may cause unnecessary distress by preparing all the equipment beforehand and out of the child's sight unless the child specifically requests to see it.
- Step-by-step, honest, age-appropriate information will be provided to Colin and his parents to increase their sense of control.
- Throughout the procedure Colin will be allowed choices, if appropriate, such as which nostril will be used. This will increase co-operation and give Colin a sense of control and reduce feelings of helplessness.
- Following the procedure Colin will be praised, with emphasis on the positive aspects of the experience and age-appropriate reward stickers or certificates should be given.

Activity of living: eating and drinking (Roper et al. 2000).

A dietician will be involved to plan a feeding regime for Colin to ensure that he has the correct fluid and nutritional intake. Feeds can be given by gravity, as a bolus or by a pump continuously (Guidelines and Audit Implementation Network (GAIN) 2015). Feeds given continuously reduce the risk of gastrointestinal symptoms but this does mean the child needs to be connected to the pump most of the time, which limits mobility. Feeds given as a bolus at meal times will help maintain normal body feeding patterns.

Goal: Colin will receive suitable enteral feeds to meet his physical and nutritional needs.

Implement and evaluate:

- When possible Colin will be fed at normal meal times.
- If Colin is able to take any food or fluid orally this should be given at the same time as the feed.
- Enteral feeding should not be an unpleasant experience for Colin.

Question 5. Describe the procedure for passing a nasogastric tube

See Table 29.1.

Table 29.1 The procedure for passing a nasogastric tube.

Action	Rationale and evidence
1. Collect the required equipment: Nasogastric tube Syringe pH indication paper Tape to secure Hydrocolloid dressing Oral fluid for older child Two gallipots Water or water-based lubricant Disposable gloves Scissors Plastic apron	When choosing a nasogastric feeding tube the size and material it is made from needs to be considered. There are two main types commonly used, polyvinylchloride (PVC) and polyurethane tubes. The PVC tubes quickly lose their flexibility when in contact with gastric secretions; these are therefore primarily used for short-term feeding as they need changing frequently according to the manufacturers' guidance (Mandal et al. 2017). The polyurethane tubes are more suitable for longer term feeding as they are softer and more flexible and can remain *in situ* for up to one month. Tubes are sized according to their internal lumen; 6, 8, and 10 French gauge (Fg) are usually used for children (Ford et al. 2010; Mandal et al. 2017). It is essential to follow the manufacturers' guidelines regarding the size of the syringe used when aspirating the tube in order to prevent damage (Guidelines and Audit Implementation Network (GAIN) 2015). When aspirating the tube the negative pressure created at the tip of the syringe is dependent on the size and type of syringe and the force exerted.
2. Wash and dry hands using recognised technique and put on plastic apron.	To prevent cross infection hands must be decontaminated immediately before each and every episode of direct patient contact or care (National Institute of Clinical Excellence (NICE) 2021a). Plastic aprons should be worn when required for a single episode of patient care and then discarded (NICE 2021:a).
3. Explain to the child and parent that you are going to pass the nasogastric tube, explain what the child should do if they wish you to stop.	Promote psychological support.
4. Clean work surface/trolley prior to placement of equipment.	Passing a nasogastric tube is a clean procedure.
5. Prepare a piece hydrocolloid dressing.	To prevent epidermal damage this should be three times the width of the tube and cover two-thirds of the child's cheek between the side of the nostril and the child's ear.
6. Cut adhesive tape and place within easy reach.	To secure adequately this should be wide enough to cover the nasogastric tube and overlap the sides sufficiently to hold it securely in place; however, it should not overlap the hydrocolloid dressing.
7. Wash and dry hands.	To prevent bacterial contamination of the tube.
8. Water/lubricant → gallipot.	To lubricate the tip of the tube.
9. Place strip of pH paper in second gallipot.	
10. Open syringe; place within easy reach.	
11. Put on disposable gloves.	To prevent bacterial contamination of the tube.
12. Remove nasogastric tube from packaging; ensure not damaged.	
13. Measure length of tube from nostril to ear, and then from ear to stomach, just past the xiphoid process. Note/mark the point on the tube or hold the tube at the calculated point and keep between the fingers of your less dominant hand.	To determine the length of tube required. Traditionally the NEX measurement (length from nose to earlobe to the xiphoid process) is used to indicate the length of tube required. A study by Taylor (2020) suggested that for paediatric gastric tube insertion, a graphic method based on height was a more accurate method for determining depth of tube insertion to reduce misplacement.
Ensure end cap of the tube is in place.	To prevent leakage of gastric contents.
14. Ask assistant (parent) to supportively hold child as appropriate to age and level of understanding.	To prevent the child moving during the procedure and provide comfort.

(Continued)

Table 29.1 (Continued)

Action	Rationale and evidence
Older children may prefer to sit up with their head supported. Babies can be wrapped in a blanket and encouraged to suck a dummy through the procedure.	
15. Select clear nostril; older children can choose which nostril. Lubricate the tip of the tube using a water-based solution. Insert tip of tube into nostril. Angle tube slightly upwards and slide backwards along the floor of the nose into the pharynx.	Consider airway maintenance in infants who are obligatory nose breathers. Lubrication reduces the risk of friction and tissue damage. Follow manufacturers' guidelines regarding type of lubrication. Follows the normal contour of the nasal passage.
16. Continue to gently feed tube downwards. As the tube passes to the back of the nose, advise child to take sips of water (if appropriate) to help the tube go down or in the case of a baby offer them a dummy. A short pause may be necessary for the tube to pass through the cardiac sphincter into the stomach.	In the case of obstruction, pull tube back and turn it slightly and advance again. If obstruction is felt again try the other nostril. The tube should be gently inserted as the child swallows as this will assist with the movement of the tube and reduce any discomfort. If at any time during this procedure the child starts to cough or their colour deteriorates the procedure should be stopped immediately and the tube removed. The most common site for resistance when passing a nasogastric tube is at the laryngeal level at the arytenoid cartilages and piriform sinuses (Mandal et al. 2017). Lateral neck pressure compresses the piriform sinuses and moves the arytenoid cartilages medially, relieving 85% of the incidences of impaction.
17. Stop when the point marked on the tube reaches the outer edge of the child's nostril.	The tube should be in the stomach.
18. Ask person assisting to hold the tube in position. Check the nasogastric tube is in the child's stomach. Remove the end cap. Using syringe aspirate a small amount of gastric contents by gently pulling back on the plunger. Detach syringe, replace end cap. Test pH of fluid using pH indicator paper, readings should be less than 5.5. (NPSA 2019. Replace aspirate in infants at risk of electrolyte imbalance. If there is difficulty obtaining aspirate, lie the child on his/her left side and encourage to swallow a small amount of oral fluid if allowed. Attempt to push the tube away from the stomach wall by inserting 1–5 ml of air down the tube using a 20 or 50 ml syringe. Try advancing or retracting the tube slightly to alter the position in the stomach.	When determining the position of nasogastric tubes insufflation and auscultation of air into the stomach is an unreliable method of checking tube position as it has been shown to give false positive results as bowel or chest sounds can be misinterpreted as evidence of gastric tube placement (Rosengarten & Davies 2021). Placing the proximal end of the tube under water and observing for bubbles on expiration runs the risk of aspirating the water on inspiration, particularly when the child is ventilated. Examining the colour of aspirate alone is not a safe indication of tube placement (Mandal et al.2017). The use of blue litmus paper turning pink/red to indicate whether aspirate is acidic, is not safe as it does not indicate the degree of acidity present. This is crucial as bronchial secretions can be slightly acidic which will turn the litmus pink. Testing the pH of aspirate is the recommended method. The NPSA (2019) recommends that feeding can commence if aspirate is below pH 5.5. However, care should be taken as the use of antacids, proton pump inhibitor drugs, or H_2 receptor antagonists can elevate the pH of the gastric contents and limit the usefulness of this test in those children receiving these therapies. If any doubt exists on the correct placement of the nasogastric tube then consider re-passing the tube or checking position by X-ray.
19. Apply hydrocolloid dressing to child and secure tube using adhesive tape.	Most children benefit from using a barrier product such as hydrocolloid dressings and transparent films to protect the skin under strong adhesive tapes (Powers 2019).
20. Document nostril used, size, date, and time of insertion. It is useful to make a note of the length of the tube extending from the nostril as this may help determine if the tube has been displaced.	PVC tubes lose their flexibility when in contact with gastric secretions and need changing frequently according to the manufacturer's guidance.

REFERENCES

Abdelhadi, R.A., Rempel, G., Sevilla, W., Turner, J.M., Quet, J., Nelson, A., RD, Rahe K, Wilhelm, R., Larocque, J., Guenter, P. (2020) 'Transitioning From Nasogastric Feeding Tube to Gastrostomy Tube in Pediatric Patients: A Survey on Decision-Making and Practice', *Nutrition in Clinical Practice*, **36**:3, Pp. 654–664.

Clarke, S. (2021) An exploration of the child's experience of staying in hospital from the perspectives of children and children's nurses using child-centered methodology. *Comprehensive Child and Adolescent Nursing*, **0**, 1–14.

Falcoski, P., Philpot, U., Tan, J., Hudson, L.D. & Fuller, S.J. (2021) Nasogastric tube feeding in linewith new dietetic guidelines for the treatment ofanorexia nervosa in a specialist children andadolescent inpatient unit: a case series. *Journal of Human Nutrition and Dietetics*, **34**, 33–41.

Ford, L., Trigg, E., Mohammed, T., Montgomery, H. & Vidler, V. (2010) *Practices in Children's Nursing: Guidelines for Hospital and Community*, 3rd edition. Edinburgh: Churchill Livingstone.

Graham, D., Paget, S.P. & Wimalasundera, N. (2019) Current thinking in the health care management of children with cerebral palsy. *Medical Journal of Australia*, **210**(3), 129–135.

Guidelines and Audit Implementation Network (GAIN) (2015) *Guidelines for caring for an infant, child, or young person who required enteral feeding*, Available at https://www.rqia.org.uk/RQIA/files/4f/4f08bb34-7955-49ea-adf1-9de807d3da66.pdf (Accessed on 1 September 2021).

Hopwood, N., Moraby, K., Dadich, A., Gowans, J., Pointon, K., Ierardo, A., Reilly, C., Syrmis, M., Frederiksen, N., Disher-Quill, K., Scheuring, N., Heves, R. & Elliot, C. (2021) Paediatric tube-feeding: an agenda for care improvement and research. *Journal of Paediatrics and Child Health*, **57**, 182–187.

Kim, H.-J., Choi, H.-N. & Yim, J.-E. (2018) Food habits, dietary intake, and body composition in children with cerebral palsy. *Clinical Nutrition Research*, **7**(4), 266–275.

Mandal, M., Bagchi, D., Sarkar, S. & Chakrabarti, P. (2017) Nasogastric tube placement- a simple yet difficult procedure- a review. *Journal of Medical and Dental Sciences*, **6**(31), 2572–2576.

National Institute of Clinical Excellence (NICE) (2020) *Nutritional Support in Adults: enteral Tube Feeding*. Available at https://pathways.nice.org.uk/pathways/nutrition-support-in-adults. (Accessed on: 1st September 2021).

National Institute of Clinical Excellence (NICE) (2021a) *Prevention and control of healthcare-associated infections overview*. Available at https://pathways.nice.org.uk/pathways/prevention-and-control-of-healthcare-associated-infections (Accessed on 1 September 2021).

National Institute of Clinical Excellence (NICE) (2021b) Babies, children and young people's experience of healthcare. Available at https://www.nice.org.uk/guidance/ng204/resources/babies-children-and-young-peoples-experience-of-healthcare-pdf-66143714734789 (Accessed on 1 September 2021).

National Patient Safety Agency (NPSA) (2019) *Guidelines for the insetion and management of enteral feeding tubes*. Available at https://www.bsuh.nhs.uk/library/wp-content/uploads/sites/8/2019/06/Guidelines-for-the-Insertion-and-Management-of-Enteral-Tubes.pdf (Accessed on 1 September 2021).

Nur, F.T., Handryastuti, S. & Poesponegoro, H.D. (2019) Feeding Difficulties in Children with Cerebral Palsy: prevalence and Risk Factor. In: *The 1st International Conference on Health, Technology and Life Sciences*, KnE Life Sciences, 206–214.

Pope, N., Tallon, M., McConigley, R., Leslie, G. & Wilson, S. (2017) Experiences of acute pain in children who present to a healthcare facility for treatment: a systematic review of qualitative evidence. *JBI Database of Systematic Reviews and Implementation Reports*, **15**(6), 1612–1644.

Powers, J. (2019) Securing Orogastic and Nasogastric Tubes in Intubated Patients. *Critical Care Nurse*, **39**(4), 61–63.

Rees, L., Shaw, V., Qizalbash, L., Anderson, C., Desloovere, A., Greenbaum, L., Haffner, D., Nelms, C., Oosterveld, M., Paglialonga, F., Polderman, N., Renken-Terhaerdt, J., Tukkola, J., Warady, B., Van de Walle, J. & Shroff, R. (2021) Delivery of a nutritional prescription by enteral tube feeding in children with chronic kidney disease stages 2-5 and on dialysis—clinical practice recommendations from the Pediatric Renal Nutrition Taskforce. *Pediatric Nephrology*, **36**, 187–204.

Roper, N., Logan, W.W. & Tierney, A.J. (2000) *The Roper-Logan-Tierney Model of Nursing: Based on the Activities of Living*. Edinburgh: Elsevier Health Sciences.

Rosengarten, L. & Davies, B. (2021) Nutritional support for children and young people: nasogastric tubes. *British Journal of Nursing*, **30**(13), 12–18.

Sadowska, M., Sraecka-Hujar, B. & Kopyta, I. (2020) Cerebral Palsy: currrent Opinions on Definition, Epidemiology, Risk Factors, Classification and Treatment Options. *Neuropsychiatric Disease and Treatment*, **16**, 1505–1518.

SCOPE (2020) *Cerebral Palsy*. Available at https://www.scope.org.uk/advice-and-support/cerebral-palsy-introduction (Accessed: 1 September 2021).

Serjeant, S. & Tighe, B. (2021) A meta-synthesis exploring caregiver experiences of home enteral tube feeding. *Journal of Human Nutrition and Dietetics*, **00**, 1–10.

Taylor, S. (2020) Methods of Estimating Nasogastric Tube Length: all, Including "NEX," Are Unsafe. *Nutrition in Clinical Practise*, **35**(5), 864–870.

CHAPTER 30

Enteral Feeding – Gastrostomy Care

Catherine Paxton

SCENARIO

Jane is a two-year-old girl who was born prematurely at 28 weeks' gestation and suffered a grade IV intraventricular haemorrhage. This has left her with an evolving cerebral palsy. Cerebral palsy is one of the most common congenital or acquired neurological impairments in children, characterised by abnormal co-ordination of movement and/or muscle tone, Panteliadis (2015). Jane lives with her parents, Lynne and Paul, and twin brother John who is meeting his developmental milestones and suffered no health problems as a result of his prematurity. Her maternal grandparents are involved with Jane's care on a daily basis.

Jane has had feeding problems since her birth, with her family devoting large parts of each day to feeding, each meal taking up to two hours to finish. This leaves them with little time to spend on other family activities. Jane was fed via a nasogastric tube for a period of time but she kept pulling this out and the family found it increasingly stressful to repass the nasogastric tube. Many of these feeding issues have been highlighted in the literature. Glasson et al. (2020) carried out a qualitative study looking at gastrostomy and quality of life, where one parent noted 'I was probably spending an hour and a half per meal, messing around with a couple of sips of a bottle, a sprinkle of food here and there' p. 972. Placement of a gastrostomy was seen as a help to quality of life for child and family, allowing less time for feeding and more for other interactions. Within their book, Sullivan (2009) further explore the complexities and practicalities of nutritional support in children with neurodisabilities.

Jane has always been smaller than her brother, with her weight and length tracking along the 0.4th centile on her UK-WHO growth chart. Information on the growth charts can be sourced on the Royal College of Paediatrics and Child Health website. Following a recent viral illness, her weight has drifted below the 0.4th centile and her oral feeding skills have deteriorated, meaning it is becoming increasingly difficult to feed Jane. She has been referred to her local children's hospital so Jane's family can discuss the possibility of her having a gastrostomy tube inserted.

At this appointment, Jane's family met the surgeon, who discussed the procedure and the nutrition nurse, who showed them a gastrostomy tube, gave them literature to take home and answered any questions the family had. They also met the dietitian to discuss possible feeding methods once the tube is inserted. The feeds can be given as a daytime bolus or as an overnight feed via a feeding pump.

The decision to proceed and allow Jane to have a gastrostomy tube inserted was a difficult one for the family to make. The decision to go ahead with insertion of a gastrostomy tube was helped by meeting the parents of a couple of other children who had had a gastrostomy tube inserted. Gunton-Bunn and McNee (2009) carried out a review of the literature looking at the psychosocial impact of gastrostomy placement and highlighted a number of issues that are important for children's nurses to consider. These issues included the quality of information they were given at time of discussing gastrostomy tubes, what helped them to make the decision, and how the gastrostomy tube impacted on life after placement. This continues to be echoed in the literature Mahant et al. (2018) outline recommendations for clinicians engaging with families when making decisions around gastrostomy feeding.

QUESTIONS

1. What is a gastrostomy tube, and name the different types of gastrostomy tubes?
2. Discuss the nursing care of Jane in relation to the first 48 hours following insertion of her gastrostomy tube.
3. How would the children's nurse prepare Jane and her family for discharge following insertion of a gastrostomy tube?

Care Planning in Children and Young People's Nursing, Second Edition. Edited by Sonya Clarke and Doris Corkin.
© 2024 John Wiley & Sons Ltd. Published 2024 by John Wiley & Sons Ltd.

ANSWERS TO QUESTIONS

Question 1. What is a gastrostomy tube and name the different types of gastrostomy tubes?

A gastrostomy tube is a feeding tube that connects the stomach with the surface of the abdominal wall. It is usually placed in children who require medium to long-term nutrition support.

In 1980, Gauderer et al. reported a technique to insert a feeding tube that did not require a laparotomy – the percutaneous endoscopic gastrostomy (PEG), which uses an endoscope to insert a gastrostomy tube. Under general anaesthetic, the endoscope is passed through the mouth, down the oesophagus and into the stomach. A light at the end of the endoscope, along with finger indentation is used to identify a suitable position in the stomach to place the tube (Figure 30.1a). The skin is cleaned and a small incision is made in the skin, a wide-bore needle is passed through the incision into the stomach. A guide wire is passed through the needle; this is grasped by forceps which is passed through the end of the endoscope (Figure 30.1b). The endoscope and guide wire are pulled up the oesophagus and out through the mouth. The PEG tube is attached to the guide wire at the mouth, the guide wire is then pulled out through the abdominal wall pulling the PEG tube into the stomach, and an endoscope is then passed to check tube position (Figure 30.1c). Figure 30.2 shows examples of PEG tubes.

This PEG tube needs to remains in *situ* until the stoma tract has healed, usually 6–8 weeks, and can then be replaced. It can be replaced with a G-tube or low-profile skin-level feeding tube more commonly called a button (see Figure 30.3). Both of these gastrostomy tubes are held in the stomach by a water filled balloon (see Figure 30.4).

Heuschkel et al. (2015) notes that a button gastrostomy lies flush with the skin, providing a more acceptable and less obtrusive way to connect an extension set and tube feeds.

All planned care should adopt an appropriate model of nursing, for example Casey (1988) and Roper et al. (2000). Casey's model looks at working in partnership with families and it is important to work with Jane's family as they will be providing her ongoing care following discharge. Coleman et al. (2003) further explore the concept of family and carer participation by looking at a practice continuum tool. This highlights an important concept in children's nursing, identifying that there will be times during Jane's care where it will be appropriate for it to be all nurse led, for example in the immediate

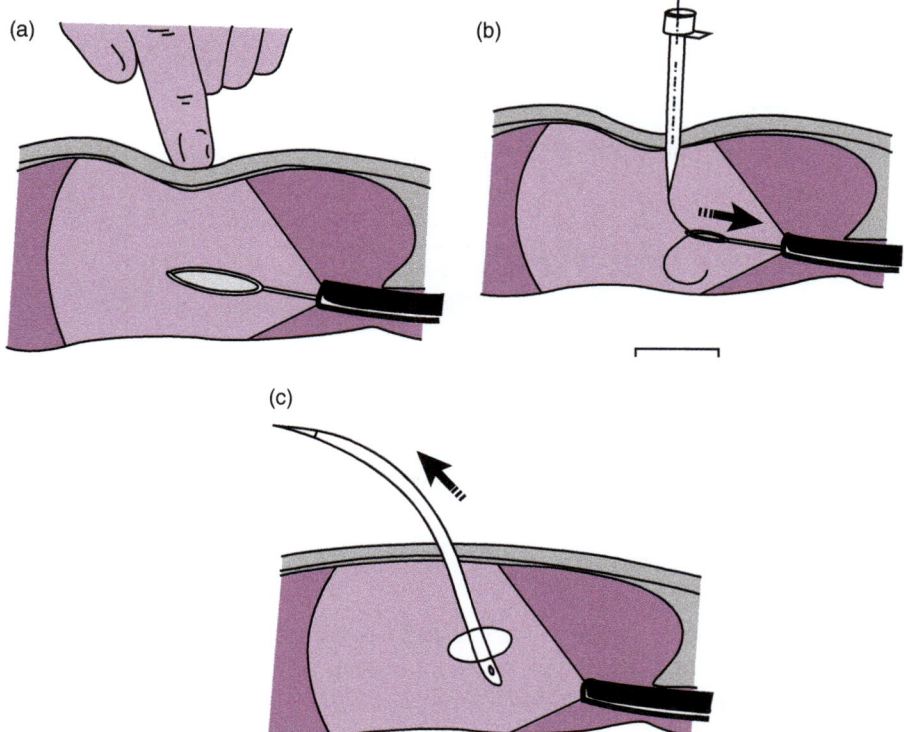

FIGURE 30.1 Percutaneous endoscopic gastrostomy tube placement (Cotton & Williams 1996). Reproduced with kind permission.

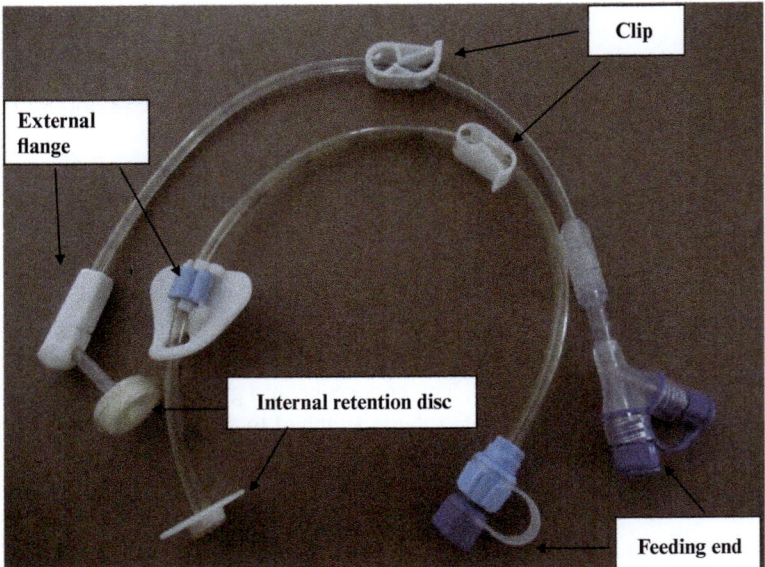

FIGURE 30.2 Percutaneous endoscopic gastrostomy (PEG) tubes and component parts.

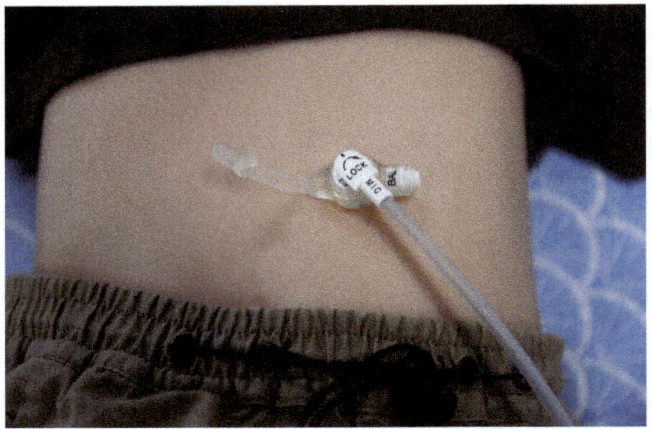

FIGURE 30.3 Low-profile skin level gastrostomy tube *in situ* (button).

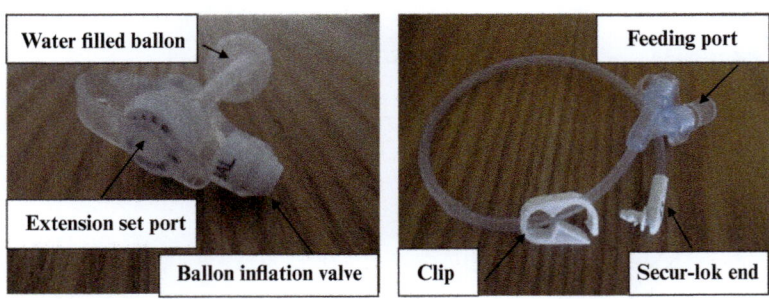

FIGURE 30.4 Low-profile button and extension set.

postoperative period, moving through to times where it is all parent or family led, for example just prior to discharge home having completed training for home enteral tube feeding. It is important though to negotiate how, and indeed how much family involvement there is on an individual family basis Watts et al. (2014). Although Roper et al. (2000) address 12 activities of daily living (see Chapter 1) this chapter will only address maintaining a safe environment, personal cleansing and dressing, and eating and drinking in relation to postoperative care and discharge planning.

Question 2. Discuss the nursing care of Jane in relation to the first 48 hours following insertion of her gastrostomy tube.

Activity of living: maintaining a safe environment.

Assess and plan postoperative interventions:

- Family-centred partnership approach to care; involve the parents when collecting Jane from recovery and return Jane to her prepared bed space. Jane's parents and grandparents to be involved in all aspects of care.

Implement postoperative interventions:

- In order to be able to manage any postoperative airway problems that may arise, ensure that the bed space has working oxygen and suction for Jane's return from theatre.
- Attach Jane to appropriate monitoring and infusion equipment as per hospital policy.
- Read medical and nursing notes, adhering to anaesthetist and surgeon's instructions.
- Record observations, TPR, SAO2 (oxygen saturations), and BP on appropriate postoperative documentation. Frequency of monitoring as per hospital protocol.

Paediatric Early Warning Scores (PEWS) charts have been introduced to aid recognition of clinical deterioration, that may occur in the post-operative period, and appropriate escalation to staff with emergency and critical care skills, Chapman and Maconochie (2019).

- Using an appropriate pain assessment tool for children with a neurodevelopmental disorder, assess and record pain score. Crosta et al. (2014) identify and review a range of assessment tools that might be used for children with cerebral palsy (see also Appendix Is this appendix still in the book and is the reference up to date? 3, RCN 2010 pain guidelines).
- Administer analgesia as required in accordance with medical prescription. Note, although insertion of a gastrostomy is a relatively simple procedure, children can experience high levels of post-procedure pain requiring regular paracetamol, non-steroidal, and occasionally opiate based medications.
- Observe gastrostomy stoma site for redness, leakage, and swelling. The early detection of complications following gastrostomy is crucial, as highlighted by the National Patient Safety Alert (2010). Adjust external fixator (see Figure 30.2) on gastrostomy tube if it appears tight.
- Hospital policy may be to attach the gastrostomy tube to a drainage bag and leave on free drainage in the immediate postoperative period to allow for drainage of gastric contents and stomach decompression.
- Provide ongoing support to Jane's family and provide explanations for all interventions.

Activity of living: eating and drinking.

Assess and plan postoperative interventions:

- To assess Jane's nutritional status using a nutrition screening tool, for example Paediatric Yorkhill Malnutrition Score (PYMS) (Gerasimidis et al. 2010). Plan how to meet Jane's nutritional requirements following insertion of her gastrostomy tube.
- To monitor and maintain Jane's hydration.

Implement postoperative interventions:

- Nil by mouth/feeding tube for first 3–12 hours, post-gastrostomy tube insertion. The timing of feed commencement varies between centres. Homan et al. (2021) suggest feeding can commence three hours after gastrostomy tube placement. The length of hospital stay is reduced in those that commence feeds earlier Peck et al. (2020).
- Administer intravenous fluids as per prescription, adhering to local hospital intravenous policy on monitoring of intravenous cannula site and infusion pump pressures.
- Commence enteral feeds according to dietician plan once medical staff have advised feeding can commence.
- Wash hands, put on gloves and apron before handling feed or setting up feed pump (see Figure 30.5). The National Institute for Health and Care Excellence (NICE) (2012) in their Healthcare-associated infections clinical guideline highlights importance of food hygiene when setting up enteral feed pumps.

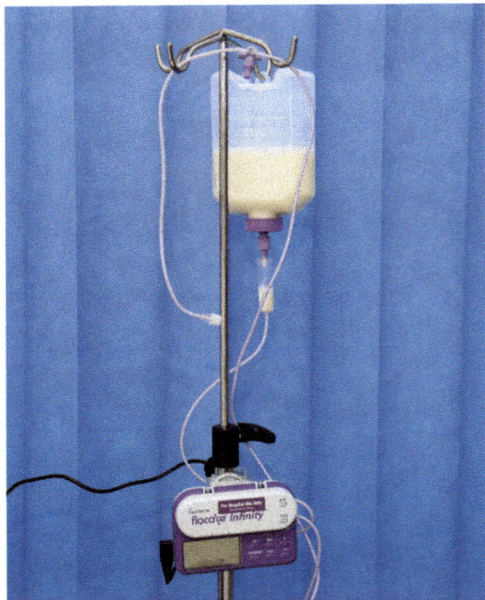

FIGURE 30.5 An enteral feed pump.

Activity of living: personal cleansing and dressing.

Assess and plan postoperative interventions:

- Assess Jane's personal cleansing and dressing requirements in partnership with her parents.
- Ensure that all equipment required to carry out Jane's personal hygiene has been collected and is close to hand.

Implement postoperative interventions:

- Maintain oral hygiene, especially while nil by mouth.
- Always wash and dry hands before handling the PEG tube.
- Put on gloves and an apron.
- Clean the PEG stoma site using gauze and sterile water or saline, this should be demonstrated to Jane's family and they should then be supervised carrying out the procedure.
- The gastrostomy stoma site should be cleaned and dried once a day.
- Avoid using any creams or talcum powder around the gastrostomy stoma site.

Evaluate all nursing interventions and document

Activity: did you do what you aimed to do and what was the outcome to reduce risk of infection?

Question 3. How would the children's nurse prepare Jane and her family for discharge following insertion of a gastrostomy tube?

Assess and plan for a safe discharge:

- Discharge planning should ideally begin on admission. Jane is assessed as clinically fit for discharge home: apyrexial, tolerating oral and gastrostomy feeds, gastrostomy site is satisfactory. Jane's family members are educated and confident they can carry out Jane's ongoing care at home.
- Identify those members of the multidisciplinary team in the community that need to be contacted and any equipment the family will require to provide ongoing care for Jane at home.

Page et al. (2021) carried out a survey of family carers looking at training and support following a child's gastrostomy placement. As well as valuing support from other parents they valued ongoing learning and support from community nurses.

Activity of living: maintaining a safe environment:

Implementation of discharge plan:

- Ensure local hospital training checklist is completed and signed; examples of these can be found on the Children with Exceptional needs website. (https://www.cen.scot.nhs.uk/training-parentscarers-and-health-care-support-staff)
- All equipment (feed pump and stand, prescribed feed, giving sets and syringes) required for discharge home is supplied.
- Jane is registered with a homecare company for ongoing feed and equipment supplies.
- Referral to children s community nurse for support and advice at home and to arrange training on use of the gastrostomy tube for staff at Jane's nursery.
- Discharge medication checked as per hospital policy, given, and administration instructions explained to the family. Paracetamol and ibuprofen for pain relief, Omeprazole and domperidone for gastroesophageal reflux as per doctor's advice.
- Doctor's letter for GP is given to Jane's family.
- Outpatient appointment arranged and given to the parents.

Activity of living: eating and drinking:

- Parents are educated and able to use the enteral feeding pump and administer bolus feeds.
- Jane is tolerating her feeds as per the dietician's feed plan. No or minimal vomiting, bowels are moving regularly without any difficulty.
- Parents know what to watch for in terms of Jane not tolerating feeds, for example vomiting, loose stools, or constipation.
- Referral to speech and language therapist for ongoing input with oral feeding skills.
- Parents have a copy of the dietician's feed plan and a contact number for their dietician.

Activity of living: personal cleansing and dressing:

- Parents are advised to dress Jane in vests with popper fasteners to keep her gastrostomy tube tucked underneath her clothing and prevent it from getting caught when being lifted.
- For the first two weeks following gastrostomy tube insertion showers are preferable to immersion baths. Jane has a bathing chair and can be sat in this to be showered.
- Parents demonstrate competent cleaning and drying of the stoma site: turning the gastrostomy tube through 360 degrees and adjustment of external fixator as required. Once home a clean cloth, unscented soap, and water should be used to clean the stoma site. In a survey of family carers Page et al. (2021) they reported that the training carried out as demonstration and practice supervised by a Healthcare Professional as 'extremely useful' when learning to care for their child's gastrostomy tube.
- Homan et al. (2021) advise that swimming is permitted but shouldn't be encouraged for two weeks post gastrostomy insertion.
- Contact nutrition nurse specialist for advice on any gastrostomy tube related complications. Common complications include leakage, blockage, overgranulation (see Figure 30.6), and infection (Townley et al. 2017).

Evaluate all nursing interventions and document

Activity: did you do what you aimed to do, and what was the outcome?

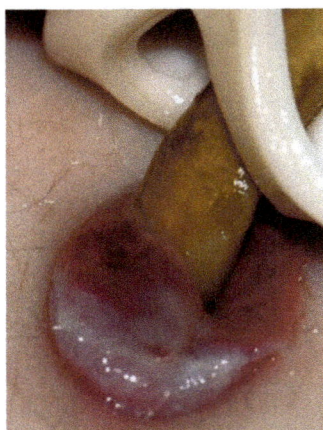

FIGURE 30.6 Overgranulation tissue at stoma site.

ADDITIONAL RESOURCES

https://www.whatwhychildreninhospital.org.uk/GT-hospital (accessed 3 Oct 2021)
https://www.whatwhychildreninhospital.org.uk/GT-home (accessed 3 Oct 2021)
https://www.oxstar.ox.ac.uk/more/supporting-parents/your-childs-gastrostomy (accessed 3 Oct 2021)
https://www.patientsafetyoxford.org/clinical-safety-programmes/previous-programmes/paediatric-gastrostomy/overview/paediatric-gastrostomy-resources/booklets-for-parents (accessed 3 Oct 2021)
https://www.nutriciaflocare.com/infinity_pump.php
www.freegopump.co.uk
https://www.nice.org.uk/guidance/cg139/evidence (accessed 3 Oct 2021)
https://www.healthcareimprovementscotland.org/previous_resources/best_practice_statement/caring_for_children_and_young_.aspx (accessed 24 Oct 2021)

REFERENCES

Casey, A. (1988) A partnership with child and family. *Senior Nurse*, **8**(4), 8–9.

Chapman, S.M. & Maconochie, I.K. (2019) Early warning score in paediatrics: an overview. *Archives of Disease in Childhood*, **104**, 395–399. 10.1136/archdischild-2018-314807. https://www.cen.scot.nhs.uk/training-parentscarers-and-health-care-support-staff (accessed 24 June 2022).

Coleman, V., Smith, L. & Bradshaw, M. (2003) Enhancing consumer participation using the practice continuum tool for family-centred care. *Paediatric Nursing*, **15**(8), 28–31. DOI: 10.7748/paed2003.10.15.8.28.c876

Cotton, P. & Williams, C. (1996) *Practical Gastrointestinal Endoscopy*, 4th edition. Oxford: Wiley-Blackwell.

Crosta, Q.R., Ward, T.M., Walker, A.J. & Peters, L.M. (2014) A review of pain measures for hospitalized children with cognitive impairment. *Journal for Specialists in Pediatric Nursing*, **19**, 109–118. doi:10.1111/jspn.12069.

Gerasimidis, K., Keane, O., Macleod, I., Flynn, D.M. & Wright, C.M. (2010) A four-stage evaluation of the Paediatric Yorkhill Malnutrition Score in a tertiary paediatric hospital and a district general hospital. *British Journal of Nutrition*, **104**(5), 751–756. DOI: 10.1017/S0007114510001121

Glasson, E.J., Forbes, D., Ravikumara, M., Nagarajan, L., Wilson, A., Jacoby, P., Wong, K., Leonard, H. & Downs, J. (2020) Gastostomy and quality of life in children with intellectual disability: a qualitative study. *Archives of Disease in Childhood*, **105**, 969–974. https://pubmed.ncbi.nlm.nih.gov/32269039 [accessed 6 March 2023]

Gunton-Bunn, C. & McNee, P. (2009) Psychosocial implications of gastrostomy placement. *Paediatric Nursing*, **21**(7), 28–31. DOI: 10.7748/paed2009.09.21.7.28.c7230

Heuschkel, R.B., Gottrand, F., Devarajan, K., Poole, H., Callan, J. & Dias, J.A. (2015) ESPGHAN position paper on management of percutaneous endoscopic gastrostomy in children and adolescents. *Journal of Pediatric Gastroenterology & Nutrition*, **60**, 131–141. https://doi.org/10.1097/mpg.0000000000000501.

Homan, M., Hauser, B., Romano, C., Tzivinikos, C., Torroni, F., Gottrand, F., Hojsak, I., Dall'Oglio, L., Thomson, M., Bontems, P., Narula, P., Furlano, R., Oliva, S. & Amil-Dias, J. (2021) Percutaneous endoscopic gastrostomy in children: an update to the ESPGHAN position paper. *Journal of Pediatric Gastroenterology & Nutrition*, **73**, 415–426. https://doi.org/10.1097/mpg.0000000000003207.

Mahant, S., Cohen, E., Nelson, K.E. & Rosenbaum, P. (2018) Decision-making around gastrostomy tube feeding in children with neurological impairment: engaging effectively with families. *Paediatrics & Child Health*, **23**(3), 209–213. doi:10.1093/pch/pxx193.

National Institute for Health and Care Excellence (2012) Healthcare-associated infections: prevention and control in primary and community care. Available from: https://www.nice.org.uk/guidance/cg139/evidence/control-full-guideline-pdf-185186701.

Page, B., Butler, S., Smith, C., Lee, A.C.H. & Vincent, C.A. (2021) Training and support for a child's gastrostomy: a survey with family carers. *British Medical Journal Paediatrics Open*, **5**, e001068. doi:10.1136/bmjpo-2021-001068.

Panteliadis, C.P., Hagel, C., Karch, D. & Heinemann, K. (2015) Cerebral Palsy: a lifelong challenge asks for early intervention. *The Open Neurology Journal*, **9**, 45–52. DOI: 10.2174/1874205X01509010045

Peck, J., Mills, K., Dey, A., Nguyen, A.T.H., Amankwah, E.K., Wilsey, A., Swan, E., Sorany, S., Karjoo, S., McClenathon, D. & Wilsey, M. (2020) Comparison of tolerance and complication rates between early and delayed feeding after percutaneous endoscopic gastrostomy placement in children. *Journal of Pediatric Gastroenterology and Nutrition*, **70**(1), 55–58. https://europepmc.org/article/med/31567888.

Roper, N., Logan, W.W. & Tierney, A.J. (2000) *The Roper-Logan-Tierney Model of Nursing: Based on Activities of Living*. Edinburgh: Elsevier Health Sciences.

Sullivan, P.B. (2009) *Feeding and Nutrition in Children with Neurodevelopmental Disability*. London: MacKeith Press.

Townley. A., Wincentak, J., Krog, K., Schippke, J., & Kingsnorth, S. (2017) Paediatric gastrostomy stoma complications and treatments: a rapid scoping review. *J Clin Nurs*. **27**(7-8):1369–1380. DOI: 10.1111/jocn.14233

Watts, R., Huaqiong, Z., Shields, L., Taylor, M., Munns, A. & Ngune, I. (2014) Family-centred care for hospitalized children aged 0-12 years: a systematic review of qualitative studies. *JBI Database of Systematic Reviews & Implementation Reports*, **12**(7), 204–283. doi:10.11124/jbisrir-2014-1683.

Care of Children and Young Persons with Endocrine Disorders

SECTION 9

Nephrotic Syndrome

Janet Kelsey

CHAPTER 31

SCENARIO

Gary, aged four years, has recently started to wake up with puffy eyes and tiredness. His abdomen is now swollen, and his urine has become frothy and reduced in amount. Gary went to his GP with both his parents where he was found to have ++++ of protein in his urine. Gary was referred to the local children's assessment unit where he was assessed and admitted to the children's ward.

QUESTIONS

1. What is nephrotic syndrome (NS)?
2. Discuss specific NS nursing care of Gary, especially during the first three days since admission to hospital.
3. Explain the normal mechanism for maintaining tissue fluid balance.
4. Describe pharmaceutical management of NS.

ANSWERS TO QUESTIONS

Question 1. What is nephrotic syndrome (NS)?

Nephrotic syndrome is a condition traditionally presenting with the classic triad of marked oedema, decreased serum albumin, and albuminuria alongside hyperlipidaemia. A syndrome is a group of signs and/or symptoms which occur together, the cause of which is not always obvious. The disease is characterised by degenerative lesions in the kidney (nephrosis). There is increased permeability of the glomeruli and consequently a high loss of plasma protein in the urine (albuminuria). Nephrotic syndrome is defined as the combination of 'significant' proteinuria (protein: dipstick 3–4+ or urine protein/creatinine ratio >0.2 g/mmol = >200 mg/mmol), hypoalbuminemia (less than 25 g/L), and generalised oedema. Primary nephrotic syndrome, also known as idiopathic nephrotic syndrome (INS), is associated with glomerular diseases intrinsic to the kidney and not related to systemic causes. The cause is not fully understood. However, it is thought that there may be an immune pathogenic response (Lane 2020; Lee 2021). Secondary nephrotic syndrome refers to an aetiology extrinsic to the kidney such as infection, conditions such as Lupis, medications and drugs for example lithium, nonsteroidal anti-inflammatory drugs, and heroin (Andolino & Reid-Adam 2015). Additionally, more than 39 genes have been associated with nephrotic syndrome and approximately 30% of children with steroid resistant disease having a genetic cause for their disease (Lane 2020).

Proteinuria is definitive of nephrosis; it occurs because of changes to capillary endothelial cells, the glomerular basement membrane, or podocytes, which normally filter serum protein selectively by size and 'charge'. Most recently molecular changes in the glomerular capillary wall have been identified as explaining the proteinuria and in minimal change disease, the increased glomerular permeability to plasma proteins, has been attributed to changes in the negative charge in the capillary wall (Cara-Fuentes et al. 2016). The result is urinary loss of macromolecular proteins, primarily albumin, but also opsonins, immunoglobulins, erythropoietin, transferring, hormone-binding proteins, and antithrombin III in conditions that cause non-selective proteinuria (McMillan 2010).

Care Planning in Children and Young People's Nursing, Second Edition. Edited by Sonya Clarke and Doris Corkin.
© 2024 John Wiley & Sons Ltd. Published 2024 by John Wiley & Sons Ltd.

The traditional explanation for oedema is known as the underfill theory, as the plasma protein concentration falls so does the colloid osmotic pressure that it exerts; therefore, fluid moves out of the capillaries and accumulates in the tissue spaces to cause oedema. The resulting fall in the blood flow through the kidneys causes them to secrete renin, an enzyme which stimulates the production of aldosterone by the adrenal cortex. This causes an increase in the re-absorption of water and salt through the kidney tubules. This re-absorption exacerbates the generalised oedema. However, in contrast the overfill theory presents the case for a defect in renal sodium handling where the increase in renal sodium reabsorption leads to salt and water retention intravascular volume expansion and subsequent hypertension (Lane 2020; Lee 2021).

Disordered lipid metabolism results in hyperlipidaemia presenting as elevated serum cholesterol and triglyceride concentrations for which the explanation has been that the liver increases protein synthesis to replace the serum proteins lost in the urine (Tao et al. 2000). Furthermore Lane (2020) reports that serum cholesterol levels have been shown to be separate to the level of albumin synthesis. It is not known if this altered lipid metabolism alters the long-term risk of atherosclerosis

Complications of nephrotic syndrome nay include thromboembolism, infection, hypertension, and acute kidney injury. Thrombosis may occur as a result of the loss of antithrombin III, and this can be exacerbated by hypovolemia. The loss of immunoglobulins increases the risk of infection and transient hypertension may be an atypical presentation and volume overload should be considered. Lee (2021) cites Gipson et al. 2009) stating that hypertension is present in 13% to 51% of children with nephrotic syndrome. Acute kidney injury risk factors include intravascular volume depletion, infection, nephrotoxic agents, and interstitial oedema (Rheault et al 2015). Risk of infection is increased due to the low immunoglobulin levels which may be as a result of impaired synthesis and possible impaired T cell function. Any number of infections can occur including peritonitis and sepsis (Lane 2020).

Children presenting with NS are likely to be lethargic, irritable, and have poor appetite; they may also have diarrhoea and abdominal pain and an upper respiratory tract infection. Blood pressure is usually normal or low. Persistent hypertension is rare in minimal change disease (MCD) or focal segmental glomerulosclerosis (FSGS) and should raise suspicion of some other form of glomerular disease such as membranoproliferative disease (Dolan & Gill 2008). Occasionally children present with gross haematuria.

Nephrotic syndrome can affect children of any age but is most common amongst school age and adolescence. Up to 90% of cases of childhood NS have MCD, the commonest glomerular disease of childhood, with a median age at presentation of four years, which is more common in males than females (ratio 3:2). Over 90% of cases with MCD will respond to steroid therapy (Hodson et al. 2009). About 80% to 90% of children with steroid-sensitive nephrotic syndrome (SSNS) have relapses (Larkins et al. 2020). Steroid responsiveness is the most important determining factor in the long-term prognosis of NS. Conditions such as FSGS and mesangiocapillary glomerulosclerosis (MCGN) account for the remaining 20% of cases of NS. These conditions tend to present in the older child and the majority do not respond to oral steroid therapy (Dolan & Gill 2008).

Question 2. Discuss specific NS nursing care of Gary, especially during the first three days since admission to hospital.

Children presenting with their first episode of NS are admitted to hospital for diagnostic assessment, nursing and medical management, and parental education. Therefore, the initial nursing assessment should be in partnership with child and family (Casey 1988), and include the following specific to NS: observation of the level of oedema – weight on admission is taken as a baseline observation. Note any swelling around the eyes, ankles, and other dependent parts and record the level of pitting – in Gary's case the scrotal area should be observed for swelling, irritation, or redness and the skin should be inspected for any evidence of breakdown. Ask Gary and his mother about his appetite, urinary output, and signs of tiredness or irritability. Assess vital signs, including capillary refill and blood pressure, and ask about recent infections. Carry out urinalysis to identify protein loss and specific gravity.

It is likely that the following problems will be identified specific to his NS:

- An excess fluid volume
- Risk of imbalanced nutrition
- Risk of impaired skin integrity
- Risk of tiredness and/or irritability
- Risk of infection
- Lack of understanding of the disease process and care planning

The NS specific goals of Gary's nursing care are therefore to relieve oedema and return fluid balance to within normal parameters, improve his nutrition, maintain skin integrity, to conserve Gary's energy, to prevent infection, and for Gary and his family to learn about the disease and the care required both in immediate future and long term. Gary will also require venepuncture as part of the investigations into his NS and should be prepared for this procedure and it should be carried out as for any child.

Activity of living: eating and drinking (Roper et al. 2000).

Problem:

- Gary has an excess fluid volume
- Gary is at risk of hypovolemia
- Risk of imbalanced nutrition

Goals:

- Gary's oedema will be reduced, and this will be evidenced by appropriate weight loss and reduced abdominal girth.
- Gary will not become hypovolaemic.
- Gary will have an adequate nutritional intake to meet his normal growth needs, evidenced by him eating 80% of his meals.

Implement and evaluate:

- Daily weighing with minimal clothing and an empty bladder to determine increase or decrease in weight as a result of either retention of fluid or successful diuresis (1L of fluid =1kg of weight).
- Recording of oral/parenteral input and measurement of output to help calculate fluid requirements and to provide a visual means of determining the degree of diuresis.
- Observation of level of oedema. To identify the presence of oedema digital pressure is applied to the swollen area; removal of digital pressure leaves a characteristic indentation or pitting of the tissues.
- If Gary has mild oedema any need for fluid restriction should be frequently evaluated.
- Test all urine for protein losses and measurement of specific gravity. Remission is determined as continuous negative protein loss.
- Observation for signs of hypovolemia to include cool peripheries, capillary refill time >2 seconds, a core-peripheral temperature gap of >2ºC, tachycardia and dizziness. Although hypotension is a late sign of hypovolemia, blood pressure should be monitored regularly with appropriate size cuff.
- Any signs of hypovolemia should be escalated immediately.
- A no-added-salt diet whilst there is >++ proteinuria, this is dependent on the level of oedema and changed as appropriate.
- Offer a balanced diet which appeals to Gary.

Activity of living: maintaining a safe environment.

Problem:

- Risk of impaired skin integrity
- Risk of infection
- Gary is at risk of thrombosis
- Risk of pulmonary oedema

Goals:

- Gary will be free from signs of infection, as evidenced by normal vital signs.
- Respiration will be within normal limits with normal respiratory sounds.
- Skin integrity will be maintained, as evidenced by his skin remaining free from breakdown with no evidence of redness or irritation.
- Gary will show no evidence of thrombosis

Implement and evaluate:

- Temperature, pulse, and respiration are measured and recorded four hourly. A rise in temperature, pulse, and respiration rates might indicate an underlying infection. The breathing rate, rhythm, and depth should be observed to identify the accumulation of fluid in pulmonary spaces and escalated in accordance with paediatric early warning scoring.
- Regular observations of oxygen saturations. Any symptoms of respiratory distress should be escalated immediately.
- Protect Gary from anyone with an infection; this includes children, staff, family, and visitors. Prevention of cross infection is important for all patients, but children with NS are at increased risk of bacterial infection, most commonly with *Streptococcus pneumoniae*. This increased susceptibility is due to urinary loss of immunoglobulins and complement components. It is therefore desirable to provide some isolation initially to prevent cross infection, though many units do not advocate such measures except where the child is on immunosuppressive drug therapy.
- Administer prophylactic antibiotics if prescribed.
- Inspect all skin surfaces regularly for breakdown; ensure Gary changes his position at a minimum of two hourly. Bathe and dry skin carefully especially in skin folds.
- Offer a scrotal support if Gary's scrotum is swollen.
- If Gary is hypovolemic then consider nursing him in anti-embolism stockings.

Activity of living: working and playing.

Problem:

- Gary will potentially be isolated from other children and not have access to his normal play activities.

Goal: Gary will conserve energy and play appropriately, as evidenced by him resting as needed and engaging in a level of play he is comfortable with.

Implement and evaluate:

- Encourage Gary to rest when he is tired. Bed rest is not encouraged as there is an increased risk of thrombosis due to the loss of proteins such as anti-thrombin 111; this might be exacerbated by hypovolaemia (Renal Clinicians Group 2005).
- Assist Gary to mobilise when he is feeling more able.

- Provide play activities appropriate to age.
- Play with Gary at his pace.

Activity of living: communication.

Problem:

- Gary and his family do not have understanding of his current illness.

Goal:

- Gary and his family will verbalise an understanding of the disease and his care needs.

Implement and evaluate:

- Ascertain current level of knowledge and understanding.
- Involve family in planning care.
- Provide a written plan of care.
- Teach the family about the use of steroids.
- Teach family about how to keep Gary in optimum health; this should include recognising signs of infection, how to respond to increasing weight either due to oedema, or the potential to become overweight following steroid therapy, how to test his urine, and respond to increasing proteinuria and advice regarding vaccinations.
- Provide Gary and his family with written information and documentation for recording protein levels prior to discharge.

Question 3. Explain the normal mechanism for maintaining tissue fluid balance.

Tissue fluid balance is maintained by the counteraction of two pressures: blood pressure and the osmotic pressure of plasma protein. This is achieved by the following processes:

1. At the arterial end of the capillaries the blood pressure is greater than the osmotic pressure. As a result, fluid is forced through the capillary walls into the tissue spaces.

2. At the venous end the osmotic pressure is greater than the blood pressure and fluid is therefore drawn into the capillary.

Normally these two opposing factors keep a steady balance of fluid in the tissues. Any factor which disturbs this equilibrium may lead to oedema.

Oedema is said to be present when there is excess fluid in the interstitial spaces. For example, sodium and water retention leads to increased blood pressure and loss of protein in the urine (proteinuria). This leads to a decrease in plasma protein (hypoproteinaemia) and therefore decreases osmotic pressure. Fluid then collects and stagnates in the interstitial space.

Question 4. Describe pharmaceutical management of NS.

Corticosteroids

Currently a 12-week initial course is recommended with the general consensus being daily steroid induction followed by alternate day maintenance and then stop. All children should be issued with a steroid warning card and advised that the medicine should be taken with food to reduce the gastrointestinal side effects. Medication may be prescribed to protect against gastric irritation during steroid treatment. However, 60–80% of steroid-responsive nephrotic children will relapse and 60% of these > five relapses. Relapses often being triggered by other illnesses. A child is considered to have relapsed if they produce >2+ proteinuria for more than 3 days and parents should be aware to contact their healthcare team.

Corticosteroids are both anti-inflammatory and immunosuppressive. The objectives of steroid therapy are to induce and maintain remission and to minimise side effects (Box 31.1). Diuresis generally occurs one to two weeks after therapy starts. This is followed by a reduction in the oedema. Prolonged steroid therapy may be associated with side effects. Refer to Box 31.2.

BOX 31.1

Corticosteroid side effects
Behavioural problems
Increased appetite
Weight gain/obesity
Acne
Hirsutism
Increased susceptibility to infection
Posterior subcapsular cataracts

Hypertension
Growth suppression
Pubertal delay
Adrenal suppression
Acute pancreatitis
Osteoporosis
Impaired glucose metabolism

BOX 31.2

Side-effects of cyclophosphamide (Dolan & Gill 2008)
Bone marrow suppression
Reversible hair loss
Gastro-intestinal upset

Haemorrhagic cystitis
Impaired fertility
Malignancy

For children who relapse frequently and are at risk of adverse effects from corticosteroids Non-corticosteroid immunosuppressive medications are used to prolong periods of remission in these children. The most recent systematic review showed that oral or IV cyclophosphamide, oral chlorambucil, levamisole, cyclosporin, and rituximab substantially reduce the incidence of relapse in children with relapsing SSNS (Larkins et al. 2020).

Antibiotics
Prophylactic penicillin may be beneficial whilst the child is oedematous and has proteinuria, but this is usually discontinued when the child goes into remission. Suspected infections should be treated promptly (NHSGGC 2017).

Albumin
The clinical indications for albumin are clinical hypovolaemia and severe symptomatic oedema. However, children should be monitored closely during administration due to the possibility of intravascular overload and pulmonary oedema (NHSGGC 2017).

Diuretics
Diuretics may be used to control oedema until remission begins, but close observation for hypovolaemia is essential as plasma volume may be present and hypovolaemic shock can result (Lane 2020).

Immunisation
Live vaccines should not be given to immunosuppressed children; all children with nephrotic syndrome should be vaccinated against pneumococcal infections. Varicella vaccination may be offered when the child is in remission and not immunocompromised (NHSGGC 2017).

REFERENCES

Andolino, T.P. & Reid-Adam, J. (2015) Nephrotic syndrome. *Pediatrics in Review*, **36**(3), 117–126. https://doi.org/10.1542/pir.36-3-117 (accessed 12 August 2021).

Cara-Fuentes, G., Clapp, W.L., Johnson, R.J. & Garin, E.H. (2016) Pathogenesis of proteinuria in idiopathic minimal change disease: molecular mechanisms. *Pediatric Nephrology*, **31**(12), 2179–2189. https://link.springer.com/article/10.1007/s00467-016-3379-4 (accessed 12 August 2021).

Casey, A. (1988) A partnership with child and family. *Senior Nurse*, **8**(4), 8–9.

Dolan, M. & Gill, D. (2008) Management of nephritic syndrome. *Paediatrics and Child Health*, **18**(8), 369–374.

Gipson, D.S., Massengill, S.F., Yao, L., Nagaraj, S., Smoyer, W.E., Mahan, J.D., Wigfall, D., Miles, P., Powell, L., Lin, J., Trachtman, H. & Greenbaum, L.A. (2009) Management of childhood onset nephrotic syndrome. *Pediatrics*, **124**(2), 747–757. https://doi.org/10.1542/peds.2008-1559.

Hodson, E.M., Willis, N.S. & Craig, J.C. (2009) Corticosteroid therapy for nephrotic syndrome in children (Review) The Cochrane Library, Issue 1. www.thecochranelibrary.com (accessed 2 September 2009).

Lane, J. (2020) Pediatric Nephrotic syndrome. E-medicine Nephrology. http://emedicine.medscape.com (accessed 12 August 2021).

Larkins, N.G., Liu, I.D., Willis, N.S., Craig, J.C. & Hodson, E.M. (2020) Non-corticosteroid immunosuppressive medications for steroid-sensitive nephrotic syndrome in children. *Cochrane Database of Systematic Reviews* Issue 4, Art. No.: CD002290. DOI: 10.1002/14651858. CD002290.pub5 (accessed 6 September 2021).

Lee, J. (2021) Children with kidney disease: an overview of pediatric primary nephrotic syndrome. *Pediatric Nursing*, **47**(3), 109–113, 123 (accessed 12 August 2021).

McMillan, J. (2010) Nephrotic syndrome Merck manuals online medical library. www.merck.com/mmpe/sec17/ch235/ch235c.html#BABDDJGD (accessed 28 September 2010).

NHSGGC (2017) Paediatrics for Health professionals. Idiopathic Nephrotic Syndrome in Children, Management. https://www.clinicalguidelines.scot.nhs.uk (accessed 6 September 2021).

Renal Clinicians Group (2005) *Guidelines for the Management of Nephritic Syndrome*. Renal Unit Royal Hospital for Sick Children. Galsgow: Yorkhill Division.

Rheault, M.N., Zhang, L., Selewski, D. T., Kallash, M., Tran, C. L., Seamon, M., Katsoufis, C., Ashoor, I., Hernandez, J., Supe-Markovina, K., D'Alessandri-Silva, C., DeJesus-Gonzalez, N., Vasylyeva, T.L., Formeck, C., Woll, C., Gbadegesin, R., Geier, P., Devarajan, P., Carpenter, S. L., Kerlin, B.A., Smoyer, W. E. (2015). AKI in Children Hospitalized with Nephrotic Syndrome. *Clinical Journal of the American Society of Nephrology*, **10** (12): 2110–2118, December. doi: 10.2215/CJN.06620615.

Roper, N., Logan, W. & Tierney, A.J. (2000) *The Roper-Logan-Tierney Model of Nursing: Based on Activities of Living*. London: Elsevier.

Tao, M., Wang, H.-P., Sun, J. et al. (2000) Progress of research on dyslipidemia accompanied by nephrotic syndrome. *Chronic Diseases and Translational Medicine*, 2020, **6** (03): 182–187. DOI: https://www.sciencedirect.com/science/article/pii/S2095882X21000220 [Accessed 6 March 2023].

CHAPTER 32

Newly Diagnosed Diabetic

Pauline Cardwell, Doris Corkin, and Lynne Robinson

SCENARIO

Miley, a six-year-old girl who is in the pre-operational stage of cognitive development (Bee & Boyd 2013), has become 'out of sorts' recently. She lives at home with her parents and her twin brothers who are 18 months old. Her parents describe Miley as normally a very energetic child, and recently as being too tired to play and more impatient than usual. They also notice that her breath is 'smelly' and she woke during the night complaining of 'a sore tummy'.

Whilst at the GP surgery, Miley has her urine tested and it is quickly identified that the sample contains glucose and ketones. Additionally, the practice nurse carries out a blood glucose test which reveals a sugar level of 22.5 mmol/L (normal range 4–7 mmol/L, National Institute for Health and Care Excellence (NICE) 2016). Dr Good, her GP, advises Miley's parents that it is likely she has diabetes and that she needs to go to hospital for further investigations and management of her condition.

Miley is referred to the children's medical ward by her GP with a provisional diagnosis of diabetes mellitus (DM). On admission to the ward Miley's parents appear anxious, distressed and demanding answers to questions. According to Miley's parents, she has been drinking excessive amounts of fluids, passing urine frequently (polyuria), losing weight and generally feeling unwell, over the last 2–3 weeks. Following further investigations in the children's ward, Miley's diagnosis of diabetes mellitus type 1 (DMT1) is confirmed with an HbA1c (111 mmol/mol) blood test that measures long-term blood glucose (normal non-diabetic HbA1c is 42 mmol/mol). In diabetes 48 mmol/mol is target (Diabetes UK), so treatment and management of disease need to be established.

WHAT IS DIABETES MELLITUS?

This is a chronic disease which is characterised by a raised blood glucose level, resulting from a lack of the hormone insulin or a resistance to insulin in the body. The disease is categorised into two main types: type 1 and type 2, which will impact on the ongoing management of the condition.

QUESTIONS

1. Explain the pathophysiology of diabetes mellitus type 1.
2. Discuss the impact of this condition for Miley and her family.
3. Outline how to monitor blood glucose levels and administer insulin.
4. Describe the information that Miley and her parents will require to manage her condition safely after discharge from hospital in relation to managing hypoglycaemia and hyperglycaemia attacks.

The proposed answer plans offer 'lists of potential responses' with limited rationale; it is therefore recommended for the individual student/healthcare professional to explore the issues through further reading. Answers are not meant to be definitive or restrictive and may be amended to facilitate changing circumstances at any time.

Care Planning in Children and Young People's Nursing, Second Edition. Edited by Sonya Clarke and Doris Corkin.
© 2024 John Wiley & Sons Ltd. Published 2024 by John Wiley & Sons Ltd.

ANSWERS TO QUESTIONS

Question 1. Explain the pathophysiology of diabetes mellitus type 1.

Diabetes mellitus type 1 (DMT1) is the most common endocrine disorder in children, which can occur at any stage of development during childhood, even during infancy, with an increasing incidence in the UK (Burns et al. 2010). Literature would suggest that the aetiology of DMT1 is not completely understood, but may be triggered by genetical or environmental factors (Gan, Albanese-O'Neil and Haller, 2012). The condition is characterised by the failure to produce insulin in the beta cells within the islets of Langerhans in the pancreas.

DMT1 relates to a deficiency of insulin production, which requires a well-balanced healthy diet, glucose monitoring, insulin injections, and exercise (Dowling 2021). A lack of insulin within the body inhibits the metabolism of carbohydrates, proteins, and fats. Insulin is required to facilitate the uptake of glucose, which is the primary energy of body cells (Axton & Fugate 2009). If the body is not able to access glucose, it then metabolises fat and proteins, which causes an increase in food intake and weight loss.

Diabetes mellitus type 2 (DMT2) is a combination of insulin deficiency and insulin resistance, and is linked to obesity or family history of DMT2, with increasing incidence in children (Mayer-Davis et al. 2018). Treatment is mainly focused on diet and exercise, although oral medication may be required.

Characteristics of DMT1 include:

- Polyuria
- Polyphagia
- Polydipsia
- Acetone breath
- Weight loss
- Abdominal pain
- Ketonuria
- Glucosuria
- Hyperglycaemia
- Lethargy
- Enuresis in toilet trained children

    (Gormely-Fleming 2021)

ACTIVITY 32.1

Explore the above medical terms and reflect upon your clinical experience of caring for a newly diagnosed diabetic child.

Question 2. Discuss the impact of this condition for Miley and her family.

Activity of living: communication and dying, as per Roper, Logan, & Tierney model of care (Holland & Jenkins 2019).

This is an overwhelming and daunting diagnosis for Miley and her family. Learning that Miley has diabetes will be difficult for her parents to come to terms with, as they may feel shock, denial, anger, fear, sadness, guilt, or responsible for their child's chronic condition (Kenny & Corkin 2013). Adapting to and managing diabetes will no doubt disrupt the normal routine within the family home and place a great strain on the family unit. The fact that DMT1 is a life-long condition which can have long-term complications, for example damage to eyes, heart, and kidneys, can be devastating for Miley's parents (Hamilton et al. 2017). Whilst this can be a stressful time for Miley and her parents their concerns should be clearly recorded and addressed as appropriate in her care plan. Service Delivery and Organisation (SDO, 2010) identify in their recommendations the importance of recording and communicating effectively care plans, by methods which are quality assured and effective in meeting patient education and self-care needs. Should problems arise around compliance with treatment of DMT1 serious life-threatening consequences may occur, such as admission to intensive care for life-saving interventions or indeed early mortality in severe cases.

Miley's parents will require ongoing education and support from the children's diabetes care team which will include the consultant paediatrician, paediatric diabetes nurse specialist, paediatric dietitian, and other professionals as required, with access to contact details. Information will be provided in verbal and written forms in a timely manner to suit Miley and her parents' needs, and they should be given the opportunity to ask questions and clarify information provided (NICE 2015, 2022). Parents should also be made aware of charities, for example Diabetes UK, as they have many valuable age-appropriate resources to help inform Miley and themselves about her condition.

ACTIVITY 32.2

Review informative resources available on: www.diabetes.org.uk
Do you know of any other resources for children and their families?

Question 3. Outline how to monitor blood glucose levels and administer insulin.

Activity of living: maintaining a safe environment as per Roper, Logan, & Tierney model of care (Holland & Jenkins 2019).

Blood glucose monitoring is a central aspect of care for Miley and her parents, to ensure treatments are ongoing and responsive to needs. This allows Miley's parents to appreciate the changes in her glucose levels in response to growth and development, illness, exercise, and changes in her lifestyle. Miley's parents must be confident in performing blood glucose monitoring and recording accurately, to assist in developing a log of Miley's response to care delivered and changes in her management regime. See plan in Box 32.1.

*Continuous Glucose Monitoring (rtCGM; real time Continuous Glucose Monitoring)

A CGM is a small waterproof sensor inserted under the skin which measures glucose in the interstitial tissue every few minutes, rather than measuring glucose levels in the blood. A reusable transmitter is then attached to the sensor for use up to 7 to 10 days (Dexcom G6). The sensor then sends glucose values to the transmitter. Unlike blood glucose testing where you get a single measurement, you get a graph of glucose levels using CGM. A CGM is particularly useful when trying to improve glycaemic control, reduce hypoglycaemic episodes and to stabilise basal rates. Ongoing real time CGM should be considered for preschool children, and children and young people who are very active (NICE, 2015). CGM's maybe considered expensive and funding will need to be obtained for continuing supplies as per local trust policy.

*Flash Glucose Monitoring (isCGM; intermittent scanned Continuous Glucose Monitoring)

Is less painful and a more convenient style of monitoring, **launched in the UK 2014** (https://www.diabetes.org.uk/). **A Free Style** glucose scanning (FGS) system is a sensor-based, factory-calibrated system that measures glucose levels in interstitial fluid (not blood) in children (aged above 4 years) with diabetes mellitus (Kotzapanagiotou et al. 2020). Flash glucose monitoring enables the glucose levels to be monitored by holding a hand held reader (or SMART phone) over a small sensor, inserted subcutaneously, usually at the top of the arm. The sensor is a small, waterproof, round disc and lasts for up to 14 days before being replaced. Children and young people should be advised to test their blood capillary glucose when a glucose reading is displayed on the reader out of normal range when hypoglycaemia or illness is detected, or if rapidly changing glucose. Trend arrows on the reader indicate whether the glucose levels are rising, decreasing, or remaining stable. A graph of glucose levels over the past eight hours are also displayed, as long as the sensor is scanned three

> **BOX 32.1 CARE PLAN**
>
> | Action: how to monitor blood sugars | Reason |
> |---|---|
> | 1. The children's nurse should be aware of Miley's plan of care and incorporate a family-centred approach (Casey 1988) in order to gain consent, parental co-operation, and involvement. | To ensure clear communication pathway is implemented. |
> | 2. The children's nurse should collect all equipment, such as electronic blood glucose meter and reagent test strip (check expiry date and ensure test strip code is compatible with glucose meter code), lancet (finger-pricking device), sharps disposing box and tissue to wipe site after obtaining blood sample. | To ensure safe practice and accurate blood glucose testing. |
> | 3. Be aware of Miley's care plan, for example check blood glucose 20–30 minutes before meals (aim for 4–7 mmol/L), at bedtime or at other times as indicated. | To monitor condition and record findings. |
> | 4. The children's nurse and Miley should wash their hands (warm water to increase capillary blood flow) and dry prior to and after procedure. Then nurse should apply gloves prior to carrying out procedure. | To prevent cross infection. |
> | 5. Ensure test strip is inserted into glucose meter and is ready to receive blood sample. Blood glucose testing involves pricking the side of Miley's finger (either second or third) using appropriate finger pricking device, to obtain small drop of blood. Bring the reagent strip to the pricked finger and touch it to the droplet of blood as per manufacturer's guidelines. Apply gentle pressure with tissue to sample site to remove excess blood. | Prevent nerve damage and ensure rotation of sites. Ensuring adequate sample for analysis. |
> | 6. Dispose of finger-pricking device or component as appropriate in sharps box as per hospital policy. Ensure blood glucose meter is cleaned between patient use. | Nurse and patient safety. |
> | 7. The children's nurse should accurately and immediately record the blood sugar result in Miley's diary and nursing care plan (NMC, 2010). Ensure doctor is informed of latest result. | Ensuring safe practice and supporting continuity of care. |
> | 8. Praise Miley for her co-operation and participation throughout the procedure and reward as appropriate, for example a badge or bravery certificate. Discuss with parents the use of reward charts in the home to support compliance with ongoing monitoring. | To promote Miley's involvement in ongoing care needs. Parental education. |

times, within eight hour periods over twenty-four hours. Flash glucose monitoring is useful to detect trends in glycaemic control, especially overnight and therefore enables changes to be made to insulin regimes.

Medical guidelines should be adhered to, regarding whether blood finger stick testing is still advised and also how often the child or young person should be testing their blood glucose in addition to scanning. There is an insulin bolus advisor within the meter but this requires a finger stick blood test and does not advise on insulin calculation from scanning the sensor. Indeed, flash glucose sensors do not continuously send glucose measurements to the reader, therefore this flash glucose monitoring should not be used as an alternative to CGM. However, flash glucose monitoring has been considered as a cost effective option to diagnose trends in glucose levels.

ADMINISTRATION OF INSULIN INJECTION

The administration of insulin injections is a complex aspect of care delivery within the multifaceted role of the children's nurse. Standards for medicine management are regulated by the Nursing and Midwifery Council (NMC 2008) and clearly highlight the nurse's responsibility to ensure safe practice when administrating medication. Abdomen, thigh, and upper arms are the most commonly used injection sites for insulin administration, which is administered at a 90-degree angle using the appropriate delivery device. These sites need to be rotated in order to prevent lipoatrophy, which will inhibit the absorption of insulin, thus leading to instability in overall condition. Ensure all equipment used to deliver insulin is used and disposed of as per manufacturer's guidelines/hospital policy.

As the NMC (2008) supports the administration of medicines by a carer, the parents should be encouraged by the children's nurse to become competent in the administration of insulin injections to Miley in the paediatric setting, thus supporting a child and family partnership approach to care (Casey 1988). Although the responsibility to ensure the insulin is administered remains with the children's nurse in the hospital setting; the nurse also needs to ensure the parents are educated and confident to deliver insulin injections as prescribed. In most cases the insulin will be delivered by a syringe, pen device, or a pump. Insulin is administered in units, and in the initial period of management the units administered may be adjusted by the doctor or diabetes nurse specialist, to achieve adequate control that gives blood glucose results pre-meals of 4–7 mmol/L. Considerations appropriate to Miley's age and stage of development should always be taken into account, with clear negotiation and support for the parents regarding Miley's ongoing care needs, for example when Miley refuses her insulin injection. The use of play therapy or distraction techniques can be a useful aid to the children's nurse in engaging Miley in her ongoing care needs.

TYPES OF INSULIN

Insulin is a protein which is used to treat DMT1 and is delivered via subcutaneous injection or pump infusion. Regimes are determined on an individual basis, requiring up to four injections per day. There are four different categories of insulin (BNFc, 2020–2021; NICE, 2016) please read:

- Rapid-acting – onset of action 15 minutes
- Short-acting – onset of action 30–60 minutes
- Intermediate-acting – onset of action approximately 1–2 hours
- Long-acting – once-daily dose to produce a constant level of insulin

Selection of insulin used is usually based on needs of child and made by the consultant in charge of care.

CALCULATION OF INSULIN DOSE

The administration of prescribed medications to children must be viewed by the children's nurse as a key aspect of nursing care that requires sound knowledge of pharmacology, numeracy skills, and the ability to communicate effectively with Miley and her family (Casey 1988; Pentin et al. 2016). To ensure accurate dosing, body weight is used more frequently for ease of paediatric calculations. In order to calculate drug doses accurately the children's nurse must be able to demonstrate an understanding of child development theory, the units of drugs in current use and approved abbreviations.

Student nurses should be involved in the procedure of drug calculation and administration as a learning tool. However, in order to meet legal, trust, and professional guidelines, student nurses should *NEVER* single check an insulin injection and administer unsupervised. As nurses administer medications on a regular basis there is the potential for errors to occur (Diggle 2022; NHS National Patient Safety Agency 2010).

STORAGE OF DRUGS

Safe storage of drugs involves both environmental and security factors, such as a lockable medicines trolley and refrigerator. Children's nurses must ensure all medicines are stored in accordance with the patient/drug information leaflet. Parents need to ensure that they have an adequate supply of insulin to meet Miley's needs and it should be stored in a refrigerator until required. Once the insulin vial/pen fill is in use it can be stored at room temperature and must be discarded after one month (Sadik 2001). As with all medicines they must be stored safely and out of the reach of children, including Miley and her twin brothers.

When in the school environment, Miley's medicines and monitoring equipment must be stored safely and appropriately to ensure continuity of care whilst in school (Diabetes UK 2011), which is supported by an individual care plan.

Question 4. Describe the information that Miley and her parents will require to manage her condition safely after discharge from hospital, in relation to managing hypoglycaemia and hyperglycaemia attacks.

Discharge plan: in order for Miley's parents to manage her condition safely after discharge from hospital it is essential to discuss, amongst other aspects of care, the management of low and high blood sugars to prevent the possibility of long-term complications, and life-threatening events occurring.

> **BOX 32.2   HYPOGLYCAEMIA**

Symptoms of hypoglycaemia

- Hunger
- Sweating
- Shaking/trembling
- Irritability
- Palpitations
- Lack of concentration
- Glazed eyes
- Mood changes – anger/aggressive behaviour
- Drowsiness
- Vagueness (Dowling 2021)

Treating hypoglycaemia

- Immediately give a sugary drink or food such as, lucozade or coke, glucose tablets, sweets, teaspoonfuls of sugar, or glucogel.
- Follow this with other long-acting carbohydrates, for example sandwiches, fruit, cereal bar, biscuits, or a meal if due.
- Seek further guidance from diabetes care team. (Abraham et al. 2018)

> **BOX 32.3   HYPERGLYCAEMIA**

Symptoms of hyperglycaemia

- Urinary frequency
- Thirst – increased
- Tiredness/lethargy
- Weight loss
- Visual disturbances – blurring (Hamilton et al. 2017)

Treatment of hyperglycaemia

- Can have a quick onset and may lead to diabetic ketoacidosis (DKA), which can be life threatening in severe cases and require hospitalisation.
- Close monitoring of blood glucose levels and recording of same (up to four times per day).
- Good adherence to dietary regime and support from diabetic care team.
- Review of insulin regime and injection technique.

Hypoglycaemia, often referred to as a 'hypo', is when the blood sugar level is low (below 3.9 mmol/L). Refer to Box 32.2 and Box 32.3. These hypos can have a rapid onset and are caused by (Abraham et al. 2018):

- A delayed/missed meal or snack
- Not enough food – especially carbohydrates
- Too much insulin has been given
- Increased activity levels

Nursing alert!

If the child is unconscious do not give anything to eat or drink, call for medical assistance immediately and stay with the child until help arrives.

Hyperglycaemia is when the blood glucose level is high (>15 mmol/L) and is linked to poor control of the condition. Causes for the high glucose levels include: missing doses of insulin/oral treatments, poor injection technique or eating a high carbohydrate diet. Physical stress can initiate extra glucose production by the body, leading to hyperglycaemia (www.diabetes.co.uk).

CHILDREN WITH DIABETES IN SCHOOL

Whilst education is an important aspect of life for children and young people, care for the child with diabetes in school must be appropriate to their needs, parallel with optimising their academic performance. Schools must adopt positive attitudes towards children with diabetes and adopt a child-centred policy which offers children and their parents support in the school environment from appropriately trained staff (Diabetes UK 2008; Spencer et al. 2013).

REFERENCES

Abraham, M.B., Jones, T.W., Naranjo, D. et al (2018) ISPAD Clinical Practice Consensus Guidelines 2018: assessment and management of hypoglycemia in children and adolescents with diabetes. *Pediatric Diabetes*, **19**(Suppl 27), 178–192. doi:10.1111/pedi.12698.

Axton, S.E. & Fugate, T. (2009) *Paediatric Nursing Care Plans for the Hospitalized Child*, 3rd edition. Upper Saddle River, NJ: Pearson Prentice Hall.

Bee, H. & Boyd, D. (2013) *The Developing Child*, 12th edition. London: Pearson.

British National Formulary for Children (BNFc) (Sept 2020–2021) *British Medical Journal*. London: PS Publishing.

Burns, M.R., Bodansky, H.J. & Parslow, R.C. (2010) Paediatric intensive care admissions for acute diabetes complications. *Diabetic Medicine*, **27**, 705–708.

Casey, A. (1988) A partnership with child and family. *Senior Nurse*, **8**(4), 8–9.

Diabetes UK (2008) *Making All Children Matter: Support for Children with Diabetes in Schools*. London: Diabetes UK.

Diabetes UK (2011) Diabetes week 2011–Let's talk Type I diabetes in schools. www.diabetes.org.uk/In_Your_Area/N_Ireland/Public-meetings.

Diggle, J. (2022) Injecting insulin safely and effectively. Promoting team work in diabetes care. S13–S16 (accessed 7th July 2022).

Dowling, L. (2021) Effective management of type 1 diabetes in children and young people. *Nursing Children and Young People*. doi:10.7748/ncyp.2021.e1310.

Gan, M.J., Albanese-O'Neill, A. & Haller, M.J. (2012) Type 1 diabetes: current concepts in epidemiology, pathophysiology, clinical care and research. *Current Problems in Pediatric Adolescent Health Care*, **42**, 269–291.

Gormely-Fleming, L. (2021) Caring for Children With Diabetes and Other Endocrine Disorders. In: Glasper, A., Richardson, J. and Randall, D. (eds). *A Textbook of Children's and Young People's Nursing*, 3rd edition. London: Elsevier, 2021, 355–356.

Hamilton, H., Knudsen, G., Vaina, C.L. et al (2017) Children and young people with diabetes: recognition and management. *British Journal of Nursing*, **26**(6), 340–347.

Holland, K. & Jenkins, J. (2019) *Applying the Rope-Logan-Tierney Model in Practice*, 3rd edition. Edinburgh: Elsevier.

Kenny, J. & Corkin, D. (2013) Childrens' nurses role in the global development of a child with diabetes. *Nursing Children and Young People*, **25**(9), 22–25.

Kotzapanagiotou, E., Tsotridou, E., Volakli, E. et al (2020) Evaluation of continuous flash glucose monitoring in a pediatric ICU setting. *Journal of Clinical Monitoring and Computing*, **34**, 843–852.

Mayer-Davis, E.J., Kahkoska, A.R., Jefferies, C. et al. (2018) ISPAD clinical practice consensus guidelines 2018: definition, epidemiology, and classification of diabetes in children and adolescents. *Pediatric Diabetes*, **19**(Suppl 27), 7–19. doi:10.1111/pedi.12773.

National Institute for Health and Care Excellence (2016) Diabetes (Type 1 and Type 2) in children and young people: diagnosis and management. NICE guideline No. 18. NICE, London.

National Institute for Health and Clinical Excellence (2015, updated 2022) Diabetes (Type 1 and Type 2) in children and young people: diagnosis and management. NICE Guideline (NG 18). https://www.nice.org.uk/guidance/ng18 (accessed 6 March 2023)

NHS National Patient Safety Agency (2010) Rapid Response Report. Safer Administration of Insulin. NPSA/2010/RRR013.

Nursing and Midwifery Council (2008) *Guidelines on the Administration of Medicine S*. London: NMC.

Nursing and Midwifery Council (2010) *Record Keeping – Guidance for Nurses and Midwives*. London: NMC.

Pentin, J., Green, M. & Smith, J. (2016) Undertaking safe medicine administration with children, part 2: essential numeracy. *Nursing Children and Young People*, **28**(7), 37–43.

Sadik, R. (2001) Case 12. Gareth Jones: three-year old with diabetes. In: Sadik, R. and Campbell, G. (eds). *Client Profiles in Nursing, Child Health*. London:Greenwich Medical Media Limited.

Service Delivery and Organisation (2010) *The organisation and delivery of diabetes services in the UK: a scoping exercise*. https://www.uk.elsevierhealth.com/a-textbook-of-childrens-and-young-peoples-nursing-9780702062322.html (accessed 6 March 2023).

Spencer, J.E., Cooper, H.C. & Milton, B. (2013) The lived experiences of young people (13-16 years) with Type 1 diabetes mellitus and their parents – a qualitative phenomenological study. *Diabetic Medicine*, **30**(1), 17–24.

https://www.diabetes.org.uk/guide-to-diabetes/diabetes-technology/flash-glucose-monitors-and-continuous-glucose-monitors (accessed 6 March 2023).

Acute Kidney Injury (AKI)

Hazel Gibson and Rosi Simpson

CHAPTER 33

SCENARIO

Twelve-year-old Jack, who lives with his mother and two siblings, was admitted to his local general hospital with abdominal pain. He had an appendectomy (see Chapter 24) for a perforated appendix.

Postoperatively his abdominal pain, nausea, and vomiting persisted. An abdominal CT scan (computed tomography) showed a pelvic collection and intravenous antibiotics were commenced.

Jack's nausea and vomiting continued despite regular antiemetics. On day 7 postoperatively he had an episode of *frank haematuria*. Following this he became *anuric* and it was noted that his intake and output record was incomplete. Blood taken at this time showed elevated levels of *urea* and *creatinine* (see Table 33.1).

A medical decision was made to transfer Jack to the regional children's hospital for further management and treatment. On admission, his serum creatinine and urea levels had increased further, his serum CO_2 level was reduced, his CRP was raised, and he had become hypertensive and remained anuric (see Table 33.1). A diagnosis of Acute Kidney Injury secondary to dehydration was made.

Table 33.1 Definitions.

Frank haematuria: the passage of blood in the urine that is visible to the naked eye.

Anuric: the failure of the kidneys to produce urine.

Urea: the main breakdown product of protein metabolism, the product that unrequired nitrogen is excreted by the body in urine.

Creatinine: a product of protein metabolism found in muscle.

CO_2: serum CO_2 indicator of respiratory/metabolic acidosis.

CRP (C reactive protein): a protein whose plasma concentrations are raised in infection and inflammatory states and in the presence of tissue damage or necrosis.

eGFR: estimated glomerular filtration rate – calculation of kidney function by the flow rate of blood filtered through the glomerular capillaries in the kidneys – see www.infokid.org.uk

QUESTIONS

1. Define acute kidney injury.
2. With reference to a model of care, identify the immediate problems when planning Jack's care.
3. Continuing with the nursing process and model of care, discuss in further detail the immediate problems identified in Jack's care plan.
4. What would indicate that Jack may require renal replacement therapy (RRT)?
5. Using the information provided give rationale for the dialysis modality chosen for Jack.
6. How would you assess if Jack is recovering his renal function?

This scenario aims to give insight into how recognition, assessment, and early intervention of predisposing factors can prevent and influence outcomes of Acute Kidney Injury (AKI). Plotz et al. (2008) observed a high incidence of significant AKI in the at-risk paediatric population.

Care Planning in Children and Young People's Nursing, Second Edition. Edited by Sonya Clarke and Doris Corkin.
© 2024 John Wiley & Sons Ltd. Published 2024 by John Wiley & Sons Ltd.

ANSWERS TO QUESTIONS

Question 1. Define acute kidney injury.

Acute renal failure (ARF) has been replaced by the term acute kidney injury (AKI) and is recognized as a clinical syndrome rarely with a sole or distinct pathophysiology (Davies 2009: Makris & Spanou 2016). Acute kidney injury (AKI) is a clinical spectrum manifested as being abrupt (within hours) sustained decrease in kidney function, encompassing injury (structural damage) and impairment (loss of function) resulting in raised serum creatinine and/or decrease in urine output from baseline (Mehta et al. 2007). RIFLE criteria for classification and staging adapted for paediatrics has been further enhanced as a diagnostic tool, by proposed modifications of staging by Acute Kidney Injury Network (AKIN 2007), Kidney Disease Improving Global Outcomes (KDIGO 2012) and NICE guidelines (2019), to standardise practice.

Paediatric – modified RIFLE (pRIFLE)

- **R** Risk
- **I** Injury
- **F** Failure
- **L** Loss – need for renal replacement therapy (RRT) >4 weeks
- **E** End-stage renal disease (ESRF), requiring dialysis >3 months

(Bellomo et al. 2004)

Paediatric – modified RIFLE (pRIFLE).

Stage	Estimated CCL	Urine output criteria
1. Risk	eCCl <25%	<0.5 mls/kg/hour for >8 hours
2. Injury	eCCl <50%	<0.5 mls/kg/hour for >16 hours
3. Failure	eCCl <75%	<0.5 mls/kg/hour for >24 hours
or	eCCl <35 ml/min/1.73 m^2	anuric for 12 hours

CCl = creatinine clearance.
(Akcan-Arikan et al. 2007).

Ricci et al. (2008), have shown that this classification is a good predictor of outcome, showing that mortality increased with worsening Rifle class. It is hoped that these new guidelines will standardise and improve diagnoses and outcomes for renal patients. Currently no studies have been able to determine exactly at what point 'renal replacement therapy' (RRT) should be initiated. This can differ widely between units and even individual practitioners.

ACTIVITY 33.1

Further reading – information for parents and carers: www.infokid.org.uk

*Acute Kidney Injury Network (AKIN 2007)
*KDIGO Clinical Practice Guideline for Acute Kidney Injury (2012)

Question 2. With reference to a model of care, identify the immediate problems when planning Jack's care.

Nursing prevention strategies, recognition of risk factors and management of AKI depend on nurse's knowledge of pathophysiology, pharmacological agents together with therapeutic clinical measures.

Activity of living: elimination (Roper et al. 1990).

Assess: Jack is anuric.

Activity of living: eating and drinking.

Assess: Jack has continued nausea and vomiting leading to dehydration. This could lead to potential problems such as:

- Over hydration – if IV fluids commenced and fluid balance is not regularly reviewed or an inability to adhere to 24-hour fluid allowance.

- Catabolism – due to reduced calorie intake and inability to tolerate oral nutrition.

- May require dietetic involvement, for example nasogastric feed, supplements/enteral feeds.

Activity of living: maintaining a safe environment.

Assess: Jack has the potential problem of fluid excess related to anuria, excessive fluid administration, and sodium and water retention.

Potential electrolyte imbalance due to:

↓ renal potassium excretion (hyperkalaemia)

↓ renal sodium excretion (hypernatraemia) Decreased sodium due to excess hydration (hyponatraemia)

Activity of living: breathing and circulation (*importance of compliance & consequences of non-adherence*).

Assess: Jack has the potential problem of pulmonary oedema due to fluid overload, and fluid retention. He has the potential problem of hypertension due to fluid overload.

Activity of living: controlling body temperature.

Assess: Jack has the potential problem of infection due to compromised nutritional status and complications due to underlying pathology

Activity of living: communication (Casey 1988).

Assess: Jack and his family are anxious due to the suddenness, severity of his illness, the potential for long-term kidney damage. Jack is almost a teenager with the potential problem of compliance/concordance.

Question 3. Continuing with the nursing process and model of care, discuss in further detail the immediate problems identified in Jack's care plan.

Activity of living: elimination.

Plan:

- To find cause of anuria and if possible restore renal function

- To prevent fluid overload

Implement:

- Weigh twice daily – morning and evening.

- Ensure bloods are taken on a daily basis to review kidney function – increase frequency if indicated – assist with same.

- Record minimum four hourly vital signs – heart rate (HR), blood pressure (BP), respiratory rate (RR). Paediatric vital signs are individualised specific to age, size and underlying medical condition:

    Assess fluid status from results

    Decreased BP, increased HR continued dehydration

    Increased BP fluid overload

    Increased RR pulmonary oedema

- Calculate individual fluid requirement and ensure accurate record completion.

Activity of living: eating and drinking.

Plan:

- To ensure required nutritional and fluid intake and prevent a catabolic state

- To reduce uraemia

- To minimise nausea and vomiting

Implement:

- Record a minimum daily weight.
- Give IV fluids as prescribed – adhere to local hospital policies and procedures for administration of intravenous fluids.
- Assist with venepuncture to retain daily bloods or more frequently as indicated.
- Liaise with dietician for daily dietetic assessment.
- Give prescribed anti-emetics as per local hospital policy for administration of medicines and monitor effect.
- Record accurate hourly intake and output to account for insensible loss (approx. 400 ml/m^2) + previous 24 hours' output and other losses.
- Offer small amounts of high calorie, low salt, low potassium, calculated protein foods – take into account personal likes and dislikes.
- Consider the need for supplementary/enteral feeding if oral nutrition cannot be tolerated.
- Provide parent and child information and explanation of dietary needs.
- Consider parental or child involvement in recording diet and oral intake.

Activity of living: maintaining a safe environment.

Plan: monitor serum potassium and reduce to a safe level.

Implement:

- Assist with the collection of a minimum of daily bloods – increase frequency if clinically indicated.
- Liaise with dietician and ensure dietary potassium restriction is adhered to in diet.
- Give prescribed medications as per hospital policy and monitor effects/side effects, for example sodium bicarbonate drives potassium from blood into the cells.
- Consider the need for ECG monitoring, depending upon serum electrolyte levels.
- Provide parental and child information on diet and potassium containing foods.
- If potassium remains elevated give explanation and information in preparation for dialysis.

Activity of living: breathing and circulation.

Plan: to reduce BP to a safe level.

Implement:

- Record a minimum of four hourly BP and HR (increase frequency if condition indicates).
- Give anti-hypertensives as prescribed as per local hospital policy and monitor effects/side effects. Withold regular ACEi/ARB if taking pre admission as may cause further deterioration of renal function. ACE/ARB should not be given as a treatment for acutely elevated blood pressure in the setting of a patient with AKI.
- Ensure parents and child are aware of their fluid allowance and the importance of compliance.
- Consider child and parents' involvement in the recording of oral fluid intake.
- Weigh to assess hydration status, that is, fluid overload may contribute to increased BP.
- If BP remains elevated provide parents and child with information and explanation if dialysis is considered. Consider age appropriate and developmental needs when providing written and verbal information.
- Involve play therapist – distraction.

NB when administering prescribed medications, the frequency and/or dose may need adjusted due to the child's reduced renal function.

ACTIVITY 33.2

Familiarise yourself with normal paediatric biochemistry/haematology/laboratory parameters: CLINICAL BIOCHEMISTRY HANDBOOK FOR PAEDIATRICS 2022 yorkhospitals.nhs.uk
https://www.yorkhospitals.nhs.uk/seecmsfile/?id=2561

Evaluation: evaluate all nursing procedures and complete relevant documentation.

Activity: did you achieve what you set out to achieve?

Question 4. What would indicate that Jack may require renal replacement therapy (RRT)?

Blood indicators

- Increased creatinine as a result of reduced excretion of waste products of metabolism.
- Decreased CO_2 indicating metabolic acidosis due to excessive loss of bicarbonate.
- Refractory hyperkalaemia (increased serum potassium level) due to reduced excretion despite optimising medical management.
- Uraemia (increased serum urea level) due to retention of nitrogenous waste.
- Falling haemoglobin level due to reduced production of hormone erythropoietin.

Clinical/physical observations

- Anuria – fluid accumulates as kidneys fail to excrete excess body water weight increases.
- Positive/negative oedema – peripheral/ pulmonary oedema due to accumulation of fluid in extravascular space which has moved from intravascular to extravascular space.
- Hypertension (blood pressure above 95th centile for height/weight) (Pediatric Hypertension Association 2006).
- Reduced appetite, nausea + / – vomiting

Jack's bloods are continually monitored, together with an accurate intake and output chart and regular observations. Unfortunately, Jack's blood pressure remains elevated and despite the importance of adhering to a fluid allowance, Jack sneaks extra oral fluids.

This results in his continued hypertension and oedema, which develops into the more serious condition of pulmonary oedema.

See Box 33.1 and Figures 33.33.1 and 33.33.2.

BOX 33.1 TYPES OF DIALYSIS

Peritoneal dialysis (PD)	Haemodialysis (HD) or Haemodiafiltration (HDF)
• Neonates – Children and Young People • Initially small fill volumes to reduce risk of leakage, respiratory compromise • Hospital and home based • Contra-indicated in abdominal surgery, anatomical problems, social situations • Uses a large surface area • Avoids sudden fluid and solute shifts • Burden of care for parent/carer	• Immediate use • Hospital based at specialist centre • Disruption to family life • Demand vascular access via double lumen central venous catheter or arteriovenous (AV) fistula • Increase fluid and dietary restrictions • Improve quality of life outcomes (HDF)

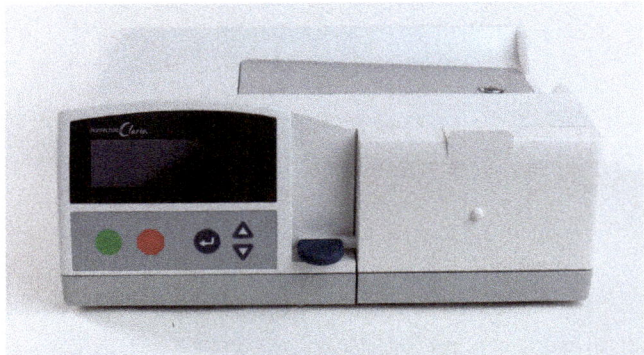

FIGURE 33.1 Home choice peritoneal dialysis machine (updated picture to be inserted).

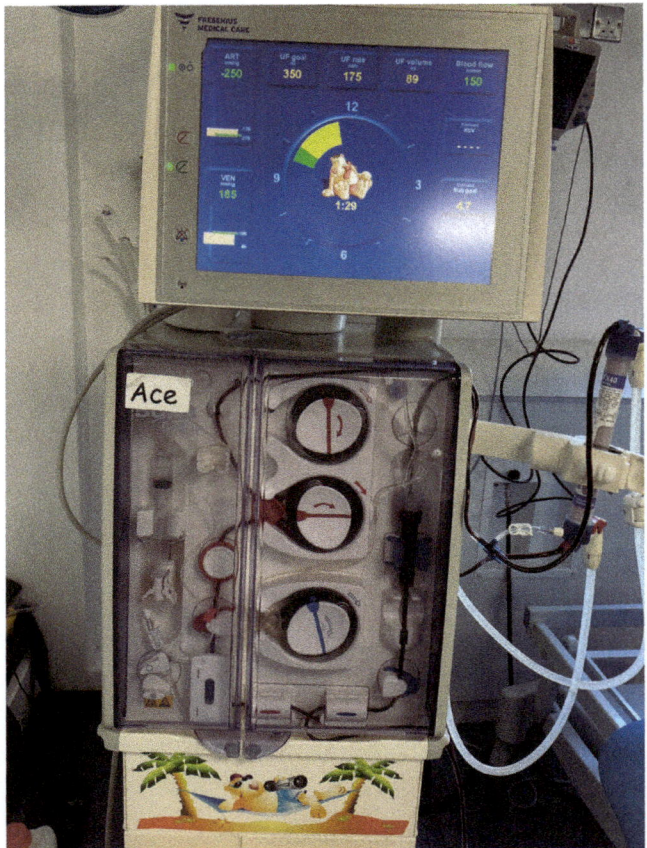

FIGURE 33.2 Haemodialysis (HD) machine (updated picture to be inserted).

Question 5. Using the information provided give rationale for the dialysis modality chosen for Jack.

Haemodialysis (HD) or Haemodiafiltration (HDF) modality of choice in AKI (Shroff et al. 2018) due to:

- Recent abdominal surgery
- Urgent normalisation of serum potassium
- Urgent removal of fluid due to pulmonary oedema and hypertension
- Allows nutritional supplements to be given during treatment

Jack receives HDF three times per week for three weeks.

Question 6. How would you assess if Jack is recovering his renal function?

Blood indicators

- Decreased serum creatinine – improved excretion of waste products of metabolism
- Decreased serum urea levels – improved excretion of nitrogenous waste
- Increased CO_2 – correction of acidosis
- Normalising level of potassium – excretion of electrolytes

Physical indicators

- Increased urinary output – reduced need for fluid removal by dialysis and fluid restriction
- Daily weight reduces
- Normalising BP – reduced need for antihypertensives
- Decreased serum urea level – increased appetite
- Ability to tolerate diet and fluids

Jack's general wellbeing improves, with increased energy levels, normalisation of BP (appropriate for age, height, and weight), and blood results returning to within normal parameters.

Preparation is made for discharge and follow-up.

REFERENCES

Acute Kidney Injury Network (AKIN) (2007) Report of an initiative to improve outcomes in acute kidney injury.

Akcan-Arikan, A., Zappitelli, M., Loftis, M.M., Washburn, K.K., Jefferson, L.S. & Goldstein, S.L. (2007) Modified RIFLE criteria in critically ill children with acute kidney injury. *Kidney International*, **71**, 1028–1035.

Bellomo, R., Ronco, C., Kellum, J.A. et al. (2004) Acute renal failure – definition, outcome measures, animal models, fluid therapy and information technology needs: the Second International Consensus Conference of the Acute Dialysis Quality Initiative (ADQI) Group. *Critical Care*, **8**(4), R204–12.

Casey, A. (1988) A partnership with child and family. *Senior Nurse*, **8**(4), 8–9.

Davies, A. (2009) Diagnosing and classifying acute kidney injury. *Journal of Renal Nursing*, **1**(1), 9–12.

Kidney Disease Improving Global Outcomes (KDIGO), (2012) Clinical practice guideline for the evaluation and management of chronic kidney disease.

Makris, K. & Spanou, L. (2016) Acute kidney injury: definition, pathophysiology and clinical phenotypes. *Clinical Biochemist Reviews*, **37**(2), 85–98.

Mehta, R., Kellum, J.A., Shah, S.V. et al. (2007) Acute Kidney Injury Network: report of an initiative to improve outcomes in acute kidney injury. *Critical Care*, **11**(2), R31.

NICE guideline (NG148) (2019) Acute kidney injury: prevention, detection and management. National Institute for Health and Care Excellence.

Plotz, F.B., Bouma, A.B., van Wijk, J.A., Kneyber, M.C. & Bokenkamp, A. (2008) Pediatric acute kidney injury in the ICU: an independent evaluation of pRIFLE criteria. *Intensive Care Medicine*, **34**(9), 1713–1717.

Ricci, Z., Cruz, D. & Ronco, D. (2008) The RIFLE criteria and mortality in acute kidney injury: a systematic review. *Kidney International*, **73**(5), 538–546.

Roper, N., Logan, W. & Tierney, A. (1990) *The Elements of Nursing*, 3rd edition. London: Churchill Livingstone.

Shroff, R., Bayazit, A., Stefanidis, C.J. et al (2018) Effect of haemodiafiltration vs conventional haemodialysis on growth and cardiovascular outcomes in children – the HDF, heart and height (3H) study. *BMC Nephrol*, **19**, 199.

www.infokid.org.uk. Information for parents and carers.

https://www.yorkhospitals.nhs.uk/seecmsfile/?id=2561.

FURTHER READING

A great resource can be sourced at infokid.org.

Care of Infants and Young Persons with Skin Conditions

SECTION 10

Infant with Infected Eczema

CHAPTER 34

Gilli Lewis and Debbie Rickard

SCENARIO

Henry is a ten-month-old infant who has been admitted to the children's ward for treatment of his infected eczema. Henry has three siblings, two of which also have eczema. Henry's father had mild eczema as a child. The family of six live in a small two-bedroom, council-owned house.

Henry is covered in lesions; he has a weeping, crusting, staphylococcal infection. He appears irritated, itchy and is crying on assessment. This is his third admission to hospital; he has previously been admitted for treatment of bronchiolitis and exacerbated eczema. Apart from eczema, Henry is physically well. He is afebrile, feeding normally, but his sleep has been affected. Henry has been bottle fed infant formula milk since birth, and he commenced solid food at six months of age; no allergic responses have been noted to date.

QUESTIONS

1. What is eczema?
2. On Henry's admission to the ward, the children's nurse will need to complete a nursing assessment, from which a nursing plan of care may be developed. Describe how the nurse would carry out this assessment.
3. Identify the key healthcare deficits/issues/problems Henry and his mother, Sharon, present with and using an appropriate model of nursing plan goals of nursing care in relation to these problems.
4. Henry has been admitted with infected eczema. Describe the nursing care plan which the children's nurse should follow to ensure Henry receives appropriate evidence-based skin care.

ANSWERS TO QUESTIONS

Question 1. What is eczema?

Eczema is a common inflammatory skin condition, affecting up to 20% of children in the UK with around 1 in 20 having severe disease (Cork et al. 2019, de Lusignan et al. 2021). Eczema has a higher incidence in infancy and childhood, but can affect individuals throughout life and is typically an episodic disease of exacerbation and remissions. Effective therapy improves quality of life for children with eczema and their parents and carers. Lack of evidence based information and support about therapy leads to poor adherence, and consequently to treatment failure (Axon et al. 2021; Cork et al. 2020; Santer et al. 2012).

Environmental and genetic influences can lead to the breakdown of the skin barrier. This makes the skin susceptible to trigger factors, including irritants and allergens, which can make eczema worse. Many cases of eczema resolve or improve during childhood, but some persist into adulthood. Some children who have eczema will go on to develop asthma and/or allergic rhinitis; this sequence of events is sometimes referred to as the 'atopic march' (Yang et al. 2020). However while evidence does exist to support the existence of the atopic march, its prevalence may be overstated (Aw et al. 2020). There can be an association with personal or family history of atopy (atopic eczema, allergic rhinitis and/or asthma).

Care Planning in Children and Young People's Nursing, Second Edition. Edited by Sonya Clarke and Doris Corkin.
© 2024 John Wiley & Sons Ltd. Published 2024 by John Wiley & Sons Ltd.

Eczema is usually characterised by epidermal changes, pruritus (itch), and lesions with indistinct borders. These lesions can appear as erythema, papules, or scales; they can present in an acute, subacute or chronic phase. Oedema, serous discharge and crusting occur with continued irritation and scratching. In chronic cases, the skin may become thickened and leathery and hyperpigmented from recurrent irritation and scratching. This is called lichenification. Chronic eczema is more likely to have distinct borders.

Affected sites vary with age (see https://dermnetnz.org/topics/atopic-dermatitis).

Infantile eczema commonly affects the face, sparing around the mouth, and later the hands, feet, and elsewhere (Halkjaer et al. 2006; Thomsen 2014).

While the underlying cause of eczema is not yet fully known it is thought to involve complex pathways including skin barrier dysfunction, altered innate or adaptive immune responses. There is increasing evidence disruption of the skin barrier function and atopy affect one another reciprocally. Eczema is a product of interplay between environmental factors and genetic susceptibility (Cork et al. 2020). As described by Leung et al. (2004), 'the skin represents the interface between the body and the surrounding environment' (p. 654).

When the skin barrier is impaired from dryness (xerosis) by genetic or environmental means and/or excoriated (in response to the pruritus from the skin xerosis) this allows bacteria, viruses, and allergens to penetrate the skin.

Historically eczema has been poorly understood and frequently under treated and there continues to be significant unmet need (Cork et al. 2020). There is no cure for eczema however effective management includes minimizing exacerbations (often referred to as *flares*) with a prevention focus supporting the patient and family to have control (Cork et al. 2020; Thomsen 2014). With the increasing prevalence of eczema, it is no longer dismissed as a trivial disorder; indeed, the impact of this chronic condition on the individual, families, and the community are increasingly being recognised (National Eczema Society 2021; Santer et al. 2012; Wan et al. 2020).

Question 2. On Henry's admission to the ward, the children's nurse will need to complete a nursing assessment, from which a nursing plan of care may be developed. Describe how the nurse would carry out this assessment.

Assessment

The initial assessment will be carried out during a family interview, in which the nurse may ask questions relevant to the care of the child. It is important to be aware that caregivers of children with eczema are often frustrated and exhausted. If possible, hospitalisation of the child should be avoided as these children are highly susceptible to infections. However, admission may sometimes be the only answer to provide intensive therapy or to relieve an exhausted caregiver.

In this interview it is important to cover the history of Henry's condition, including treatments that have been recently tried and any known allergens or triggers. It is useful to include a review of the home environment and daily routine. The nurse should evaluate Henry's mother's knowledge of eczema.

To aid management of eczema in children, the children's nurse should take detailed clinical and drug histories that include:

- Age of onset, pattern, and severity of the eczema
- Response to previous and current treatments
- Understanding of treatments and how these are used/implemented
- Possible trigger factors (irritant and allergic)
- The impact of the eczema on Henry his parents and siblings
- Dietary history including any dietary manipulation or restrictions
- Growth and development
- Personal and family history of atopic conditions (such as asthma and hay fever)

In addition to the interview, data collection about Henry must include vital signs, and height and weight to assess growth. Observing general nutritional state and a complete examination of all body parts, with careful documentation of the eruptions and their location and size. It is helpful to touch the skin to assess skin integrity; rough skin is an indicator of skin dryness. Unaffected areas, as well as those that are weeping and crusted, should be documented to assist review of progress.

It may be necessary to reassess when Henry is physically better, and Sharon is not so exhausted (physically and/or emotionally).

Question 3. Identify the key healthcare issues/problems Henry and his mother, Kate, present with and using an appropriate model of nursing plan goals of nursing care in relation to these.

Identified problems

- Impaired skin integrity related to lesions and inflammatory process
- Risk of serious infection related to broken skin and lesions
- Acute pain related to intense itching, irritation, and broken skin
- Disturbed sleep pattern related to itching and discomfort
- Incomplete knowledge of caregivers related to disease condition and treatment

Model of nursing

Anne Casey's model of nursing (Casey 1993) guides nurses to work in partnership with children and their families. The philosophy behind the model is that the best people to care for the child are the family, with help from various professional staff. After all, following discharge from hospital, it is the family who will provide the ongoing care at home.

However, forming a partnership of care is not simple, and requires skill and sensitivity. Negotiating care is discussed by Anne Casey in her model. The ability to negotiate care is an underestimated skill, which is essential if nurses are to come alongside families/caregivers in true partnership when planning care for children.

The nurse, in this case, will need to discuss the identified problems and possible goals of nursing care with Sharon.

Goals for Henry:

1. Improving and maintaining skin integrity; minimising flares
2. Preventing infection of skin lesions
3. Maintaining comfort, relief of itch
4. Improving sleep patterns
5. Enabling normal growth and development

Goals for Kate/other caregivers:

1. Increasing knowledge about the condition
2. Increasing evidence-based knowledge about management of the condition
3. Improving confidence and competence in providing skin care

Question 4. Henry has been admitted with infected eczema. Describe the nursing care plan which the children's nurse should follow to ensure Henry receives appropriate evidence-based skin care.

The nursing care plan will be based on the problems identified during assessment, and the goals as discussed with Kate and stated above.

Improving and maintaining Henry's skin integrity, minimising flares

1. The ultimate aim of treatment is to maintain skin integrity and minimise flares by replacing moisture and reducing inflammation. The key to helping maintain skin integrity is to moisturise.

2. Henry needs a daily skin care routine which should be incorporated into his usual daily routine. Discuss Henry's current skin care routine with Kate.

Using emollient

- Emollients should form the basis of eczema management (Cork et al. 2003; Lindh & Bradley 2015), and generally should always be used. However, this is dependent on the severity of eczema and the flares.

- Emollients are moisturisers, which have emulsifiers and/or humectants, which affect the permeability barrier function of skin (Hon et al. 2018; van Zuuren et al. 2017).

- Clinical experience has shown that the amount of emollient used is important in bringing about an improvement in eczema (Cork et al. 2003; Salvati et al. 2021). Emollients should be used in larger amounts and more often than other treatments. Other treatments such as topical steroids do not replace emollients; they must always be used in conjunction with emollients unless condition is mild. (Applying emollient on top of topical steroid works well). Emollients improve efficacy of steroids and reduce flares. Emollients should be used in response to symptoms and prophylactically in response to known triggers.

- The nurse needs to ascertain that Kate understands the use of emollients, as part of Henry's skin care routine. Any misunderstandings and gaps in knowledge can then be discussed and offer online resources such as videos (https://www.youtube.com/watch?v=nj4JSWGL5KQ. Guy's and St Thomas' NHS Foundation Trust YouTube video).

- The nurse should show Kate how to apply emollients, including how to smooth emollients onto the skin rather than rubbing them in. Kate should be advised that regular application of emollients is a way that she can help her child and relieve his symptoms.

- Proven improved clinical response to effective emollient use motivates individuals, families, and health professionals to continue with emollient use in eczema management (Barfield et al. 2017; Cork et al. 2003).

Topical corticosteroids, such as hydrocortisone

- Henry will require topical corticosteroid treatment.

- The nurse should ensure Kate is aware topical corticosteroids need to be applied to areas of active eczema, which may include areas of broken skin. Potency of steroid required depends on response along with severity and age.

- Topical steroids should be applied only to the red areas, including the face, as prescribed. This helps to reduce redness and inflammation. If the skin is still itchy despite being well hydrated this may indicate the need for a topical steroid as there may be an inflammatory response in the skin not visible to the eye. Additionally in darker skin redness is not always easily identified and steroid may need to be applied to hyperpigmented or lichenified skin (National Eczema Society 2021).

- The prescribed topical steroid should be applied daily after bathing to all inflamed areas of skin. Depending on potency of the steroid used, once daily is usually adequate.

- It is important to discuss the benefits and harms of treatment with topical corticosteroids with Kate, emphasising that the benefit outweighs possible harm when used correctly. The harms of using topical steroid is usually a common concern for parents. Evidence for several years now is appropriate use of topical steroids is safe (Axon et al. 2021; Siegfried et al. 2016). It is important for parents to know the potency of the topical steroid that is used. Hydrocortisone is extremely mild and there are likely to be little or no side effects from use. Poor adherence to therapy is usually the cause of exacerbations of eczema, rather than simply severity of disease. Poor adherence to therapy can occur for several reasons, including misunderstanding of topical preparations, such as topical steroids, and their use and potential side effects (Smith et al. 2010). Poorly managed eczema can damage the skin as much as overuse of topical steroids.

- Potent topical corticosteroids should not be used in children aged less than 12 months of age without specialist paediatric or dermatological supervision.

Topical calcineurin inhibitors (TCIs)

TCIs work by altering the immune system and have been developed to provide a steroid-sparing alternative for treating eczema. Topical tacrolimus and pimecrolimus are not recommended for the treatment of mild atopic eczema or as first-line treatments for eczema of any severity; topical tacrolimus and pimecrolimus are also not recommended for children under two years of age. In time these recommendations may change.

Wet wrap therapy (WWT)

- Henry may benefit from the use of WWT. If Kate is not familiar with this treatment, the nurse would need to explain its use and demonstrate its application. Then later, the nurse could watch Kate apply the wet wraps to evaluate if Kate needs more instruction, information, or encouragement to provide this therapy if required when Henry is discharged home.

- Wet wrap therapy involves the application of wet elasticated viscose tubular bandages as occlusive dressings, either to the whole body (limbs and trunk)–'wet wrapped', or only to the worst affected areas (e.g. two limbs). An emollient is applied thickly to the skin with two bandages applied, the first wet after being soaked in water, the second dry. The water in the dressings helps to rehydrate the skin, and improves inflammation. Wet wrap therapy can be effective for hard to control eczema and/or intolerable itching (pruritus) (Devillers & Oranje 2006). Wet wraps also create a mechanical barrier against scratching, which allows improved healing of excoriated lesions and some protection against infection and environmental allergens. The absorption of topical medications is increased by the hydration and occlusion provided by the wet wraps (Janmohamed et al. 2014). However, severely infected eczema is contraindicated with wet wraps (van Os-medendorp et al. 2020).

- With a greater understanding of safety and efficacy of topical steroids there is less need for wet wrapping or localized dry wrapping may instead be helpful. Dry wrapping is with one piece of tubifast which is easier to use but emollient will need to be applied regularly beneath the wrap.

Preventing infection of skin lesions

- *Staphylococcus aureus* colonisation/infection is commonly associated with disease severity in children with eczema and is well recognised as a trigger for exacerbating eczema (Khadka et al. 2021, Kim & Kim 2019).

- Sharon should be taught how to recognise the signs and symptoms of bacterial infection with staphylococcus and/or streptococcus (multiple pustules, angry cherry red, and painful skin). Eczema failing to respond to effective therapy, or rapidly worsening eczema (fever and malaise), indicates the need to seek prompt medical attention. Recognition of early signs and symptoms may prevent exacerbations and/or recurrent infections. Weeping or crusting is not necessarily a sign of infection rather it is likely serous ooze from dry skin. To assess apply an ointment emollient 2–3 times in 10–15 minutes. If not infected the skin integrity will improve within 20–30 minutes.

- Kate should obtain new supplies of topical eczema medications after treatment for infected eczema because products in open containers can become contaminated with microorganisms and act as a source of infection.

- Systemic or oral antibiotics that are active against *Staphylococcus aureus* and streptococcus should be administered to treat widespread bacterial infections of eczema. However mild clinically infected eczema does not need treatment with antibiotics (Francis et al. 2017).

- Antiseptics such as triclosan or chlorhexidine may be prescribed, at appropriate dilutions for bathing or showering, as adjunct therapy to decrease bacterial load in children who have recurrent infected or exacerbated eczema. Long-term use should be avoided. There is evidence that dilute bleach baths as a cheap antimicrobial may reduce bacterial colonisation . However, as bleach is a drying agent, it should not be used daily except when managing an acute exacerbation.

Preventing re-infection

- The nurse will admit Henry and family into an isolation room/ward to prevent cross infection in hospital. It should be explained this is for Henry's protection, as he is susceptible to infections. (It is also for the protection of other children who may be at risk of infection from Henry.)

- The nurse will administer oral or intravenous antibiotics to Henry if prescribed.
- If there are open lesions, the nurse must use aseptic techniques to prevent infection. Ideally the use of gloves is minimal as touch is a form of communication.

Maintaining comfort, relief of itch

- The nurse should plan soothing baths (see below) before nap/bedtime.
- Itch is often due to skin dryness; regular use of emollient usually will relieve this.
- Emollient should be applied whenever the skin is dry, red or itchy.
- Oral antihistamines are frequently prescribed for children with eczema to eliminate itch. The rationale is this acts on the H1 receptor to decrease histamine release and therefore eliminates itch (this is not the cause of itch in eczema unless it is an allergic response). In addition, the older antihistamines may have a sedative effect, which may assist with sleep in the short term (clinicians are moving away from this due to the ongoing side effects and risks with use). However, there is no evidence of the efficacy of antihistamines in reducing itch in children with eczema (Matterne et al. 2019).
- Cotton, loose fitting clothing is recommended to cause least irritation when eczema is exacerbated.
- Henry's nails should be cut short and filed, to minimise damage from scratching.
- Distraction – ensure both Henry and Kate have toys and books to entertain them. This will help to prevent Henry from continually scratching and ease the loneliness and boredom from being in isolation in hospital.

Bathing

- Daily baths are regarded as the mainstay for infants and young children.
- Tepid baths are no longer recommended. There is no evidence to support their use. In fact, it is suggested that the vasodilation created by a warm bath aids absorption of emollient in the water (Ren et al. 2021). Antiseptic baths need to be a minimum of 10 minutes duration (Barnes & Greive 2013), which is more likely to be tolerated with a warm bath.
- Henry should be placed into a warm bath, with a soap substitute like emulsifying ointment melted in hot water first. There is no evidence using bath additives routinely assists eczema management (Santer et al. 2018). However, for acute exacerbated eczema adding emollient to the bath can be effective. As there is a staphylococcal infection present, antiseptic bath oil (like Oilatum Plus or QV Flare Up) ideally is added to the water *in addition* to the emollient.
- Apply creams and ointments immediately after the bath to maximise absorption. Apply thinly not sparingly and in one direction.

For Kate, the nursing plan goals are:

- Increasing knowledge about disease process.
- Increasing knowledge about management of the disease and its rationale.
- Improving confidence and competence in providing skin care.

Education

- This is a key part of the nursing care plan for Henry. The aim here is to provide Kate with enough information and confidence so she can provide effective skin cares herself. The aim is to transfer the power of knowledge from the nurse to the parent.
- Following a discussion with Kate, gaining an understanding of her knowledge, the nurse should spend time educating Kate about eczema and its treatment. She/he should provide information in verbal and written forms, with practical demonstrations which may be via online resources. Modelling care by nursing staff is invaluable.

- The nurse will need to assess Kate's ability to take in this information, that is, it may need to be done in short episodes with demonstrations of care and an arrangement to complete education by the end of hospitalisation, with follow-up by paediatric community nurses following discharge and/or following attendance to a nurse eczema clinic, if available.

- When discussing treatment options with Kate the nurse should tailor the information they provide to suit Henry and Kate's cultural practices relating to Henry's cares.

- The nurse should at all times be positive and supportive in their education. If Kate is willing, the nurse should encourage her to provide the skin care for Henry, as discussed, under supervision initially and then on a daily basis. This should increase Kate's confidence and competence in providing appropriate skin care for Henry.

- Assess Kate's energy levels: is she sleep deprived? Does she need a break, assistance with Henry's care or even time to spend with his siblings? Encourage involvement of Kate's partner and other family or social supports in Henry's care, so that the responsibility does not rest solely with Kate.

- Encourage Kate to ask questions particularly if she does not see the expected improvement.

- Nurses are increasingly recognised as the health professional to enable effective management of eczema (Cork et al. 2003; van Os-medendorp et al. 2020). The key to effective management of eczema is education and support with an individual plan that empowers the individual and/or family to successfully self-care.

Evaluation

Finally, it will be important for the nurse to evaluate all planned care for Henry and his mum, Kate, and then re-plan care to address any remaining or ongoing healthcare or knowledge needs.

REFERENCES

Aw, M., Penn, J., Gauvreau, G.M., Lima, H. & Sehmi, R. (2020) Atopic march: collegium internationale allergologicum update 2020. *International Archives of Allergy and Immunology*, **181**(1), 1–10. https://www.karger.com/Article/FullText/502958 [Accessed 6 March 2023].

Axon, E., Chalmers, J.R., Santer, M., Ridd, M.J., Lawton, S., Langan, S.M., Grindlay, D., Muller, I., Roberts, A., Ahmed, A., Williams, H.C. & Thomas, K.S. (2021) Safety of topical corticosteroids in atopic eczema: an umbrella review. *BMJ open*, **11**(7), e046476. https://doi.org/10.1136/bmjopen-2020-046476 [Accessed 6 March 2023].

Barfield, A., Brown, H., Pernell, P., & Woodard, J. (2017) Effectiveness of emollient therapy in pediatric patients with atopic dermatitis. *Journal of the Dermatology Nurses' Association*, 5/6, **9**(3), 123–128. https://doi.org/10.1097/JDN.0000000000000297 [Accessed 6 March 2023].

Barnes, T.M. & Greive, K.A. (2013) Bleach baths for atopic eczema. *Australasian Journal of Dermatology*, **54**, 251–258. https://pubmed.ncbi.nlm.nih.gov/23330843 [Accessed 6 March 2023].

Casey, A. (1993) The development and use of the partnership model of nursing care. In: Glasper, E.A. and Tucker, A. (eds). *Advances in Child Health Nursing*. London: Scutari Press.

Cork, M.J., Britton, J., Butler, L., Young, S., Murphy, R. & Keohane, S.G. (2003) Comparison of parent knowledge, therapy utilization and severity of atopic eczema before and after explanation and demonstration of topical therapies by a specialist dermatology nurse. *The British Journal of Dermatology*, **149**(3), 582–589. https://pubmed.ncbi.nlm.nih.gov/14510993 [Accessed 6 March 2023].

Cork, M.J., Danby, S.G. & Ogg, G.S. (2020 December). Atopic dermatitis epidemiology and unmet need in the United Kingdom. *The Journal of Dermatological Treatment*, **31**(8), 801–809. doi: 10.1080/09546634.2019.1655137. Epub 2019 Oct 21. PMID: 31631717; PMCID: PMC7573657.

de Lusignan, S., Alexander, H., Broderick, C., Dennis, J., McGovern, A., Feeney, C. & Flohr, C. (2021) The epidemiology of eczema in children and adults in England: a population-based study using primary care data. *Clinical and Experimental Allergy: Journal of the British Society for Allergy and Clinical Immunology*, **51**(3), 471–482. https://doi.org/10.1111/cea.13784 [Accessed 6 March 2023].

Devillers, A.C. & Oranje, A.P. (2006) Efficacy and safety of 'wet-wrap' dressings as an intervention treatment in children with severe and/or refractory atopic dermatitis: a critical review of the literature. *The British Journal of Dermatology*, **154**(4), 579–585. https://doi.org/10.1111/j.1365-2133.2006.07157.x [Accessed 6 March 2023].

Francis, N.A., Ridd, M.J., Thomas-Jones, E., Butler, C.C., Hood, K., Shepherd, V., Marwick, C.A., Huang, C., Longo, M., Wootton, M. & Sullivan, F.CREAM Trial Management Group (2017) Oral and topical antibiotics for clinically infected eczema in children: a pragmatic randomized controlled trial in ambulatory care. *Annals of Family Medicine*, **15**(2), 124–130. https://doi.org/10.1370/afm.2038 [Accessed 6 March 2023].

Halkjaer, L.B., Loland, L., Buchvald, F.F., Agner, T., Skov, L., Strand, M. & Bisgaard, H. (2006) Development of atopic dermatitis during the first 3 years of life: the Copenhagen prospective study on asthma in childhood cohort study in high-risk children. *Archives of Dermatology*, **142**(5), 561–566. https://doi.org/10.1001/archderm.142.5.561 [Accessed 6 March 2023].

Hon, K.L., Kung, J., Tsang, K., Yu, J., Lee, V.W. & Leung, T.F. (2018) Emollient acceptability in childhood atopic dermatitis: not all emollients are equal. *Current Pediatric Reviews*, **14**(2), 117–122. https://doi.org/10.2174/1573396313666170605080034 [Accessed 6 March 2023].

Janmohamed, S.R., Oranje, A.P., Devillers, A.C., Rizopoulos, D., van Praag, M.C., Van Gysel, D., Goeteyn, M. & de Waard-van der Spek, F.B. (2014) The proactive wet-wrap method with diluted corticosteroids versus emollients in children with atopic dermatitis: a prospective, randomized, double-blind, placebo-controlled trial. *Journal of the American Academy of Dermatology*, **70**(6), 1076–1082. https://doi.org/10.1016/j.jaad.2014.01.898 [Accessed 6 March 2023].

Khadka, V.D., Key, F.M., Romo-González, C., Martínez-Gayosso, A., Campos-Cabrera, B.L., Gerónimo-Gallegos, A., Lynn, T.C., Durán-mckinster, C., Coria-Jiménez, R., Lieberman, T.D. & García-Romero, M.T. (2021) The skin microbiome of patients with atopic dermatitis normalizes gradually during treatment. *Frontiers in Cellular and Infection Microbiology*, **11**, 720674. https://doi.org/10.3389/fcimb.2021.720674 [Accessed 6 March 2023].

Kim, J.E. & Kim, H.S. (2019) Microbiome of the skin and gut in atopic dermatitis (AD): understanding the pathophysiology and finding novel management strategies. *Journal of Clinical Medicine*, **8**(4), 444. https://doi.org/10.3390/jcm8040444 [Accessed 6 March 2023].

Leung, D.Y., Boguniewicz, M., Howell, M.D., Nomura, I. & Hamid, Q.A. (2004) New insights into atopic dermatitis. *The Journal of Clinical Investigation*, **113**(5), 651–657. https://doi.org/10.1172/JCI21060 [Accessed 6 March 2023].

Lindh, J.D. & Bradley, M. (2015) Clinical effectiveness of moisturizers in atopic dermatitis and related disorders: a systematic review. *American Journal of Clinical Dermatology*, **16**(5), 341–359. https://doi.org/10.1007/s40257-015-0146-4 [Accessed 6 March 2023].

Matterne, U., Böhmer, M.M., Weisshaar, E., Jupiter, A., Carter, B. & Apfelbacher, C.J. (2019) Oral H1 antihistamines as 'add-on' therapy to topical treatment for eczema. *The Cochrane Database of Systematic Reviews*, **1**(1), CD012167. https://doi.org/10.1002/14651858.CD012167.pub2 [Accessed 6 March 2023].

National Eczema Society (2021) https://eczema.org/information-and-advice/living-with-eczema/skin-pigmentation/?

Ren, W., Xu, L., Zheng, X. et al. (2021) Effect of different thermal stimuli on improving microcirculation in the contralateral foot. *BioMed Eng OnLine*, **20**, 14. https://doi.org/10.1186/s12938-021-00849-9 [Accessed 6 March 2023].

Salvati, L., Cosmi, L. & Annunziato, F. (2021) From emollients to biologicals: targeting atopic dermatitis. *International Journal of Molecular Sciences*, **22**(19), 10381. https://doi.org/10.3390/ijms221910381 [Accessed 6 March 2023].

Santer, M., Burgess, H., Yardley, L., Ersser, S., Lewis-Jones, S., Muller, I., Hugh, C. & Little, P. (2012) Experiences of carers managing childhood eczema and their views on its treatment: a qualitative study. *The British Journal of General Practice: The Journal of the Royal College of General Practitioners*, **62**(597), e261–e267. http://doi.org/10.3399/bjgp12×636083 [Accessed 6 March 2023].

Santer, M., Rumsby, K., Ridd, M.J., Francis, N.A., Stuart, B., Chorozoglou, M., Roberts, A., Liddiard, L., Nollett, C., Hooper, J., Prude, M., Wood, W., Thomas-Jones, E., Becque, T., Thomas, K.S., Williams, H.C. & Little, P. (2018) Adding emollient bath additives to standard eczema management for children with eczema: the BATHE RCT. *Health Technology Assessment (Winchester, England)*, **22**(57), 1–116. https://doi.org/10.3310/hta22570 [Accessed 6 March 2023]

Siegfried, E.C., Jaworski, J.C., Kaiser, J.D. & Hebert, A.A. (2016) Systematic review of published trials: long-term safety of topical corticosteroids and topical calcineurin inhibitors in pediatric patients with atopic dermatitis. *BMC Pediatrics*, **16**, 75. https://doi.org/10.1186/s12887-016-0607-9 [Accessed 6 March 2023].

Smith, S.D., Hong, E., Fearns, S., Blaszczynski, A. & Fischer, G. (2010) Corticosteroid phobia and other confounders in the treatment of childhood atopic dermatitis explored using parent focus groups. *The Australasian Journal of Dermatology*, **51**(3), 168–174. https://doi.org/10.1111/j.1440-0960.2010.00636.x [Accessed 6 March 2023]

Thomsen, S.F. (2014) Atopic dermatitis: natural history, diagnosis, and treatment. *ISRN Allergy*, **2014**, 354250. https://doi.org/10.1155/2014/354250 [Accessed 6 March 2023].

van Os-medendorp, H., Deprez, E., Maes, N., Ryan, S., Jackson, K., Winders, T., De Raeve, L., De Cuyper, C. & Ersser, S. (2020) The role of the nurse in the care and management of patients with atopic dermatitis. *BMC Nursing*, **19**(1), 102. https://doi.org/10.1186/s12912-020-00494-y [Accessed 6 March 2023].

van Zuuren, E.J., Fedorowicz, Z. & Arents, B. (2017) Emollients and moisturizers for eczema: abridged Cochrane systematic review including GRADE assessments. *The British Journal of Dermatology*, **177**(5), 1256–1271. https://pubmed.ncbi.nlm.nih.gov/28432721 [Accessed 6 March 2023].

Wan, J., Takeshita, J., Shin, D.B. & Gelfand, J.M. (2020) Mental health impairment among children with atopic dermatitis: a United States population-based cross-sectional study of the 2013-2017 National Health Interview Survey. *Journal of the American Academy of Dermatology*, **82**(6), 1368–1375. https://doi.org/10.1016/j.jaad.2019.10.019 [Accessed 6 March 2023]

Yang, L., Fu, J. & Zhou, Y. (2020) Research progress in atopic march. *Frontiers in Immunology*, **11**, 1907. https://doi.org/10.3389/fimmu.2020.01907 [Accessed 6 March 2023].

Bakaa, L., Pernica, J. M., Couban, R. J., Tackett, K. J., Burkhart, C. N., Leins, L., Smart, J., Garcia-Romero, M. T., Elizalde-Jiménez, I. G., Herd, M., Asiniwasis, R. N., Boguniewicz, M., De Benedetto, A., Chen, L., Ellison, K., Frazier, W., Greenhawt, M., Huynh, J., LeBovidge, J., ... Chu, D. K. (2022). Bleach baths for atopic dermatitis. Annals of Allergy, Asthma & Immunology, 128(6), 660–668.e9. https://doi.org/10.1016/j.anai.2022.03.024

CHAPTER 35

Burns Injury

Doris Corkin and Lydia Webb
(acknowledge Idy Fu)

SCENARIO

Ka Man, a 13-year-old girl, emigrated from China five years ago with her parents and a younger brother Ka Wai, aged 8. She was studying form 1 in a local secondary school two km from home. The family lived in a small rented apartment in one of the crowded districts on Hong Kong Island. Ka Man had sustained superficial and deep partial-thickness burns to her right lower leg and right foot respectively, from a tilted pot of boiled soup while she was helping her mother carry the pot to the dining room where she tripped over. She was sent to the nearby A & E department immediately, accompanied by her mother. She remained conscious and orientated but was very restless and complaining of severe pain over her right leg.

When Ka Man arrived at the hospital, her temperature was 35.8°C, blood pressure: 80/50 mmHg, pulse: 128 beats/min, respiration rate: 36 breaths/min and SpO_2: 90%. Her right lower leg was swollen and large blisters were found. She was put on oxygen therapy at 6 L/min via a face mask and intravenous fluid infusion was commenced. Ka Man was also given a dose of IV morphine to relieve her pain. Blood sample was taken for laboratory studies – complete blood count, renal and liver function tests, and blood gas analysis. After a thorough assessment by the A & E physician, Ka Man was transferred to the burns unit for close observation and further management.

Three days after admission, Ka Man was gradually recovering from the burn injury, with stable haemodynamics and satisfactory urine output. The oedema had subsided over her right lower leg and epithelialisation started to take place. However, the right foot remained pale and some necrotic tissues were found at the wound surface. After being reassessed by the surgeon, Ka Man was scheduled for debridement and grafting surgery of her right foot with split-thickness skin grafts harvested from her left anterior thigh.

On initial presentation, it is important that the nurse and/or doctor ascertains and notes the extent of 'first aid' that Ka Man received after the injury. From the scenario we are told she attended the Emergency Department immediately which would make one wonder if any first aid was initiated. The severity of a burn and the patient's clinical outcome has been shown to improve when appropriate 'first aid' is given – that is, running cool water over the affected area for twenty minutes (Griffin et al. 2020). Therefore, it is important that, as healthcare providers, nurses are actively involved in educating parents on the importance of first aid in burns (Naumeri et al. 2019) so Ka Man's parents are better equipped should an accident such as this one happen again.

QUESTIONS

1. How should burn injuries be classified in children?
2. Discuss the immediate nursing assessments for Ka Man in relation to her burn injury.
3. Develop a nursing care plan for Ka Man during the resuscitation phase (first 24–48 hours) of a burn injury.
4. Explain the specific nursing care for managing the grafted and donor wounds of Ka Man postoperatively.

Care Planning in Children and Young People's Nursing, Second Edition. Edited by Sonya Clarke and Doris Corkin.
© 2024 John Wiley & Sons Ltd. Published 2024 by John Wiley & Sons Ltd.

Question 1. How should burn injuries be classified in children?

The severity of a burn injury is assessed by the percentage of surface area affected (the extent of injury) and the degree of involvement of the epidermis, dermis, and underlying structures (the depth of injury). Indeed, the deeper the injury the greater the number of layers that are damaged. The seriousness of the injury is also determined by other important factors such as the age of the child, the location of the wound, the general health of the child, and the presence of respiratory involvement or any associated conditions. A burn injury that accounts for 10% of the total body surface area (TBSA) can be life threatening in small children with any delayed or inappropriate treatment (Ray et al 2022).

Superficial (first-degree) burns involve damage of the epidermis. The protective functions of skin remain intact and therefore systemic infections are rare. The injury often results in redness of skin, with pain as the predominant symptom, and the wound usually heals in 5–10 days without scarring.

Partial-thickness (second-degree) burns are injuries to the second layer of skin, the dermis. The seriousness of a partial-thickness burn depends on how much of the dermis has been injured. These wounds are painful and extremely sensitive to temperature changes, exposure to air, and light touch because the nerve endings remain intact. Superficial partial – thickness wounds appear moist and mottled, pink or red, and blanch when pressure is applied. There are usually blisters present (see Box 35.1). Deep partial-thickness wounds appear dry and whitish in colour but do not blanch. A superficial partial-thickness wound usually heals spontaneously in approximately 14 days with varying degree of scarring, whereas a deep and large partial thickness burn is generally best treated with excision and grafting to reduce risk of hypertrophic scarring and contracture.

Full-thickness (third-degree) burns are serious injuries involving the entire epidermis and dermis and extending into the subcutaneous tissue. Wound colour varies from red to tan, waxy white, brown, or black, with a dry, leathery appearance. These wounds are rarely painful because the nerve endings are damaged as well as the sweat glands and hair follicles. However, a partial-thickness burn is often present at the periphery of a full-thickness wound; therefore, the child is not pain free. As the epidermis and entire dermis are destroyed, re-epithelialisation is not possible; thus surgical excision and grafting are required for wound healing.

BOX 35.1 CARE OF BLISTERS

Taken from *Clinical Practice Guidelines on Burns*, the Royal Children's Hospital Melbourne (2010).

The care of blisters depends on their size and location. Blisters are usually left alone if they are not large and not obstructing the dressing. If large bulbous blisters are present that are obstructing a dressing or causing restriction to local circulation, the blisters should be punctured and fluid aspirated for better dressing application.

If the fluid inside the blisters become opaque and infection is suspected, the blister epidermis should be removed completely. Loose epidermis from broken blisters may be debrided with caution as bleeding can occur when part of the blister remains attached to the skin.

Full-thickness (fourth-degree) burns are injuries involving underlying structures such as muscle, fascia, tendon, and bone. These wounds have the same characteristics as third-degree burns.

Question 2. Discuss the immediate nursing assessments for Ka Man in relation to her burn injury.

In partial thickness burns, water, plasma proteins, and electrolytes are lost through the damaged tissues. The release of inflammatory and vasoactive mediators activated by the burn injury increases the capillary permeability, causing shifting of fluid from the vascular compartment to the interstitial space, resulting in further fluid loss. When intravascular volume continues to decrease without correction, hypovolaemic shock develops. The nurse therefore needs to assess Ka Man's blood pressure, pulse rate, and capillary refill every 30–60 minutes in order to detect hypovolaemic shock promptly. Urinary function should also be monitored hourly to ensure fluid resuscitation is adequate for tissue perfusion, which is indicated by maintaining a urine output of 1.0–1.5 ml/kg/hour (Pham et al. 2008). As the thermoregulatory function of the skin is impaired and body heat is lost from the burnt surfaces, the nurse should monitor Ka Man's temperature for hypothermia every hour until stable.

The conscious level of Ka Man should be assessed regularly to identify possible neurological complications resulting from altered electrolyte balance, in which the child may present with confusion, weakness, and seizures. Neurovascular assessment of the affected limb must be performed hourly to rule out circulatory obstruction caused by compartment syndrome, particularly in circumferential burns, which is characterised by changes in colour and/or temperature, absence of distal pulse, loss of sensation, and deep throbbing pain.

Furthermore, the extent of injury should be assessed and the percentage of burnt areas estimated using the Lund & Browder Chart (Table 35.1) as a baseline to gauge wound healing process. The Rule of Nines method (Table 35.2) is not recommended for small children as the rates of growth in the head, thigh and lower leg vary across different age groups (Orgill 2009). However, it is useful as a rough estimate until the Lund & Browder chart can be used.

For example, 1% TBSA (total body surface area) is estimated to be roughly the size of the patient's hand (Grunwald & Garner 2008). Therefore, it is important to note that under-and over-estimating TBSA can lead to mistreatment and further problems (Ray et al, 2021–2022). Over-

Table 35.1 The Lund and Browder method for assessing percentage of burn injury in children.

Surface area (anterior and posterior)	Age				
	0–12 month	1–4 year	5–9 year	10–15 year	> 15 year
Head	19%	17%	13%	11%	9%
R & L thighs	5.5% × 2	6.5% × 2	8% × 2	8.5% × 2	9% × 2
R & L lower legs	5% × 2	5% × 2	5.5% × 2	6% × 2	6.5% × 2
Neck	2%				
Trunk	26%				
R & L upper arms	4% × 2				
R & L lower arms	3% × 2				
R & L hands	2.5% × 2				
R & L buttocks	2.5% × 2				
R & L feet	3.5% × 2				
Genitalia	1%				

R = right-sided; L = left-sided.

Table 35.2 The Rule of Nines method for assessing percentage of burn injury in adults.

Surface area	Anterior	Posterior
Head & neck	4.5%	4.5%
Torso	18%	18%
R & L legs	9% × 2	9% × 2
R & L arms	4.5% × 2	4.5% × 2
Genitalia	1%	–
Total	100%	

R = right-sided; L = left-sided.

estimation of TBSA in a burn greater than 10% will lead to over-treatment with resuscitation fluids which can result in compartment syndrome and pulmonary oedema (Dulhunty et al. 2008; Klein et al. 2007). On the other hand, if the TBSA is underestimated and the child does not receive sufficient resuscitation fluids, the burn can convert to deeper tissues and the child can be left with kidney failure and/or multi-organ failure (Oda et al. 2006).

The nurse should assess the pain intensity of Ka Man regularly and monitor the effectiveness of analgesics given. Hyperventilation may develop as a result of severe pain and anxiety in the burnt child; therefore, respiration rate and pattern should be assessed hourly to observe for respiratory complications. Changes in respiratory function and gas exchange are characterised by restlessness, irritability, increased work of breathing, and alterations in blood gas values. In addition, the nurse needs to assess the tetanus status and allergy history of the child.

Question 3. Develop a nursing care plan for Ka Man during the resuscitation phase (first 24–48 hours) of a burn injury.

See Table 35.3.

Table 35.3 Nursing care plan for Ka Man with burn injury

Nursing diagnosis (see Chapter 1)	Expected outcome	Nursing interventions/rationales
Fluid volume deficit related to fluid loss from damaged skin and increased capillary permeability.	Ka Man will maintain adequate fluid hydration status with stable haemodynamic parameters.	1. Monitor Ka Man's vital signs, urine output, mental state, skin turgor and moisture of mucous membrane *to determine adequacy of fluid replacement.*
		2. Administer intravenous fluids as ordered by doctor, and check for patency of IV line *to ensure adequate replacement for fluid loss.*
		3. Weight Ka Man daily at the same time *to rule out urinary retention or excessive diuresis.*
		4. Monitor laboratory results (e.g. potassium, sodium, haemoglobin, haematocrit) *to detect fluid and electrolyte imbalance.*
		5. Keep an accurate record of Ka Man's intake and output daily *to monitor for fluid balance.*
Risk for altered tissue perfusion related to oedema of the affected limb.	Ka Man will have optimal circulation to the affected limb without neurovascular complications.	1. Check distal pulse and sensation of the affected limb and monitor closely for signs and symptoms of circulatory obstruction *to observe for development of compartment syndrome.*
		2. Elevate the affected limb 20 to 30 degrees *to promote venous return and reduce leg swelling.*
		3. Remove restrictive clothing on the affected limb *to prevent circulatory obstruction.*
		4. Avoid applying restrictive or pressure dressings over inured limb *to prevent obstruction of blood flow.*
		5. Perform Doppler examination if diminished distal pulse is noticed *to detect circulatory obstruction early.*
		6. Teach Ka Man to report any abnormal feelings in the affected limb *to allow early detection of neurovascular complications.*
Acute pain related to tissue destruction and exposed nerve endings at the skin surface.	Ka Man will report decreased level of pain with more restful periods.	1. Assess Ka Man's pain level every hour using age-appropriate assessment tool *to determine the need for pain medication.*
		2. Administer pain medication at regular intervals when indicated *to achieve better pain control and prevent occurrence of severe pain.*
		3. Determine the best route for administering analgesics and assess for effectiveness *to ensure maximal absorption and adequate pain relief.*

(Continued)

Table 35.3 (Continued)

Nursing diagnosis (see Chapter 1)	Expected outcome	Nursing interventions/rationales
		4. Monitor Ka Man's vital signs, emotional state, appetite, activity level, and sleep pattern *to collect data regarding level of pain she is experiencing*.
		5. Offer breakthrough analgesics as necessary prior to wound dressing changes *to reduce discomfort*.
		6. Use a bed cradle *to avoid bed linen from pressing on the affected limb*.
		7. Handle the injured limb carefully and gently *to minimise discomfort and prevent unnecessary injuries*.
		8. Explain all procedures beforehand *to reduce anxiety-associated pain*.
		9. Employ age-appropriate, non-pharmacological pain relief strategies, for example music, television, games *to distract Ka Man from pain*.
		10. Allow Ka Man to participate in self-care activities as appropriate, for example bathing, removing dressing *to promote a sense of control in pain management*.
		11. Encourage parents to visit and stay with Ka Man as needed *to help comfort and support her recovery*.
		12. Teach Ka Man to touch/stroke the unaffected areas *to provide physical contact and promote comfort*.
		13. Educate Ka Man and her family on the characteristics of pain from a burn wound and their role in pain management *to promote family-centered care and effective coping*.
Impaired skin integrity related to thermal injury.	Ka Man will demonstrate no signs of wound infection and reduction in the size of burn wounds.	1. Implement standard precautions vigilantly when caring for Ka Man *to prevent cross infections*.
		2. Cleanse all burnt surfaces thoroughly and regularly with normal saline, and debride devitalised skin as necessary *to decrease risk of infection and promote healing*.
		3. Employ aseptic technique when performing dressing changes *to prevent infection*.
		4. Use appropriate wound dressing materials *to reduce dressing change and unnecessary disturbance to wounds*.
		5. Handle wound dressing with care during removal *to prevent damaging the newly-formed tissues*.
		6. Apply topical antimicrobial preparation as ordered by doctor (e.g. silver sulfadiazine) *to decrease risk of infection*.
		7. Start hydrotherapy treatment when haemodynamics are stable, using disinfected bathing equipment *to promote removal of devitalised tissues and colonised micro-organisms*.
		8. Administer prophylactic antibiotics as prescribed by doctor if indicated and observe for side effects of medication *to reduce the risk of infection*.
		9. Consider the use of temporary skin substitute *to protect the wounds, promote healing and reduce pain*.
		10. Monitor for signs and symptoms of wound infection (fever, changes in amount, colour, or odour of drainage) and educate Ka Man to report any abnormalities promptly *to allow early recognition and treatment*.
		11. Offer high-protein, high-calorie meals to Ka Man as tolerated or commence enteral (N/G) feeding if indicated *to augment nutritional requirements for wound healing*.
		12. Administer supplementary vitamins and minerals as ordered by doctor *to facilitate tissue regeneration*.
		13. Collect wound swabs for culture if symptomatic *to monitor the course of infection*.

Table 35.3 (Continued)

Nursing diagnosis (see Chapter 1)	Expected outcome	Nursing interventions/rationales
Ineffective thermoregulation related to damaged skin barrier and increased body heat loss through evaporation from burnt surfaces.	Ka Man will maintain a normal body temperature of 37 ± 0.5°C.	1. Monitor Ka Man's temperature hourly until stable, then every 2–4 hourly *to ensure early detection and treatment of hypothermia.* 2. Observe for any chills or shivering *to identify signs of hypothermia.* 3. Maintain a warm environment and avoid unnecessary exposures of the body *to prevent excessive heat loss.* 4. Warm the IV fluids prior to administration if indicated, *to offset expected heat loss.* 5. Keep the water temperature for hydrotherapy at 36.7°C and limit the procedure time to 20 minutes *to prevent excessive heat loss and reduce stress.* 6. Use a thermal insulating blanket with a bed cradle over the injured limb if necessary *to reduce radiant heat loss and increase body temperature.*
Impaired physical mobility related to pain and impaired joint movement.	Ka Man will achieve optimal physical functioning with minimal complications.	1. Keep the right foot at 90 degrees with the use of assistive devices (e.g. splint, foot board) *to maintain a functional position and minimise deformity.* 2. Perform ROM exercises every four hours for 15 minutes or as tolerated with adequate analgesic cover *to increase muscle tone and prevent joint stiffness.* 3. Use appropriate wound care method (refer to Box 34.2) and avoid tight bandaging over the affected limb *to reduce restriction in joint movement.* 4. Assist Ka Man to change position regularly and use pressure-relieving devices to support bony areas *to prevent pressure sore formation.* 5. Teach Ka Man to perform active ROM exercises to unaffected extremities and ambulate as soon as feasible *to maintain optimal joint and muscle functions.* 6. Encourage participation in self-care activities *to increase mobility and improve morale.* 7. Administer analgesics before any strenuous activities *to reduce pain and increase activity tolerance.* 8. Consider early physiotherapy consultation for rehabilitation planning *to minimise level of disability.*
Disturbed body image related to alteration in appearance and mobility.	Ka Man will express her concerns on altered physical appearance and demonstrate acceptance to the burn injury.	1. Observe Ka Man for significant behavioural and/or emotional changes *to identify depressive symptoms for early interventions.* 2. Provide opportunities for Ka Man and her family to discuss the possible outcomes of injury *to allay fear and increase coping.* 3. Be honest with Ka Man and her family, providing relevant information on the recovery process *to build a trusting relationship.* 4. Encourage Ka Man to participate in wound care *to improve acceptance of the altered physical appearance.* 5. Convey positive attitude and offer appropriate coping strategies *to enhance acceptance of the injury.* 6. Promote independence in self-care activities as much as condition allows *to increase sense of control and improve self-esteem.*

Axton & Fugate 2009; Hockenberry et al. 2005; Sadik & Campbell 2001; Severe Burn Injury Service Model of Care, NSW Department of Health (2004); Speer 1999.

BOX 35.2

The 'closed (occlusive) method' for burn wound (Smeltzer et al. 2008)

1. All dressing changes need to be carried out aseptically with adequate pain relief prior to the procedure.
2. The burn wounds should be covered with sterile non-adherent dressing, then gently wrapped with bandage circumferentially in a distal-to-proximal manner.
3. Do not allow any two burnt surfaces to come in contact (e.g. between digits, skin folds) to promote webbing of digits and prevent contractures.
4. The dressing that covers a burn wound must be about 2 cm thick to be effective for absorbing exudates and preventing it from reaching the surface where it can become infected.
5. The amount of wound exudate determines the frequency for dressing change.

Question 4. Explain the specific nursing care for managing the grafted and donor wounds of Ka Man postoperatively.

All wounds should be kept clean and dry postoperatively. The children's nurse should assess both wound sites regularly for excessive bleeding as haemorrhage is one of the most important complications after grafting surgery (Kagan et al. 2009; Orgill 2009). A sterile non-adherent dressing is used to cover the skin donor site, which is often kept intact for 3–5 days if no complications develop. A split-thickness skin graft harvest involves the epidermis and superficial (papillary) dermis, thus the donor wound at the left thigh normally heals spontaneously within 7–14 days.

For the grafted (recipient) site, small sutures may be used to secure the graft to the excised wound bed. The wound is covered with occlusive non-adherent dressing (often impregnated with antibiotic ointment to reduce bacterial proliferation) which may be removed on the fourth or fifth postoperative day, depending on the surgeon's practice. Graft detachment may result if there is haematoma formation or bacterial contamination at the wound site. The nurse should monitor the grafted area closely for any abnormalities.

Other factors that may cause graft failure include peripheral oedema and mechanical shearing forces (Kagan et al. 2009). Therefore, Ka Man must be advised to stay in bed for 7–10 days with her right foot splinted and leg elevated to maintain functional positioning, reduce the risk of graft loss due to movement and facilitate adhesion of graft to the wound bed. The children's nurse should handle Ka Man's operated leg with care and protect the grafted site from any pressure or trauma. Ka Man should also be informed not to perform any exercise or activity that stretches the graft or puts it at risk for trauma for 3–4 weeks. The nurse should monitor Ka Man's pain level more closely after surgery and provide additional analgesics to her if needed to achieve effective pain control.

REFERENCES

Axton, S. & Fugate, T. (2009) *Pediatric Nursing Care Plans for the Hospitalized Child*, 3rd edition. Upper Saddle River, NJ: Pearson Prentice Hall.

Dulhunty, J.M., Boots, R.J., Rudd, M.J. et al. (2008) Increased fluid resuscitation can lead to adverse outcomes in major-burn injured patients, but low mortality is achievable. *Burns*, **34**(8), 1090–1097. doi:10.1016/j.burns.2008.01.011.

Griffin, B.R., Frear, C.C., Babl, F., Oakley, E. & Kimble, R.M. (2020) Cool running water first aid decreases skin grafting requirements in pediatric burns: a cohort study of two thousand four hundred ninety-five children. *Annals of Emergency Medicine*, [online] **75**(1), 75–85. doi:10.1016/j.annemergmed.2019.06.028.

Grunwald, T.B. & Garner, W.L. (2008) Acute burns. *Plastic and Reconstructive Surgery*, [online] **121**(5), 311e. doi:10.1097/PRS.0b013e318172ae1f.

Hockenberry, M.J., Wilson, D. & Winkelstein, M.L. (2005) *Wong's Essentials of Paediatric Nursing*, 7th edition. St Louis: Mosby.

Kagan, R.J., Peck, M.D., Ahrenholz, D.H. et al. (2009) *Surgical Management of the Burn Wound and Use of Skin Substitutes*. Chicago: American Burn Association.

Klein, M.B., Hayden, D., Elson, C. et al (2007) The association between fluid administration and outcome following major burn: a multicenter study. *Annals of Surgery*, **245**(4), 622–628. doi:10.1097/01.sla.0000252572.50684.49.

Naumeri, F., Ahmad, H.M., Yousaf, M.S., Waheed, K. & Farooq, M.S. (2019). Do parents have knowledge of first aid management of burns in their children? A hospital based survey. JPMA. *The Journal of the Pakistan Medical Association*, [online] **69** (8), 1142–1145. Available at: https://pubmed.ncbi.nlm.nih.gov/31431768 (accessed 6 March 2023).

NSW Department of Health (2004) *NSW Severe Burn Injury Service–Model of Care.* www.health.nsw.gov.au/pubs/2004/burninjurymoc.html.

Oda, J., Yamashita, K., Inoue, T. et al (2006) Resuscitation fluid volume and abdominal compartment syndrome in patients with major burns. *Burns*, **32**(2), 151–154. doi:10.1016/j.burns.2005.08.011.

Orgill, D.P. (2009) Excision and skin grafting of thermal burns. *The New England Journal of Medicine*, **360**(9), 893–901.

Pham, T.N., Cancio, L.C. & Gibran, N.S. (2008) American Burn Association practice guidelines burn shock resuscitation. *Journal of Burn Care and Research*, **29**(1), 257–266.

Ray, W.C., Rajab, A., Alexander, H. Chmil B., Rumpf R.W., Thakkar R., Viswanathan M., Fabia R. (2022) A 1% TBSA chart reduces math errors while retaining acceptable first-estimate accuracy. *Journal of Burn Care & Research*, **43**(3), 665–678. doi:10.1093/jbcr/irab192. PMID: 34665849; PMCID: PMC9113823. (accessed 6 March 2023).

Royal Children's Hospital Melbourne (2010) *Clinical Practice Guidelines on Burns* https://www.rch.org.au/clinicalguide/guideline_index/Burns (accessed 6 March 2023).

Sadik, R. & Campbell, G. (2001) *Client Profiles in Nursing: Child Health.* London: Greenwich Medical Media.

Smeltzer, S.C., Bare, B.G., Hinkle, J.L. & Cheever, K.H. (2008) *Brunner & Suddarth's Textbook of Medical-Surgical Nursing*, 11th edition. Philadelphia: Lippincott Williams & Wilkins.

Speer, K.M. (1999) *Pediatric Care Planning*, 3rd edition. Springhouse, PA: Springhouse Corporation.

CHAPTER 36

Children with Complex Needs

Julie Chambers and Doris Corkin

SCENARIO 1

During a 20-week scan, Mum was first informed by hospital radiographer that her unborn child had brain abnormalities; a diagnosis of Holorosencephaly (HPE) was later confirmed at 28 weeks (7 months pregnant) via Magnetic Resonance Imaging (MRI) scan. Baby Penny was later born via Caesarean section (C-section) surrounded by a Paediatric Team. As her breathing was causing healthcare staff great concern, Penny needed to be immediately transferred to the local Neonatal Intensive Care Unit (NICU). There Penny was, surrounded by monitors and leads, while her distressed parents looked on in disbelief. A different world with medical terminology, language that was strange and difficult to comprehend. Penny's condition improved, then into the Special Care Baby Unit (SCBU) before getting home at six weeks old.

Having spent three weeks at home, Penny became unwell, with difficulty in feeding, and developed bronchiolitis followed by severe epilepsy. Admitted to the regional Paediatric Intensive Care Unit (PICU) then nine weeks old, Penny had various investigations, revealing she had an unstable Sodium level in her blood. According to Mum, the PICU staff were amazing, establishing very good communication and trusting relationships.

However, over the last five years, Penny's transition from hospital to community services has not always been straight forward, with much frustration along the way, especially when trying to articulate the holistic care and support the family need, within the home setting (Carter et al. 2016).

SCENARIO 2

Four-year old Leo, was born a healthy baby and appeared to meet his milestones and thereafter sadly, his parents noticed that he was not maintaining these and losing developmental ground. Upon further investigation with the medical team, a diagnosis of Infantile Onset Pome Disease was diagnosed.

ACTIVITY 36.1

Please see links: **National Institute of Neurological Disorders;** https://www.ninds.nih.gov; **Child Neurology;** https://rarediseases.info.nih.gov; rarediseases.org/videos/pompe-disease/ for further information.

Care Planning in Children and Young People's Nursing, Second Edition. Edited by Sonya Clarke and Doris Corkin.
© 2024 John Wiley & Sons Ltd. Published 2024 by John Wiley & Sons Ltd.

QUESTIONS

1. What is Holorosencephaly (HPE) and how is this disorder diagnosed?
2. What is Infantile Onset Pompe Disease (IOPD) and how is this diagnosed?
3.a Why may a child with Pompe Disease or Holorosencephaly have difficulty breathing?
3.b Explain non-invasive ventilation.
3.c Explain the use of a BiPAP machine in the home.
4. Discuss the importance of communication by healthcare professionals when caring for a child and/or young person with a life-limiting condition, in the community setting.
5. Using the Roper, Logan & Tierney model in practice devise a care plan for Penny addressing the importance of Touch and Mouth care.

ANSWERS TO QUESTIONS

Question 1. What is Holorosencephaly (HPE) and how is this disorder diagnosed?

Holorosencephaly (HPE) is a cephalic disorder, which ranges in severity based on the degree of anatomic abnormality, in which the forebrain (prosencephalon) of the embryo fails to develop into two hemispheres, that is, the right and left halves of the brain (Zantow et al. 2021).

Prognosis is dependent on the degree of fusion or malformation of the brain along with the other health complications that may be present. The brain does not deteriorate over time however often other life threatening conditions can be present. In moderate to severe cases there is likely to include spastic quadriparesis, athetoid movements, endocrine disorders, hypernatremia, and respiratory and neurological issues such as epilepsy (see National Institute of Neurological Disorders).

Causes of HPE remains undetermined, though important family members have genetic counselling. Often it seems no specific cause or may involve mutations in the gene encoding of the SHH protein which is involved with the development of the central nervous system (Wallis & Muenke 2000).

Question 2. What is Infantile Onset Pompe Disease (IOPD) and how is this diagnosed?

Pompe disease, first identified in 1932, has a variable and different progression and onset age. This multi-systemic hereditary disease is rare. Early onset after birth within 12 weeks is usually characterised with cardiac issues, which is due to heart enlargement and generalised muscle weakness. Life expectancy is very limited if untreated (within first two years of life).

This disease has been classified as Infantile Pompe, is inherited in an autosomal recessive genetic pattern, which means that healthy parents can have an affected child. Pompe disease is also known as Acid alpha glucosidase GGA, deficiency glycogen storage disease (GSD 11) see NORD (National Organization for Rare Diseases) link video/pompe-disease.

This multifaceted disease is one of the 15 known glycogen storage disorders (GSD) where there is abnormality in glycogen synthesis and glycogen breakdown. In 2006, enzyme replacement therapy (ERT) became an approved treatment (Bay et al. 2019).

Treatment of this disease is symptomatic and supportive. A team approach is needed such as cardiology, endocrine, respiratory, neurology, nursing, and allied Health Professionals such as Occupational Therapist, Speech and Language Therapist, and Physiotherapist.

Question 3. (a) Why may a child with Pompe Disease or Holorosencephaly have difficulty breathing?

Activity of living: breathing.

Infants and children with a life-limited condition such as Leo with Pompe Disease or Penny with Holorosencephaly, will have symptoms that are difficult for their families and health professionals to manage. Leo and Penny can have difficulty with their breathing especially when there are feeding difficulties. Two main functions of the respiratory system are:

- To provide a large area for gas exchange between air and circulating blood.
- To move air to and from gas-exchange surfaces of the lungs.

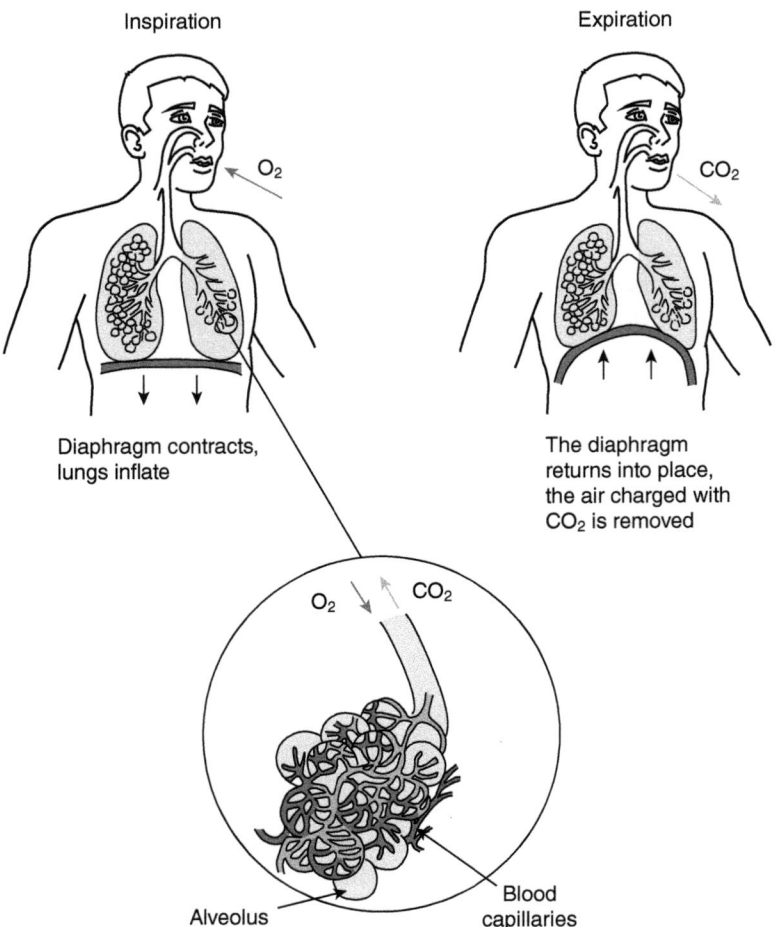

FIGURE 36.1 Gas exchange within the lungs (Reproduced with kind permission of Philips Respironics). (prev ed 35.2).

The two lungs are different: the right has three lobes and the left has two lobes, while the diaphragm acts as the floor of the thoracic cavity. When breathing, the respiratory muscles contract and the air inhaled passes through the upper airways, nose, trachea, and bronchus to alveoli in the lungs, where gas exchange takes place (see Figure 36.1) – carbon dioxide (CO_2) is eliminated and replaced with oxygen (O_2).

Bronchus obstruction and muscle (intercostal and accessory) weakness are the two main causes of breathing difficulties in these patients, affecting the respiratory system. Regarding bronchus obstruction – carbon dioxide stays within the alveoli causing breathlessness and frequent coughing (Respironics 2008).

Question 3. (b) Explain non-invasive ventilation.

Activity of living: breathing (Roper et al. 1996).
Non-invasive ventilation is the term used to describe how a ventilator delivers air to the person's lungs under pressure. The ventilator assists in keeping the small airways and air sacs inflated in the lungs. When the person breathes in the airflow is strongest, so that as much air as possible is taken in. When the person breathes out the airflow is reduced but the pressure remains positive. This is known as bi-level positive airway pressure (BiPAP) and is prescribed by a doctor to help keep the airways open, allowing more air to enter and leave the lungs (GOSH 2017). This type of ventilation assists the person when breathing, working with them and not against. The 'non-invasive' term means that the ventilation process is achieved using a mask. The mask can either fit over both mouth and nose or just the nose. Non-invasive ventilation reduces the effort of breathing and enables the child's respiratory requirements to be maintained.

In summary, non-invasive ventilation therapy can improve lung function, increase oxygen intake, on expiration ensures more efficient flushing out of carbon dioxide, improve overall wellbeing and can reduce hospital readmissions.

Question 3. (c) Explain the use of a BiPAP machine in the home.

Activity of living: Maintaining a safe environment (Roper et al. 1996). As with all medical devices, equipment should be handled with care and damp dusted weekly. Do not store equipment on the floor, and unplug prior to cleaning (see Figure 36.2). A BiPAP machine should be serviced at least yearly.

Care of Mask and Headgear

Always wash the patient's face prior to putting the mask on to minimise build-up of grease from facial pores. The mask should then be cleaned daily with a damp cloth. Remove mask shell or cushion pad weekly and wash in warm soapy water, rinse in clear water and allow to air dry. The mask should be renewed yearly. Hand wash headgear every week and replace when there appears to be loss of tension, remembering not to tumble dry.

Care of Tubing

Weekly washing of connection tubing in warm soapy water is encouraged, rinsed in clear water, and allowed to air dry as recommended. The tubing should be replaced yearly or sooner if needed.

Care of Filters

The BiPAP unit has white filters: the white ultra-fine filter should be changed monthly or sooner if dirty, and the grey pollen filter must be washed weekly in warm soapy water and towel dried completely before putting back into machine.

Please adhere to manufacturer guidelines and community trust policies.

Question 4. Discuss the importance of communication by healthcare professionals when caring for children and young people with a life-limiting condition, in the community setting.

Activity of living: communication (Roper et al. 1996).

Effective communication is an essential professional competency that is developed over time. For parents to receive the news that their son or daughter may have a life-limiting condition must be a real nightmare. A life-threatened diagnosis can create a mix of emotions, such as confusion, anger, and frustration. Indeed, the worry and fear must be overwhelming; therefore, the family living with the consequences of such news need to know that cohesive supportive services are in place which will enable them as a family to 'live' a life that is as full and complete as possible. Ensuring the choice and opportunity of being cared for at home surrounded by loved ones is important within a multidisciplinary family-centred approach to their individual care needs (Casey 1995). Well-established multidisciplinary team-working was seen as instrumental in the smooth transition of moving children, with complex needs, from hospital to home (RCN 2011).

(a)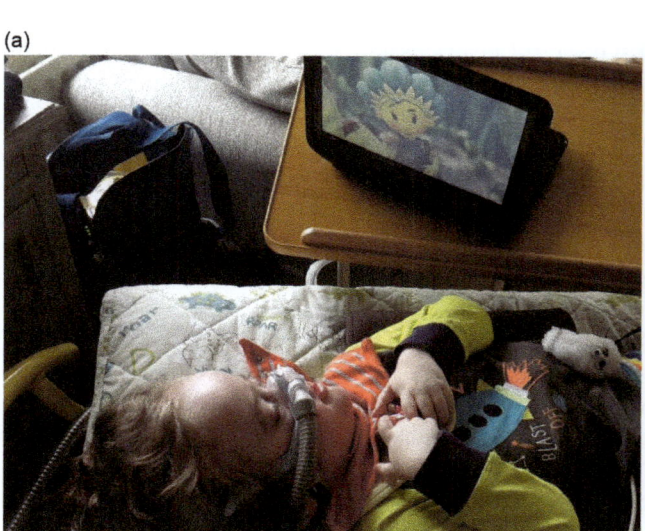

(b)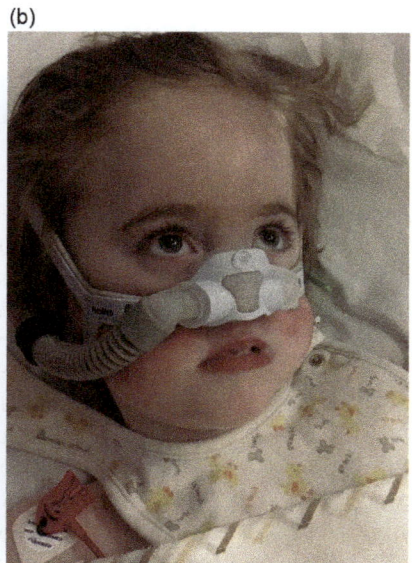

FIGURE 36.2 a and b Leo attached to his BiPAP machine (Reproduced with kind parental permission).

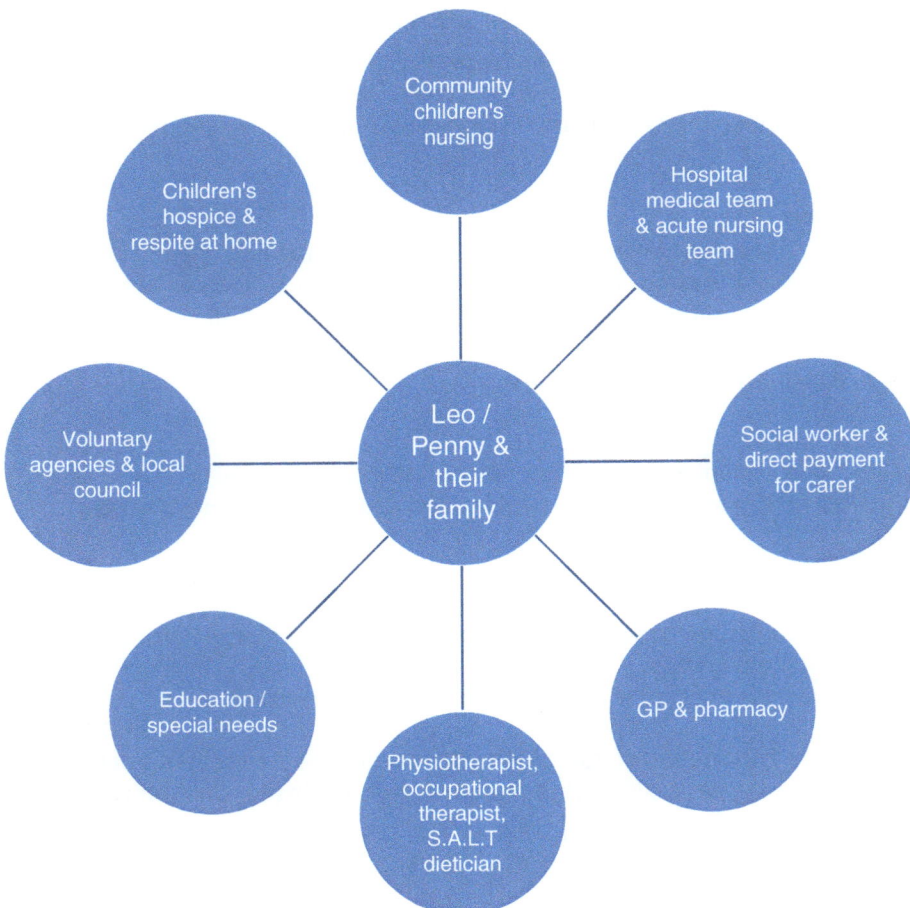

FIGURE 36.3   Demonstrating those involved in multidisciplinary team working.

Furthermore, parents and extended family should be able to concentrate on their needs and comfort, confident that the best possible care is available to them through the support of an experienced multidisciplinary team (see Figure 36.3). Young people and their parents are often frustrated when local healthcare organisations fail to share relevant information appropriately, particularly when a nursing care package is between children to adult services. Healthcare professionals need to be actively involved with parents and carers in order to avoid a lack of co-ordination within the complexity of services. Parents may be the most powerful advocates for their young people, but they may need to strengthen their voice at times and have the opportunity to speak of their experiences and needs (DH 2010).

The preferred location of caring for Penny and Leo with their life-limiting condition is the family home, with her parents receiving adequate professional support. The ultimate aim is to ensure that both Penny, Leo, and their families can establish a trusting relationship with healthcare workers, despite the intrusion of technology and equipment they should not experience a lack of privacy in their home. Family Nursing is a clinical competence linking theory to practice and should benefit all involved (Gutierrez-Aleman et al. 2021). The families of those affected by life-limiting conditions may experience financial hardship, so healthcare professionals should ensure these families do not feel isolated or abandoned in hour of need.

All parents who take on the responsibility of providing complex care in their home need to feel competent, confident, and well supported, as the availability of respite care can be limited (Corkin et al. 2006). For parents to remain the principle carers, they may have to learn complex nursing skills in order to assume 24-hour responsibility (Corkin & Chambers 2007). Community children's nursing services need to be gradually transformed and local services developed in order to support care packages in the home (DH, 2011).

Question 5. Using the Roper, Logan, & Tierney model in practice devise a care plan for Penny addressing the importance of Touch and Mouth care.

Activities of living: Maintaining a safe environment; Communication.

Prior to devising a care plan to address Penny's needs, it is important to identify what issues should be considered in relation to 'affective touch' (see Figure 36.4):

- Lifespan
- Dependence
- Factors affecting personal cleansing and dressing Roper et al. (1996)

Well known that 'affective touch' is crucial for a healthy physical and psychological development from birth to death, a key component in developing secure attachment (Bremner & Spence 2017). Although touch is the largest sense organ in the body, it has been the most neglected and recently researched (Field 2014). For example, foot and hand massage therapies could facilitate better comfort and health for Penny.

All individuals must be cared for 'holistically'; therefore, the activities of living such as Breathing; Eating and Drinking can be an issue, depending on the health problem of the individual.

Oral care for Penny could be affected by the following: lifespan and dependence. Factors can be further divided into:

- Psychological
- Socio-cultural
- Environmental

Roper et al. (1996)

The completion of oral care for patients is one of the most important nursing interventions. Oral mucositis and tooth decay could have a detrimental effect on Penny's wellbeing, including infection, pain, poor nutrition, and treatment delays. Oral care is a fundamental aspect in nursing care, and it

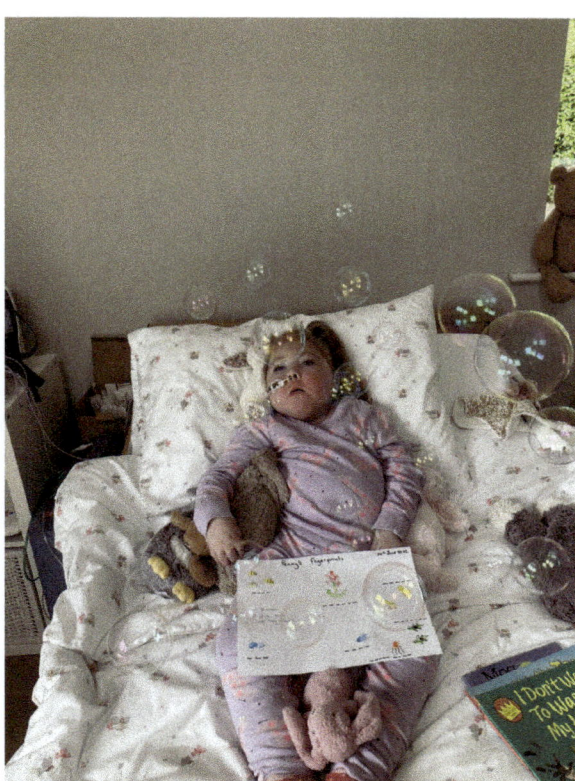

FIGURE 36.4 Penny (Reproduced with kind parental permission).

is essential that mouth care be carried out effectively, according to Morley and Lotto (2019). Children's nurses have a duty and a challenge to prevent and reduce any side effects through the appropriate oral care regimes and assessment. Literature however has demonstrated that nurses can lack this knowledge surrounding oral mucositis, its assessment, and its treatment (Costello & Coyne 2008).

Participation of Children and Young People

The views of children and their families are important, for use in the planning, delivery, and review of services (NICCY 2006). Children and young people have a right to participate in their care planning and healthcare professionals have a responsibility to facilitate this. Participation in decisions that affect children as individuals requires a child-centred approach with continuous dialogue, especially around good assessment, which is the foundation of effective care planning. A young person's perspective is crucial when assessing their needs, wishes, and feelings. Care planning requires the involvement, participation, and contribution of everyone involved in the child's life, including the child and his or her parents and should be based on a holistic assessment of the child's needs.

Based on professional experience, the authors feel it is important to note that when a parent wants to talk about a problem, they do not always want us as healthcare professionals to fix it – they may just want us to actively 'listen' and demonstrate we care. Important to make caring visible, valued, and supported. Community children's nursing has developed considerably in recent years and the future looks set for further changes and developments, driven not only by a modernising workforce but also by professional and economic factors.

Although the nursing profession has played and will continue to play a vital role in the COVID-19 response, responding to this ongoing pandemic has often required rapid changes, risk management and prioritisation, in order to meet demands, whilst ensuring the care we provide continues to be of the highest quality and standard (Southhall et al. 2020).

Indeed, the parents of these children and young people have reported that isolation and lack of contact from healthcare professionals has been one of their biggest fears throughout this unprecedented time. Experiences and excellence in community care need to be valued, celebrated, and shared, focusing on the identification, assessment, and management of these life-limited children and young people.

Colleagues, remember to tell parents, children, and young people what they are doing right, as it will help them feel valued and strengthen partnership. Every child's life is a special gift – as parents we evolve, learn, and change as our children teach us so much more than we will ever teach them.

REFERENCES

GOSH NHS Foundation Trust March (2017) Bilevel positive airway pressure (BPAP) non-invasive ventilation https://www.gosh.nhs.uk/conditions-and-treatments/procedures-and-treatments/bilevel-positive-airway-pressure-bpap-non-invasive-ventilation (accessed 6 March 2023).

Bay, L.B., Denzler, I., Durand, C. et al (2019) Infantile-onset Pompe disease: diagnosis and management. *Archivos Argentinos de Pediatria*, **117**(4), 271–278.

Bremner, A.J. & Spence, C. (2017) The development of tactile perception. *Advancement in Child Development and Behavior*, **52**, 227–268.

Carter, B., Bray, L., Sanders, C. & Van Miert, C. (2016) 'Knowing the places of care', How nurses facilitate transition of children with complex healthcare needs from hospital to home. (accessed 6 March 2023) *Comprehensive Child & Adolescent Nursing*, **39**(2), 139–153.

Casey, A. (1995) Partnership nursing: influences on involvement of informal carers. *Journal of Advanced Nursing*, **22**, 1058–1062.

Corkin, D. & Chambers, J. (2007) Community children's nursing in Northern Ireland. *Paediatric Nursing*, **19**(1), 25–27.

Corkin, D.A.P., Price, J. & Gillespie, E. (2006) Respite care for children, young people and families – are their needs addressed? *International Journal of Palliative Nursing*, **12**(9), 422–427.

Costello, T. & Coyne, I. (2008) Nurses' knowledge of mouth care practices. *British Journal of Nursing*, **17**(4), 264–268.

Department of Health (2010) *Achieving Equity and Excellence for Children*. London: DH.

Department of Health (2011) *NHS at Home: community Children's Nursing Services*. www.dh.gov.uk/publications

Field, T.M. (2014) *Touch in Early Development*. London: Psychology Press.

Gutierrez-Aleman, T., Esandi, N., Pardavila-Belio, M. et al (2021) Effectiveness of educational programs for clinical competence in family nursing: a systematic review. *Journal of Family Nursing*, **27**(4), 255–274.

Morley, H.P. & Lotto, R.R. (2019) An exploration of student nurses' views of oral health care in the hospitalised child: a qualitative study. *Nurse Education in Practice*, **38**, 79–83.

NICCY (Northern Ireland Commissioner for Children & Young People) (2006) *A Northern Ireland Based Review of Children and Young People's Participation in the Care Planning Process*. Belfast: NICCY.

Philips Respironics (2008) *My BiPAP Ventilator, My Helpful Guide*. Chichester: Philips Respironics.

Roper, N., Logan, W. & Tierney, A. (1996) *The Elements of Nursing*, 4th edition. London: Churchill Livingstone.

Royal College of Nursing (2011) *Healthcare Service Standards in Caring for Neonates, Children and Young People*. London: RCN. www.rcn.org.uk/direct (accessed 6 March 2023).

Southhall, S., Taske, N., Power, E. et al (2020) Spotlight on COVID-19 rapid guidance: NICE's experience of producing rapid guidelines during the pandemic. *Journal of Public Health*, **43**(1), e103–e106.

Wallis, D. & Muenke, M. (2000) Mutations in holoproscencephaly. *Human Mutations*, **16**(2), 99–108.

Zantow, E., Bryant, S., Pierce, S.L. et al (2021) Prenatal diagnosis of middle interhemispheric variant of holoprosencephaly: report of two cases. *Journal Clinical Ultrasound*, **49**, 765–769.

CHAPTER 37

Sickle Cell Disease

Debbie Omodele, Danielle Edge, and Doreen Crawford

SCENARIO

Anita is a 15-year-old girl with sickle cell disease (SCD) who was brought to Accident & Emergency (A&E) with pain in her chest, radiating to her abdomen. She also presented with slight yellowing of her eyes, fever, and a slight cough. Mum reported that Anita was caught in heavy rain two days ago on her way back from school and was concerned her oral intake had reduced over the last 48 hours. On examination, she was in obvious pain and was crying. Her temperature was 38.9 degrees, she complained of a sharp pain in her abdomen particularly when breathing in. She scored her pain an 8 out of 10 and despite a dose of paracetamol an hour ago her pain did not subside. Refer to Box Activity 37.1.

ACTIVITY 37.1

1. Define what sickle cell disease (SCD) is
2. Understand genetic transmission, traits and new-born screening
3. Describe the treatment and long-term management of SCD

INTRODUCTION

Question 1. What Is Sickle Cell Disease?

This chapter will explore the care of a patient with sickle cell disease (SCD), which is the most common genetic anomaly in the UK today, affecting over 1 in every 2000 live births (De et al. 2019; SCD standards, 2019). It is an autosomal recessive disorder and causes very significant morbidity and mortality. SCD predominantly affects people with African, Caribbean, and Mediterranean ancestry, however, with the ever-growing diversity of the population and inter-racial families, it can affect people of any race and ethnicity. SCD results from the presence of a mutated form of haemoglobin, haemoglobin S (HbS). The main symptoms of sickle cell disease are anaemia and episodes of severe pain, but there are a number of other complications such as stroke, acute chest syndrome, priapism, and jaundice. SCD is a chronic long term life-limiting condition, knowledge of SCD is therefore important for the children's nurse as the disease has serious implications for the quality of life (QoL) and the life chances of children (Baker et al. 2021).

Question 2. Genetic Inheritance, Carrier, and Screening.

A comprehensive review of genetics is beyond the scope of this chapter however SCD is known as an autosomal recessive disorder which means that both copies of an affected gene must be present to cause the condition (Davies & Meimaridou 2020). People with only one defective allele in the gene are known as carriers of the sickle gene. When both parents are carriers, there is a 25% chance that a child will inherit two copies of the gene (one from each parent) and develop disease.

The chance of the child inheriting one normal and one abnormal copy of the gene, so they are also a carrier of the disease, is 50%, and the chance of them inheriting no affected copy of the gene is 25%. In both these instances, the child will not inherit the condition. Each pregnancy will have a 1 in 4 chance of the offspring having the condition (Davies & Meimaridou 2020).

All pregnant women are offered screening for SCD and other unusual haemoglobins and therefore make an informed decision to either accept or decline screening. The parents of all newborn infants born in the UK are offered screening for SCD as part of the Newborn Blood Spot Programme (2018), which identifies conditions that can affect a child's long-term health or survival. This is important because early management greatly reduces the serious symptoms the disease can cause.

Question 3. Diagnosis Treatment and Long-term Management of SCD.

Newborn screening is important as a method of early detection which triggers prompt referral into the specialist care pathway and timely follow-up allowing infants to be seen at a paediatric clinic by three months of age (Sickle Cell Disease in Childhood 2019). This allows for prophylactic treatment with antibiotics (penicillin/erythromycin) to be offered and initiated by three months of age which has shown to improve quality of life by reducing the risk of infections (Cober & Phelps 2010). Diagnosis could also be made antenatally via prenatal diagnosis (PND), which is offered to couples at risk of having a baby with a significant haemoglobinopathy or via a simple venepuncture blood test for those who have not undergone screening for whatever reason.

The hallmarks of SCD include episodes of severe pain. Pain in SCD is unpredictable and often recurrent episodes due to vaso-occulsive crises, with CYP experiencing more acute episodes than chronic pain seen in the adult population (Inusa 2016). Therefore, it is essential for children's nurses and HCP's to understand the principles of achieving effective pain management by targeting and keeping patients within the therapeutic window of prescribed analgesia, maximising its effects.

Ongoing management of CYP with SCD includes regular follow-up hospital appointments, encouraging adherence to treatment, immunisations including additional pneumococcal vaccinations from the age of 2 years old, while supporting, educating, and empowering families to become experts with managing their child's care. Other long-term preventative measures to improve quality of life include regular blood transfusion therapy for stroke prevention and hydroxycarbamide for managing frequency and severity of a sickle cell crisis (Sickle Cell Disease in Childhood 2019).

Listening to the CYP and families voice about their ongoing experience is essential to long term management of SCD. Foster and Ellis (2018) systematic review highlighted the need for support for the CYP that is collaborative across health, education, and families. Refer to Box Activity 37.2.

ACTIVITY 37.2

Further reading into genetic inheritance and screening Linked antenatal and newborn screening programme https://www.gov.uk/government/publications/handbook-for-sickle-cell-and-thalassaemia-screening/newborn-screening#linked-antenatal-and-newborn-screening-programme

Further reading into Haemoglobinopathies and management Understanding haemoglobinopathies https://www.gov.uk/government/publications/handbook-for-sickle-cell-and-thalassaemia-screening/understanding-haemoglobinopathies

---

This introduction to SCD has considered what the disease is, the genetics and population screening for SCD, and treatment and management of the long-term condition. The content within this chapter will explore the case study and focus on aspects of care planning needs and questions to consider when caring for a child presenting in a SCD crisis. Finally, we will take a look to the future and consider what new treatment research might provide and further education healthcare professionals need to deliver CYP's the best evidence-based care. Box Activity 37.3.

ACTIVITY 37.3

Questions to consider for the scenario:

1. Effective pain management is essential in care planning for children with SCD – How would you assess and manage Anita's pain?

2. Fever in a child with SCD could indicate an infection, but also be linked to their disease excacerbation – consider the use of sepsis screening tools and how these aid our recognition of a deteriorating child.

3. Maintaining adequate hydration is crucial for patients with SCD – How do we maintain good hydration and manage this for Anita's acute admission?

ANSWER TO QUESTION 1

Throughout this section the nursing process has been used to structure the care process for Anita (Yura & Walsh 1978). Threaded throughout is the consideration of the young person's voice and family-centred care (NICE 2021b).

Pain Management

Activity of living: maintaining a safe environment – pain management as per Roper, Logan, & Tierney model of care (Holland & Jenkins 2019), see Chapter 1 for further reading.

Assessment

An acute painful crisis is a medical emergency therefore, your initial assessment of Anita's pain would be to assess the location and intensity of her pain using an age-appropriate pain tool and documenting her pain score on a pain assessment chart.

Anita self-reported a pain score of 8 out of 10 and as pain is a subjective experience, self-report is preferred whenever possible (Twycross et al. 2015). According to the World Health Organisation (WHO) pain ladder (2018), her pain is classified as severe therefore, the primary goal for the children's nurse is to administer strong fast acting opioids within 30 minutes (NICE 2012). Consider analgesia already taken before her presentation and document vital signs including sedation score (AVPU) on a national PEWs chart which also allows the nurse to assess the adequacy of analgesia regularly.

Common triggers such as sudden temperature changes, infection, dehydration, and stress/over exertion are likely contributors to a child with SCD presenting in pain. The children's nurse should be aware of possible triggers including other acute complications that could present during a painful crisis for example, acute chest syndrome, as this will enable prompt identification and management.

Most painful crisis are managed at home; however, uncontrollable pain requires hospital management. Therefore, children's nurses should never underestimate pain experienced. Understanding CYP pain scores, including factors that may influence pain expression for example, past experiences is key to achieving pain control (Collins et al. 2020).

Planning

Pain management is an essential part of Anita's care and should include SMART goals and monitoring tools to ensure interventions are effective. A proactive approach should be taken therefore, children's nurses must escalate sub-therapeutic doses of analgesia prescribed, advocating for dose optimisation, to prevent further escalation of her pain. Recognition of potential side effects from opioids is key to avoiding a deterioration of Anita's health which moves away from the desired goal. The goal is to keep Anita within the 'analgesic corridor' therefore, analgesia should be administered within 30 minutes of arrival to A&E with an aim to achieve pain control within 60 minutes (regular evaluation of implementation is essential. See Figure 37.1 and Box Activity 37.4.

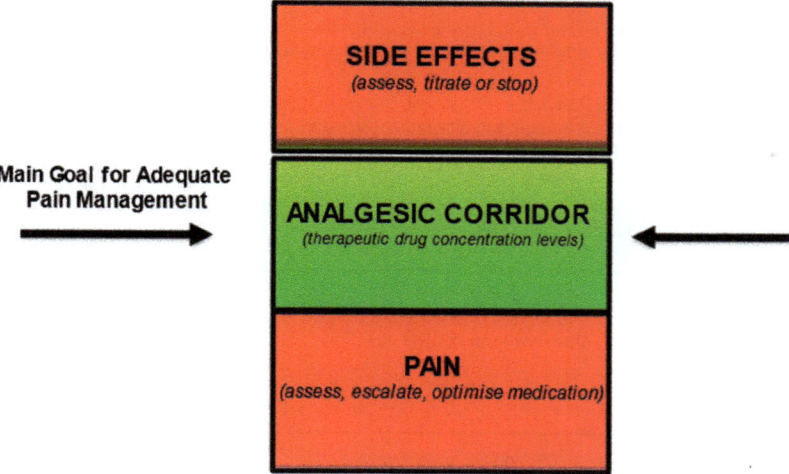

FIGURE 37.1 Analgesic corridor. Image adapted from Macintyre and Stephan (2007).

> **ACTIVITY 37.4**
>
> For further reading into recommendations for acute sickle cell pain crisis, review: NICE Introduction | Sickle cell disease: managing acute painful episodes in hospital | Guidance | NICE https://www.nice.org.uk/guidance/cg143/chapter/Introduction
> Sickle cell society standards care https://www.sicklecellsociety.org/resource/pain-management-guidelines-sickle-cell

Implementation

Managing Anita's pain within the early stages of her presentation is crucial for effective pain management and involving her in decisions made will provide a person-centered approach to her care. The use of locally agreed protocols is also key towards achieving effective and timely pain control (see example in Figure 37.2). Monitoring patients should include sedation and pain score to assess effectiveness of administered analgesia. This is especially important for CYP at risk of opioid toxicity for example, patients who are opioid naïve. It is therefore essential for nurses to have a working knowledge and understanding of specific opioid monitoring (Telfer & Kaya 2017) including mandatory observations and escalating risks promptly.

Anita's complaint of chest pain must be investigated and a high index of suspicion of acute chest syndrome (ACS) must be maintained in combination with mandatory close monitoring once adequate opioids have been administered and throughout her admission. An incentive spirometer should also be started to reduce the risk of ACS (Ahmad et al. 2011). Children's nurses should also consider a combination of non-pharmacological approaches to pain for example, the use of a Bair hugger heat pack, as this often provides additional relief. Supplementary medication such as oral analgesia (paracetamol and ibuprofen), antihistamines and lactulose should also be included in Anita's care and management.

Evaluation

A reassessment of Anita's vital signs and pain score should be repeated frequently, listening to her assessment of how effective the last intervention was. Ineffective pain control should be promptly escalated to both the medical and pain team who may recommend an opioid patient-controlled analgesia (PCA). This is especially important within the first few hours of presentation/admission.

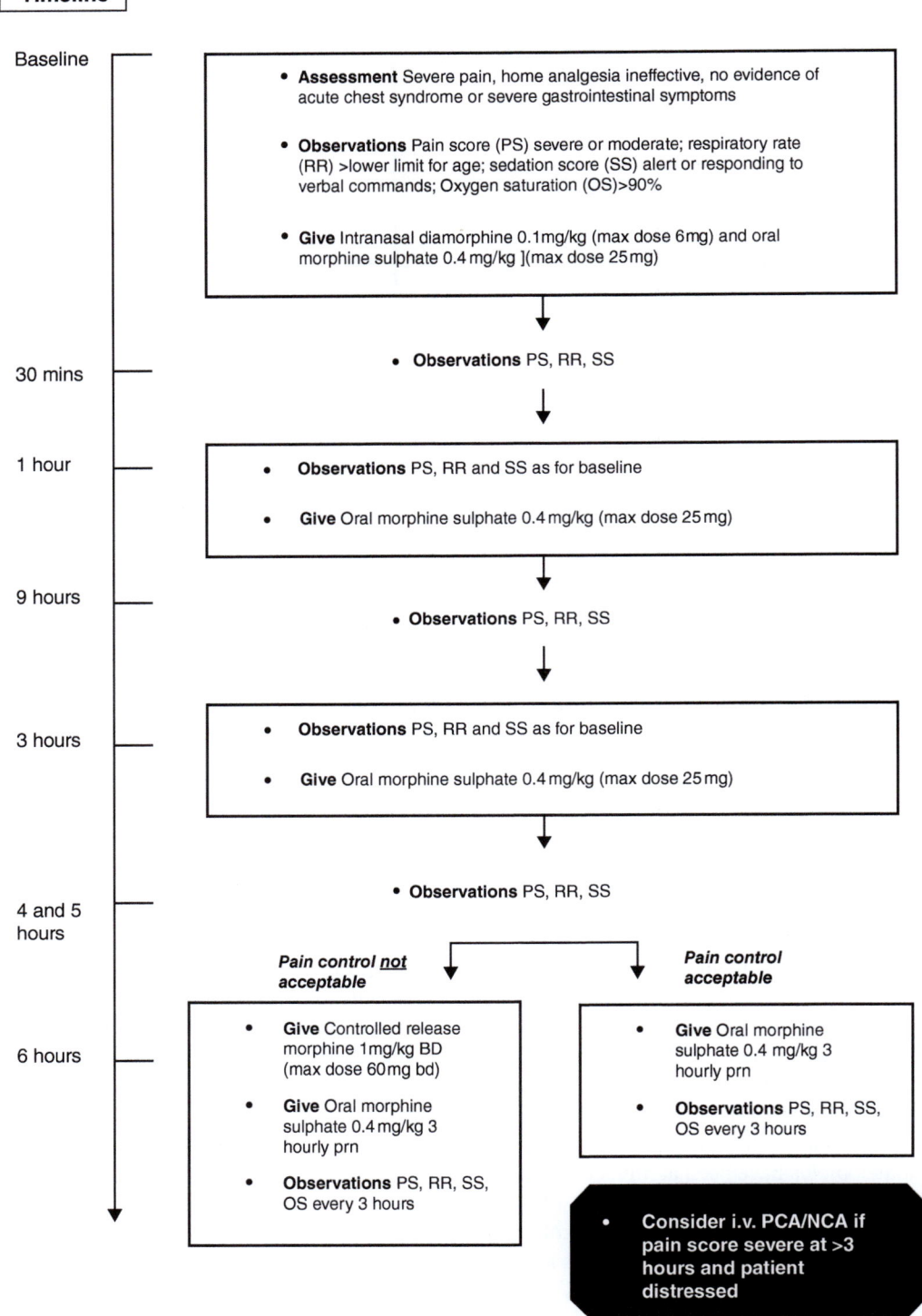

FIGURE 37.2 Sickle Cell Disease Timeline. Image adapted from Telfer et al. (2014).

FEVER

ANSWER TO QUESTION 2

Exploring Anita's fever would be a key part of planning her care. When aligning to activities of daily living model: controlling temperature as per Roper, Logan, &Tierney model of care can be used (Holland & Jenkins 2019). When considering a fever of 38.9 in any child, we should think sepsis and more so for a child with SCD. Children with SCD are at increased risk of infections partly due to hyposplenism (SCD standards 2021). With infection being the most common cause of death resulting from sickle cell disease (McCance & Huether 2019). However, a child presenting with a pain crisis may have a fever and no obvious signs of infection, it may be difficult to differentiate between acute bone infarction due to sickling (SCD standards 2021).

When undertaking the initial assessment considering history of presentation, observations and if there are any signs of infection are important to attempt to establish the cause of the fever to act appropriately. The use of a sepsis screening tool will aid decision making and selecting the correct tool for the age of the patient. Refer to Box Activity 37.5.

ACTIVITY 37.5

Review the sepsis screening tools used to aid our assessment and treatment of a child, what changes if any would be needed when caring for a child with SCD?
   Home–Sepsis Trust https://sepsistrust.org/
   Recommendations | Sepsis: recognition, diagnosis and early management | Guidance | NICE https://www.nice.org.uk/guidance/ng51/chapter/Recommendations

Following the sepsis guidelines can help aid quick and responsive treatment of sepsis, with the sepsis trust highlighting the gaining of intravenous access, taking bloods including cultures, administering intravenous antibiotics (IVAB), fluid bolus, and senior clinician review (NICE 2017). It is important that all children with SCD continue to have their prophylactic penicillin, unless another antibiotic is given to treat an infection (NICE, 2021a).

HYDRATION

ANSWER TO QUESTION 3

Activity of living model: see eating and drinking as per Roper, Logan, & Tierney model of care (Holland & Jenkins 2019). Dehydration can prolong painful episodes, therefore ensuring adequate hydration for Anita is an important aspect of her care plan. Unless there is obvious clinical and laboratorial evidence of dehydration associated with the vaso-occlusive episode, then hyper hydration may need to be prescribed (Sickle Cell Disease in Childhood 2019). Anita presented with yellowing of her eyes, signs of jaundice. Hydration encourages good blood flow and although jaundice occurs due to a breakdown in red blood cells, hydration helps the liver and kidneys flush out toxins (McCance & Huether 2019). The management for Anita should consist of:

- IV access and fluids should be commenced at maintenance rates
- A fluid chart should be commenced with both input and output
- Fluid balance should be calculated at least 12 hourly to correct dehydration and avoid overload
- Continue to encourage good oral intake.

Looking Forward to the Future

This chapter has addressed the care of newborns, children, and young people with sickle cell disease and acute presentations of their disease. Now we must look to the future of HCP's understanding of SCD and caring for CYP's and their families. The sickle cell societies inquiry 'No one's listening' (2021), highlighted substandard care and avoidable deaths of patients living with SCD. Raising concerns around health inequalities and access to care, this report made a number of recommendations that have led to a review of the care sickle cell patients receive and the education of HCP's (The sickle cell society, 2021). Your role as a children's nursing student and registered children's nurse is to ensure you can deliver safe and effective care for CYP's with SCD. To do that healthcare staff need appropriate training and education, HEE have recently launched a campaign to raise HCP's awareness of the disease and e-learning (HEE elfh Hub (e-lfh.org.uk)).

Treatment options often take a therapeutic approach such as a regular blood transfusion regime, however this is not always effective. Hydroxycarbamide is an approved oral drug that modifies the clinical severity of SCD, by reducing the frequency and severity of a sickle cell crisis and disease complications (Nevitt et al. 2017). Hydroxycarbamide remains the best option for disease modification and currently the only drug approved for children with SCD from as young as 12 months (Wang et al. 2011, Baby HUG trial). As a result, CYP will have reduced hospital admissions, improved educational achievement and a better QoL (Adesanya et al. 2021). However, other treatment alternatives exist, Crizanlizumab was recently approved in 2021 for patients 16 years and over, and has been suggested to significantly reduce the frequency of a sickle cell crisis (NICE 2021a). Data is being collected to assess its long-term effectiveness.

Options that offer prospects of a cure include a bone marrow transplant which involves replacing abnormal stem cells with HLA typed donor cells and only performed when benefits outweigh risks (Ashorobi & Bhatt 2022). If successful, the patient is cured from the symptoms however, the genotype remains; carrying a risk of passing the gene down to offspring. Gene therapy on the other hand aims to replace a defective gene with a normal one correcting the abnormal sickle gene (Olowoyeye & Okwundu 2020).

At 15 years old, transition into adult services should be discussed as part of Anita's care plan for the future. Transition is a supportive process that aims to gradually prepare teenagers for the transfer of care from children to adult services (Badawy 2022). This enables the development of independence with managing their health, empowering them to build self-advocacy and self-efficacy skills. Taking a multi-disciplinary and integrated family approach reduces the risk of teenagers and their families' disengaging from essential services (NICE 2016) and promotes an effective smooth and seamless transition. Refer to Box Activity 37.6.

ACTIVITY 37.6

Reflect on all you have read within this chapter and the impact sickle cell disease has on children, young people, and their family on everyday life:

- Consider how as part of our role as children's nurses we can support CYP to ensure that their disease does not interrupt their education and socialisation.

- How can you ensure the CYP's voice is heard within their care?

Actively listening to the CYP's voice about their ongoing care of SCD is crucial, as the immense pain that children experience can negatively affect their quality of life. Being aware of the impact their disease has on all aspects of their life, such as schooling, missing education, and psychosocial is important.

REFERENCES

Adesanya, O., Stockley, C., Anuruegbe, O. & Koodiyedath, B. (2021) Hydroxycarbamide therapy amongst children with homozygous sickle cell disease in large district general hospital – a quality improvement project. https://adc.bmj.com/content/archdischild/106/Suppl_1/A352.1.full.pdf

Ahmad, F.A., Macias, C.G. & Allen, J.Y. (2011) The use of incentive spirometry in pediatric patients with sickle cell disease to reduce the incidence of acute chest syndrome. *Journal of Pediatric Hematology/Oncology*, 33(6), 415–420.

Ashorobi, D. & Bhatt, R. (2022). Bone Marrow Transplantation in Sickle Cell Disease. https://www.ncbi.nlm.nih.gov/books/NBK538515

Badawy, S.M. (2022) Empowering children and adolescents with sickle cell disease: a transition journey to adult care. *Lancet Haematol*, **9**(8), e562.

Baker, E., Crawford, D. & Davis, K. (2021) Biological basis of child health 10: function and formation of blood and common blood disorders in children. *Nursing Children and Young People* **12**, e1278.

Cober, M.P. & Phelps, S.J. (2010) Penicillin prophylaxis in children with sickle cell disease. *Journal of Pediatric Pharmacology and Therapeutics*, **15**(3), 152–159.

Collins, P.J., Renedo, A. & Marston, C.A. (2020) Communicating and understanding pain: limitations of pain scales for patients with sickle cell disorder and other painful conditions. *Journal of Health Psychology*, **27**(1), 103–118.

Davies, K. & Meimaridou, E. (2020) Biological basis of child health 1: understanding the cell and genetics. *Nursing Children and Young People*, **32**(3), 33–43.

De, D., Blackmore, A. & Taylor, H. (2019) Enhancing the care of patients with sickle cell disease. *Nursing Standard*, **34**(10), 29–34.

Foster, N. & Ellis, M. (2018) Sickle cell anaemia and the experiences of young people living with the condition. *Nursing Children and Young People*, **30**(3), 36–43.

Holland, K. & Jenkins, J. (2019) *Applying the Roper-Logan-Tierney Model in Practice*, 3rd edition. Elsevier.

Inusa, B. (2016) Sickle Cell Disease - Pain and Common Chronic Complications, IntechOpen, London. 10.5772/62012.

Macintyre, P.E. & Stephan, A. (2007) *Schug Acute Pain Management: A Practical Guide*, 5th edition. Elsevier Health Sciences.

McCance, K.L. & Huether, S.E. (2019) *Pathophysiology: The Biologic Basis for Disease in Adults and Children*, 8th edition. Amsterdam: Elsevier.

Nevitt, S.J., Jones, A.P. & Howard, J. (2017) Hydroxyurea (hydroxycarbamide) for sickle cell disease. *Cochrane Database of Systematic Reviews*, **4**(4), 20.

NICE (2012) Sickle cell disease: managing acute painful episodes in hospital. Available: Overview | Sickle cell disease: managing acute painful episodes in hospital | Guidance | NICE

NICE (2016) Transition from children's to adults' services for young people using health or social care services NICE guideline NG43, recommendation 1.2.1.

NICE (2017) Sepsis: recognition, diagnosis and early management. Overview | Sepsis: recognition, diagnosis and early management | Guidance | NICE.

NICE (2021a) Crizanlizumab for preventing sickle cell crises in sickle cell disease https://www.nice.org.uk/guidance/ta743.

NICE (2021b) Overview | babies, children and young people's experience of healthcare | guidance | NICE https://www.nice.org.uk/guidance/ng204/chapter/Recommendations [Accessed 6 March 2023].

Olowoyeye, A. & Okwundu, C.I. (2020) Gene therapy for sickle cell disease. Cochrane Database of Systematic Reviews, Issue 11. https://www.cochranelibrary.com/cdsr/doi/10.1002/14651858.CD007652.pub7/full#CD007652-abs-0002 [Accessed 6 March 2023].

Sickle Cell Disease in Childhood (2021) Standards and Recommendations for Clinical Care. https://www.sicklecellsociety.org/paediatricstandards [Accessed 6 March 2023]

Sickle Cell Society (2021) https://www.sicklecellsociety.org/about-sickle-cell

Telfer, P., Bahal, N., Lo, A. & Challands, J. (2014) Management of the acute painful crisis in sickle cell disease: a re-evaluation of the use of opioids in adult patients. *British Journal of Haematology*, **166**(2), 157–164.

Telfer, P. & Kaya, B. (2017) Optimizing the care model for an uncomplicated acute pain episode in sickle cell disease. *Hematology American Society of Hematol Education Program*, **2017**(1), 525–533.

Twycross, A., Voepel-Lewis, T., Vincent, C., Franck, L.S. & von Baeyer, C.L. (2015) A debate on the proposition that self-report is the gold standard in assessment of pediatric pain intensity. *Clinical Journal of Pain*, **31**(8), 707–712.

Wang, W.C., Ware, R.E., Miller, S.T., Iyer, R.V., Casella, J.F., Minniti, C.P., Rana, S., Thornburg, C.D., Rogers, Z.R., Kalpatthi, R.V., Barredo, J.C., Brown, R.C., Sarnaik, S.A., Howard, T.H., Wynn, L.W., Kutlar, A., Armstrong, F.D., Files, B.A., Goldsmith, J.C., Waclawiw, M.A., Huang, X. & Thompson, B.W. (2011) BABY HUG investigators. Hydroxycarbamide in very young children with sickle-cell anaemia: a multicentre, randomised, controlled trial. *Lancet*, **14,377**(9778), 1663–1672. https://pubmed.ncbi.nlm.nih.gov/21571150.

World Health Organization (2018) *WHO Guidelines for the Pharmacological and Radiotherapeutic Management of Cancer Pain in Adults and Adolescents*. Geneva: WHO.

Yura, D. & Walsh, M.B. (1978) *The Nursing Process: Assessing, Planning, Implementing and Evaluating*. New York: Appleton Century Crofts.

Hydroxyurea treatment is transforming the lives of children with sickle cell disease in the Liverpool area. https://www.sicklecellsociety.org/hydroxyurea-treatment-transforming-lives-children-sickle-cell-disease-liverpool-area

The Sepsis trust UK (2020) Sepsis screening tool acute assessment. Available: Sepsis-Acute-12–1.3.pdf (sepsistrust.org)

RESOURCES

CHAPTER 38

Transition from Children's to Adults' Services

Claire Kerr

Adequate planning and smooth transition of healthcare services for children and young people approaching adulthood are important, particularly for those with long-term conditions. All young people experience challenges during the teenage years, such as physical and psychological changes, education, employment and living arrangement options, increased personal responsibility, and a move towards adulthood. Young people with long-term health conditions may also be taking increased responsibility for their own healthcare, typically against a backdrop of changes in service provision and provider(s). This chapter addresses young people's transition from children's to adults' healthcare services and focuses on transition for children and young people with cerebral palsy as an exemplar condition.

DEFINITIONS

A generic definition of transition is 'the process or a period of changing from one state or condition to another' (Oxford Learner's Dictionaries 2022). Some examples of transition in healthcare services for children and young people (and their families) include:

- from a neonatal unit to a ward setting;
- from a ward to home, possibly with the support of community-based and/or specialist services;
- from intensive care to the ward;
- from hospital to hospital;
- from hospital/home to a palliative setting;
- Transferring between specialist teams, for example between neuro-disability, genetics and endocrine services.

However, within children and young persons' healthcare, transition most commonly refers to the transfer of services from paediatric teams to adults' services. Transition, in this context, has been defined as 'the purposeful, planned movement of adolescents and young adults with chronic physical and medical conditions from child-centred to adult-oriented healthcare systems' (Campbell et al. 2016). Further, the National Institute for Health and Care Excellence (NICE) define transition as 'the process of moving from children's to adults' services. It refers to the full process including initial planning, the actual transfer between services, and support throughout' (NICE 2016).

Cerebral palsy is an umbrella term for a group of lifelong disorders of movement and posture. Defined as 'a group of permanent disorders of the development of movement and posture, causing activity limitation that are attributed to non-progressive disturbances that occurred in the developing foetal or infant brain. The motor disorders of cerebral palsy are often accompanied by disturbances of sensation, perception, cognition, communication, and behaviour, by epilepsy, and by secondary musculoskeletal problems.' (Rosenbaum et al. 2007). It is the commonest cause of physical disability in childhood, affecting approximately one in 500 children in high-income countries (McIntyre et al. 2022). Survival of people with severe cerebral palsy has improved in recent decades (Blair et al. 2019). The Northern Ireland Cerebral Palsy Register (NICPR) recently reported that over 90% of people with cerebral palsy survive into adulthood (McConnell et al. 2021). This means that most children with cerebral palsy will require transition planning and, for some young people with severe cerebral palsy, co-ordination of many different healthcare specialities will be required during the transition process.

Care Planning in Children and Young People's Nursing, Second Edition. Edited by Sonya Clarke and Doris Corkin.
© 2024 John Wiley & Sons Ltd. Published 2024 by John Wiley & Sons Ltd.

Despite agreed principles in relation to what constitutes good transitional care, there remain challenges in implementation within practice. A sudden move to adults' services, with no time for preparation or support, can lead to children and young people and families losing confidence and disengaging with services (Watson et al. 2011). Lack of information about the transition process and future adult services is a known barrier to successful transition (Freeman et al. 2018). An important report from the Care Quality Commission (CQC 2014) on transition to adult services for young people with complex physical health needs noted that 'young people and families are often confused, and at times distressed by the lack of information, support and services available to meet their complex health needs.' Refer to Box Activity 38.1.

> **ACTIVITY 38.1**
>
> Read the summary of the Care Quality Commission's 2014 report, 'From the pond to sea' Available at: https://www.cqc.org.uk/sites/default/files/CQC_Transition%20Report_Summary_lores.pdf

For young people with cerebral palsy, who may have complex healthcare needs, difficulties with transition are possible due to the range of services required and the co-ordination of these. Indeed, these difficulties 'are compounded' by differences in the funding and organisation of child and adult services. For example, in the UK and Ireland, care co-ordination in childhood is typically managed by a paediatrician (Solanke et al. 2018), but after discharge from children's services, young people rely increasingly on general practitioners (GPs) (National Confidential Enquiry into Patient Outcome and Death [NCEPOD] 2018; Tuffrey & Pearce 2003). However, in a recent study in Ireland, only 10% of young people with cerebral palsy reported that their GP had received a discharge letter about them (Ryan et al. 2022). The limited involvement of GPs in transition planning (Colver et al. 2020) and limited training of adult healthcare professionals in conditions with childhood onset, such as cerebral palsy, are known barriers to successful transition (Kolehmainen et al. 2017; Tuffrey & Pearce 2003). Transition from child to adult health services for young people with cerebral palsy has been shown to coincide with a decrease in visits to specialist and coordinated services, difficulties accessing clinical care (Roquet et al. 2018) and an increase in unmet health needs (Solanke et al. 2018).

In addition to these significant issues with the healthcare system and staff training, problems with transition may also exist in relation to the paediatric team, the young person and the family/carers (Tuffrey & Pearce 2003). For example, paediatricians may be reluctant to move young people on to adult services, especially if they believe those services to be lesser than the care the young person has received to date. The young person may feel 'abandoned' by their paediatric team, who they may have known for most of their life and will require time to navigate and build rapport and trust with a new team/teams in adult services (Bagatell et al. 2017; NCEPOD, 2018). Indeed, some parents may perceive a 'loss of control' as the young person enters adulthood and assumes increasing autonomy over their healthcare (Tuffrey & Pearce 2003), although interestingly, Ryan et al. (2022) reported that the majority of both young people (90%) and parents (81%) agreed that they were involved at an appropriate level in the young person's care.

Many young people with cerebral palsy do not experience practices that are thought to improve the experience and outcomes of transition (Ryan et al. 2022) despite clear recommendations from substantive programmes of research (Colver et al. 2020) and robust systematic review evidence (Campbell et al. 2016). Further, significant reports highlight:

- Issues with transition for young people with neuro-disabling conditions (Care Quality Commission [CQC] 2014; The National Confidential Enquiry into Patient Outcome and Death 2018).

- Recognition of the need to promote better transitional healthcare and provide training in transitional healthcare (Gleeson 2018; Royal College of Paediatrics and Child Health 2018; Royal College of Physicians 2015).

These reports and publication of UK transition guidelines by the National Institute of Health and Care Excellence in 2016 suggests that improving the experience and outcomes of transition should be a priority for everyone working with children, young adults, and their families. Refer to Box Activity 38.2.

ACTIVITY 38.2

Identify 1–2 issues that 'may be encountered' during transition by each of the following groups:

- The paediatric healthcare team
- The adult healthcare team
- The young person
- The young person's parents/carers

TRANSITION GUIDELINES

Early planning for the transfer from children's to adults' services can lead to a better experience of transition for children and young people by allowing a more gradual process, in which children and young people have more time to be involved in decisions and more time to adjust to changes in their future care.

In 2016 NICE published guidelines on transition from children's to adults' services for young people. These guidelines are important as they apply across the full spectrum of health and social care, from service users to commissioners of services, developed following a rigorous evidence review and consideration by experts, including people with lived experience. The recommendations in the NICE guidelines on transition from children's to adults' services for young people using health or social care services are structured under five key areas (NICE, 2016). These are summarised in the following sections to provide a comprehensive overview of how healthcare professionals, including nurses, can support young people's experiences of transition.

OVERARCHING PRINCIPLES OF TRANSITION

The overarching principles of transition put the young person and their carer's at the heart of the process, aligning with the principles of person and family centred care that prevail in paediatric healthcare (O'Connor et al. 2019; Uniacke et al. 2018). Children and young people, and their carer's, should be involved in transition service design, delivery and evaluation. In practical terms, this could mean that children and young people co-produce transition policies, strategies and resources in partnership with service organisations. Children and young people could also provide feedback as to whether the services they received were useful.

Overall, the transition support that is provided to children, young people, and their carers should be developmentally appropriate, strengths-based, and person-centred:

- Recent advances in neuroimaging indicate that between age 11 and 25 years, young people's brains change considerably (Colver & Longwell 2013). Developmentally appropriate transition support takes account of the biological, psychological, and social development of young people. It ensures that young people are informed about their care and are supported to actively participate in this process (Farre et al. 2015). Ongoing consideration of the young person's maturity, cognitive ability, psychological status, social and personal circumstances, communication needs, caring responsibilities, and needs in relation to their long-term condition is required (National Institute for Health and Care Excellence 2016).

- Strengths-based transition support focuses on what is positive and possible for the young person. It draws on the strengths of the young person, working with those that support them (practitioners, family members, carers, and others), to achieve the young person's preferred outcomes (National Institute for Health and Care Excellence 2016).

- Person-centred transition support treats the young person as an equal partner in the transition process. It fully involves the young person and their family or carers in the planning, implementation and review of all relevant transition outcomes, including but not limited to, health and wellbeing, education and employment, independent living and housing, and community inclusion.

In relation to overarching principles of transition, it is recommended that children's and adults' services should work together, proactively plan for transition, share safeguarding information and check the young person is registered with a GP.

TRANSITION PLANNING

There are five detailed areas in the NICE guidelines in relation to recommendations for transition planning (National Institute for Health and Care Excellence 2016). They are:

a) *Timing and review*: Transition planning should start at age 13–14 years, should be developmentally appropriate and reviewed at least annually. Transition planning meetings should involve the young person, their family/carers and all practitioners that support the young person (including the GP) and inform a transition plan (National Institute for Health and Care Excellence 2016).

b) *Named worker*: A single practitioner should take on a co-ordinating role in the young person's transition planning and support. This person could be from any healthcare background but should have a meaningful relationship with the young person. The NICE guidelines specify that the named worker will holistically support the young person and their family during transition for a minimum of six months before and after transfer and will hand over their responsibilities as named worker to someone in adult services. The named worker will ensure the young person is provided with support in relation to the aspects of transition shown in Figure 38.1.

c) *Involving young people*: Young people should be offered help, such as mentoring, coaching, advocacy, or peer support, to become involved in transition planning. A range of tools should be made available to help young people communicate effectively with practitioners.

d) *Building independence*: Information about building and maintaining social, leisure and recreational networks, including information about non-statutory services and peer support groups, should be included in transition planning. Young people with long-term conditions should be helped to manage their own condition (National Institute for Health and Care Excellence 2016).

e) *Involving parents and carers*: The young person should be regularly asked about how they would like their parents and carers to be involved during transition and when they have moved to adult services. Similarly, transition should be discussed with parents and carers to understand their expectations with adult's services by having the opportunity to raise concerns and queries separately from their parents or carers (National Institute for Health and Care Excellence 2016).

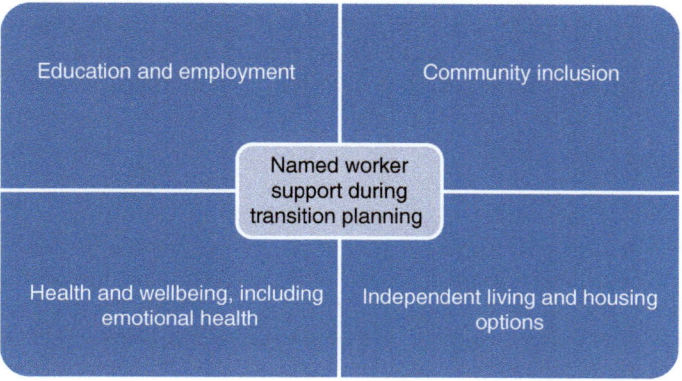

FIGURE 38.1 Aspects of transition that a named worker will offer support with during transition planning.

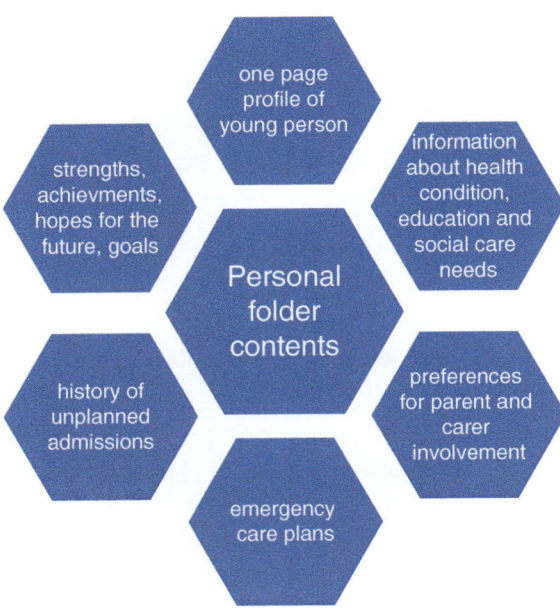

FIGURE 38.2 Information that could be included in a young person's personal folder that they share with adult services to plan transition.

SUPPORT BEFORE TRANSFER

The NICE guidelines recommend that a practitioner from the relevant adult services meets the young person before they transfer from children's services and that a contingency plan is in place if the named worker leaves their position, thus ensuring consistent transition support is available (National Institute for Health and Care Excellence 2016). Indeed children and adults' services should give young people and their families' accessible information about what to expect from services and what support is available to them. Children's services should consider working with the young person to create a personal folder that they share with adults' services. Information that could be included in the personal folder is detailed in Figure 2. The named worker will help the young person become familiar with adults' health and social care services they may potentially use. Refer to Figure 38.2.

SUPPORT AFTER TRANSFER

Overall, the support after transfer is aimed at stability and continuity of care for the young person. For example, the NICE guidelines state that the young person should see the same healthcare practitioner in adults' services for the first two attended appointments after transfer and that the same social worker should be involved throughout the transition process (National Institute for Health and Care Excellence 2016). If the young person does not meet or engage with adult services (after transfer) the adult service should follow up with the young person, their family, and relevant healthcare professionals including the GP. If there is any continued dis-engagement the young person should be referred back to the transition named worker who will review the transition plan with the young person to help them use the service or identify an alternative way to meet their support needs.

SUPPORTING INFRASTRUCTURE

As recommended, it is important to ensure that there is ownership and accountability for development and implementation of transition strategies and policies in both children and adults' services (National Institute for Health and Care Excellence 2016). Service managers should ensure availability of developmentally appropriate services to support transition, such as age-banded clinics. Managers should also consider that young people in receipt of care from multiple medical specialities benefit from care co-ordination from a single healthcare professional. Services should consider use of advocacy to support young people after transfer, and youth forums to provide feedback on services and identify gaps in transitional care. Service provision should be evaluated using data from different agencies and stakeholders. Refer to Box Activity 38.3.

> **ACTIVITY 38.3**
>
> Reflect upon the descriptions of developmentally appropriate healthcare, strengths-based transition support and person-centred care.
>
> How might you embed these principles in the care you provide for young people?

CONCLUSION

The 2016 NICE guidelines provide a comprehensive framework for transition from children's to adults' services. Although the transition named worker has a pivotal role, there are opportunities for all members of the healthcare team, the young person, their family and carers as well as community and voluntary agencies, to positively influence the experience of transition and the transfer of care to adult services. In providing timely, developmentally appropriate information and support, that involves the young person and their parents and carers and fosters independence, it is hoped that the young person is empowered to manage their condition and successfully transfer to adult health and care services. Refer to Box Activity 38.4.

> **ACTIVITY 38.4**
>
> Try these out! Using your knowledge about the overarching principles of transition, map out the key points that, from your perspective, warrant further discussion and possible inclusion in transition planning for the two young people described below. How could you facilitate the involvement of the young person and their family in that process? What adult services might they require?
>
> Case Study 1: *Amy, aged 15 years, has bilateral spastic cerebral palsy and lives with her parents and two younger siblings in a single storey bungalow in the countryside, approximately three miles from the nearest town. She can manage her own personal care although has some restriction in fine motor tasks, but can transfer independently and uses a powered wheelchair to get around. Amy has no communication issues, is regularly reviewed by her paediatrician, paediatric orthopaedic surgeon, community physiotherapist, and occupational therapist and specialised wheelchair and seating service, as she has a scoliosis. She attends her local secondary school and has a part-time classroom assistant to help with physical tasks. Amy has a good group of friends in school, but would like to increase her opportunities to socialise outside school and in the future hopes to go to university to study social policy, although her parents are anxious about her ability to live independently away from home.*
>
> Case study 2: *Zach, aged 17 years, has dystonic cerebral palsy and is unable to sit or move independently. He has a profound learning disability and is gastrostomy fed due to unsafe swallow. Zach has recurrent chest infections resulting in several unplanned hospital admissions over the past two years. He attends a specialist school for children and young people with complex disabilities where he regularly receives a range of allied health services and nursing care that have been co-ordinated by the same community paediatrician for the past 15 years. Zach also attends a tertiary neurodisability service for specialised tone management.*

REFERENCES

Bagatell, N., Chan, D., Rauch, K.K. & Thorpe, D. (2017) "Thrust into adulthood": transition experiences of young adults with cerebral palsy. *Disability and Health Journal*, **10**(1), 80–86. https://doi.org/10.1016/j.dhjo.2016.09.008.

Blair, E., Langdon, K., McIntyre, S., Lawrence, D. & Watson, L. (2019) Survival and mortality in cerebral palsy: observations to the sixth decade from a data linkage study of a total population register and National Death Index. *BMC Neurology*, **19**(1), 111. https://doi.org/10.1186/s12883-019-1343-1.

Campbell, F., Biggs, K., Aldiss, S.K., O'Neill, P.M., Clowes, M., McDonagh, J., While, A. & Gibson, F. (2016) Transition of care for adolescents from paediatric services to adult health services. *Cochrane Database of Systematic Reviews*, **4**, Cd009794. https://doi.org/10.1002/14651858.CD009794.pub2.

Care Quality Commission. (2014) From the pond into the sea: children's transition to adult health services. https://www.cqc.org.uk/sites/default/files/CQC_Transition%20Report_Summary_lores.pdf (accessed 9 September 2022).

Colver, A. & Longwell, S. (2013) New understanding of adolescent brain development: relevance to transitional healthcare for young people with long term conditions. *Archives of Disease in Childhood*, **98**(11), 902–907. https://doi.org/10.1136/archdischild-2013-303945.

Colver, A., Rapley, T., Parr, J.R., McConachie, H., Dovey-Pearce, G., Couteur, A.L., McDonagh, J.E., Bennett, C., Maniatopoulos, G., Pearce, M.S., Reape, D., Chater, N., Gleeson, H. & Vale, L. (2020) Facilitating transition of young people with long-term health conditions from children's to adults' healthcare services - implications of a 5-year research programme. *Clinical Medicine (London, England)*, **20**(1), 74–80. https://doi.org/10.7861/clinmed.2019-0077.

Farre, A., Wood, V., Rapley, T., Parr, J.R., Reape, D. & McDonagh, J.E. (2015) Developmentally appropriate healthcare for young people: a scoping study. *Archives of Disease in Childhood*, **100**(2), 144–151. https://doi.org/10.1136/archdischild-2014-306749.

Freeman, M., Stewart, D., Cunningham, C.E. & Gorter, J.W. (2018) "If I had been given that information back then": an interpretive description exploring the information needs of adults with cerebral palsy looking back on their transition to adulthood. *Child: Care, Health and Development*, **44**(5), 689–696. https://doi.org/10.1111/cch.12579.

Gleeson, H. (2018) Guidance on training in adolescent and young adult health care (including transition). London: Joint Royal Colleges of Physicians Training Board. https://www.jrcptb.org.uk/sites/default/files/Guidance%20on%20training%20in%20Adolescent%20and%20Young%20Adult%20Health%20Care%20August%202018.pdf (accessed 21 October, 2022) https://www.oxfordlearnersdictionaries.com/definition/american_english/transition (accessed 12 September 2022)

Kolehmainen, N., McCafferty, S., Maniatopoulos, G., Vale, L., Le-Couteur, A.S. & Colver, A. (2017) What constitutes successful commissioning of transition from children's to adults' services for young people with long-term conditions and what are the challenges? An interview study. *BMJ Paediatrics Open*, **1**(1), e000085. https://doi.org/10.1136/bmjpo-2017-000085.

Lea, D., Bradbery, J. (2022) *The Oxford Advanced Learner's Dictionary*. UK: Oxford University Press 10th edition.

McConnell, K., Livingstone, E., Perra, O. & Kerr, C. (2021) Population-based study on the prevalence and clinical profile of adults with cerebral palsy in Northern Ireland. *BMJ Open*, **11**(1), e044614. https://doi.org/10.1136/bmjopen-2020-044614.

McIntyre, S., Goldsmith, S., Webb, A., Ehlinger, V., Hollung, S.J., McConnell, K., Arnaud, C., Smithers-Sheedy, H., Oskoui, M., Khandaker, G., Himmelmann, K. & Global CP Prevalence Group* (2022). Global prevalence of cerebral palsy: a systematic analysis. Developmental Medicine and Child Neurology, 10.1111/dmcn.15346. Advance online publication. https://onlinelibrary.wiley.com/doi/10.1111/dmcn.15346 [Accessed 6 March 2023]

The National Confidential Enquiry into Patient Outcome and Death. (2018) Each and Every Need. London. https://www.ncepod.org.uk/2018cn.html (accessed 12 September 2022).

National Institute for Health and Care Excellence. (2016) Transition from children's to adults' services for young people using health or social care services. NICE Guideline [NG43]. https://www.nice.org.uk/guidance/ng43 (accessed 9 September 2022).

Northern Ireland Cerebral Palsy Register https://www.qub.ac.uk/research-centres/NorthernIrelandCerebralPalsyRegister (accessed 9 September 2022).

O'Connor, S., Brenner, M. & Coyne, I. (2019) Family-centred care of children and young people in the acute hospital setting: a concept analysis. *Journal of Clinical Nursing*, **28**(17–18), 3353–3367. https://doi.org/10.1111/jocn.14913.

Roquet, M., Garlantezec, R., Remy-Neris, O., Sacaze, E., Gallien, P., Ropars, J., Houx, L., Pons, C. & Brochard, S. (2018) From childhood to adulthood: health care use in individuals with cerebral palsy. *Developmental Medicine and Child Neurology*, **60**(12), 1271–1277. https://doi.org/10.1111/dmcn.14003.

Rosenbaum, P., Paneth, N., Leviton, A., Goldstein, M., Bax, M., Damiano, D., Dan, B. & Jacobsson, B. (2007). A report: the definition and classification of cerebral palsy April 2006. *Developmental Medicine and Child Neurology* Suppl, **109**, 8–14.

Royal College of Paediatrics and Child Health. (2018) Facing the future: standards for children with ongoing health needs. London https://www.rcpch.ac.uk/sites/default/files/2018-04/facing_the_future_standards_for_children_with_ongoing_health_needs_2018-03.pdf (Accessed 21 Oct 2022).

Royal College of Physicians. (2015) On the margins of medical care: why young adults and adolescents need better healthcare. London https://www.rcplondon.ac.uk/file/2366/download (accessed 21 October 2022).

Ryan, J.M., Walsh, M., Owens, M., Byrne, M., Kroll, T., Hensey, O., Kerr, C., Norris, M., Walsh, A., Lavelle, G. & Fortune, J. (2022). Transition to adult services experienced by young people with cerebral palsy: a cross-sectional study. Developmental Medicine and Child Neurology, 10.1111/dmcn.15317. Advance online publication. https://onlinelibrary.wiley.com/doi/10.1111/dmcn.15317 [Accessed 6 March 2023]

Solanke, F., Colver, A. & McConachie, H. & Transition collaborative group (2018) Are the health needs of young people with cerebral palsy met during transition from child to adult health care? *Child: Care, Health and Development*, **44**(3), 355–363. https://doi.org/10.1111/cch.12549.

Tuffrey, C. & Pearce, A. (2003) Transition from paediatric to adult medical services for young people with chronic neurological problems. *Journal of Neurology, Neurosurgery, and Psychiatry*, **74**(8), 1011–1013. https://doi.org/10.1136/jnnp.74.8.1011.

Uniacke, S., Browne, T.K. & Shields, L. (2018) How should we understand family-centred care? *Journal of Child Health Care for Professionals Working with Children in the Hospital and Community*, **22**(3), 460–469. https://doi.org/10.1177/1367493517753083.

Watson, R., Parr, J.R., Joyce, C., May, C. & Le Couteur, A.S. (2011) Models of transitional care for young people with complex health needs: a scoping review. *Child: Care, Health and Development*, **37**(6), 780–791. https://doi.org/10.1111/j.1365-2214.2011.01293.x.

Bereavement Support

CHAPTER 39

Una Hughes and Patricia McNeilly

This chapter is dedicated to the memory of Breige Morgan, Community Children's Nurse, who previously co-authored this chapter.

INTRODUCTION

The death of a child is a devastating loss for parents, siblings, and the wider family and circle of friends. When a family has lost a child or is about to lose their child, the fact that we, as professionals, provide compassionate care may be one of the things that helps to ease their pain. Where possible, family participation in advanced care planning some time before the child's death, can help to ensure that families have as much choice and control as possible around the care provided in the period leading up to and after the death. However, this is not always possible where an unexpected or sudden death has occurred or when the family have been unable or reluctant to engage in such conversations. Parents vary greatly in their preparedness for the death of their child with some parents unable to think or plan ahead in this way (Bogetz et al. 2020).

Regardless of circumstances, bereavement support is an integral part of paediatric palliative care provision (Together for Short Lives 2019 and the quality of this support can have an impact on the family's grieving process and lives for years to come. A multifaceted family centred, partnership approach to providing paediatric palliative care at this stage is very much fundamental to meeting the needs of the child, their parents, siblings, and extended family (Gill et al. 2021). Each family's bereavement journey is unique, therefore approaches must be family led and individualised. This chapter aims to: (1) provide a brief background of bereavement theory to enable practitioners to better understand the complexities of the bereavement journey (2) set out families' experiences of the loss of a child and (3) identify the practical issues that we, as healthcare professionals, can address to help support the family after a child has died using a fictitious case study.

WHAT IS BEREAVEMENT?

When offering bereavement support it is useful to define the terms bereavement, grief, and mourning See Figure 39.1. Definitions of bereavement, grief and mourning

Following bereavement parents often initially engage in traditional mourning rituals and part of the bereavement process is adapting (at least to some extent) to a new reality (Kochen et al. 2020), however this may take a lifetime (Edelman 2021) and parents may never stop mourning the loss of their child. There will be moments years after the child's death when the parents' grief may be triggered, for example, at key points in time when they wonder what their child's future may have held. Grief is not constant, it ebbs and flows as does the ability to cope with the loss. Knowledge of bereavement theory can help practitioners to develop an understanding of what families are going through. Traditionally the theory by Kübler-Ross (1969) described as the five stages of grief – denial, anger, bargaining, depression, and acceptance, started a narrative on

---

Bereavement is the loss of someone
Grief is the personal emotional response to a death
Mourning is the action taken to express the loss

FIGURE 39.1 Defintions of bereavement, grief and mourning.

Care Planning in Children and Young People's Nursing, Second Edition. Edited by Sonya Clarke and Doris Corkin.
© 2024 John Wiley & Sons Ltd. Published 2024 by John Wiley & Sons Ltd.

death, dying, and grief (Bregman 2019). However, the theory has been widely criticised and led some people to believe that they were not grieving in the 'right' way (Devine 2017). More modern theorists have focused less on a linear process or one that suggests a final resolution of grief. Stroebe and Schut (2016), for example, describe a 'Dual Process Model of Coping with Bereavement' (DPM), where people oscillate between a loss orientated process and a restoration orientated process. In loss orientated moments the bereft person is focussed on the person who has died and they may experience feelings of sadness, anger, or loneliness. Restoration orientated processes are about distraction from grief and allowing a break from the pain of loss. Stroebe and Schut (2016) suggest that moving between these two processes allows the person to face reality and deal with their grief a little at a time. Other theorists have explored the continuing bond between the parent and their deceased child and the significant part this plays throughout parents' lives (Klass 2017). In practice, parents want to find meaningful and personal ways to remember their child and build lasting memories.

The grief that families feel is a natural response to death and is a very personal and individual experience. Reactions to a child's death are affected by many things, including the relationship with the child, the type of death, whether it was expected or sudden, personality types, gender, culture, religious outlook, or past experience. Unlike many aspects of healthcare, grief cannot be fixed, but it must be acknowledged, and support offered.

WHAT ARE FAMILIES' EXPERIENCES FOLLOWING THE DEATH OF A CHILD?

Families' experiences following the loss of a child are reported in numerous research studies. Whilst unique and individual, feelings of intense sadness, tearfulness, and a longing for their child are commonly expressed across studies. Parents frequently recount their experiences in terms of the last days before the death, at the time of death and the period after (Kenny et al. 2020) highlighting the importance of anticipatory grief. Despite the recent culture shift around shared parenting, mothers and fathers often grieve differently. Fathers still tend to avoid sharing their feelings and are less likely to seek and reach out for social support. Coping mechanisms also differ with fathers coping in practical terms, for example, by returning to work and engaging with household or other physical tasks (McNeil et al. 2021). Some parents develop what is known as Prolonged Grief Disorder (PGD) that necessitates specialist psychological intervention. This can manifest as major depression or post-traumatic stress affecting daily functioning for more than six months and is more common in mothers than fathers (Baumann et al. 2020).

Denhup (2019) found that parents talked of their suffering after the death of their child as indescribable and unlike any other bereavement. Poor communication, insufficient information, not being involved in their child's care, and differences in care goals added to this suffering. Parents in a study by Cacciatore et al. (2019) identified what helped at the time of the death of their child and after. They recounted that compassion shown by professionals, openness and honesty, flexibility and individualised care, and clinical competence were very highly valued.

While the experiences of bereaved parents are unique, so too are those of siblings. Many factors may influence grief reactions and outcomes for bereaved children. For example, their age and stage of development, parenting styles, and family cultures, the relationship they had with their sibling and their involvement in the period leading up to the death and beyond. Most bereaved children in a study by Brooten and Young (2017) talked of fears and worries seven months after the sibling's death, most often around their parents or other siblings getting a terminal illness or dying. Children may experience sadness, behavioural issues, sleep disturbance, separation anxiety, or may feel different from other children. Support mechanisms and services have been developed for bereaved siblings. For example, weekend camps and group activities have been shown to have positive effects (McNeil et al. 2021). However, these rely on parents' and professionals' recommendations and are not always available.

Others close to the family can experience grief at the loss of the child depending on their relationship to the child and parents. For example, grandparents experience their own loss in addition to the devastation they feel for their adult child (Tatterton & Walshe 2019). This grief can sometimes be unacknowledged.

Nurses are well placed to support the family following the death of a child, particularly when they know the family well. A multi-agency, partnership approach is required – however, each family is unique and will vary greatly in terms of the support that they desire and need. It is vital to ensure that care at this stage is led by the family, who will have their own support mechanisms, in addition to external support provided by health care professionals. General principles of support can include the ABC'S model (see Figure 39.2).

HOW CAN WE SUPPORT THE FAMILY?

Remember your ABCs

- Ask – if you're not sure what to do ask the parents – is there is anything else you should be doing for them
- Be – be there, be available (and tell the parents that you are available)
- Care – be caring and show empathy
- Stop – look and listen – give the parents your time – do you need to consider anything else?

FIGURE 39.2 Remember your ABCs.

CASE STUDY AMY

Amy was a two-year-old girl who died at home following an undiagnosed condition characterised by global developmental delay and frequent seizures. She had an older brother and sister. Amy's dad (Ian) was working long hours to support the family and mum (Helen) had given up work to care for her and her siblings. Her condition had been deteriorating over the past six months and she had numerous hospital admissions. Following discussion with her Consultant Amy's parents decided that there should be no further active intervention and the focus of care should be to support her through the end of life phase in the home setting. This was Helen's first experience of impending death, and she was very worried about her own response to Amy's death. A multi-disciplinary, multi-agency approach was facilitated and after several weeks of supportive care, Amy died peacefully at home.

Family members close to Amy, along with her Community Children's Nurse (CCN) were present when Amy died. Amy's G.P., consultant, staff from the hospital, CCN Team and hospice made contact with Helen and Ian, visited or attended the funeral. Helen appeared to cope well at the time of the funeral despite her fears about facing Amy's death. The CCN and hospice nurse made a combined visit one week following Amy's funeral. Helen was very angry with Ian at this time. He had returned to work, and she felt he was 'getting on with things'. Meanwhile she was trying to cope with her own grief, the increasingly difficult behaviour of Michael (6yrs) and Annabel (3½yrs), who had been toilet-trained but was now requiring nappies.

The following case study and text that follows, sets out an example of how the Community Children's Nurse, along with the Children's Hospice Community Nurse Specialist may provide ongoing practical, emotional, and informational support.

In the case study Amy's parents had time to build up a relationship with the CCN and the Hospice Team and make decisions and prepare for her death. Not all childhood deaths are predicted, sometimes there is very little or no time to build relationships with parents before the child's death. Initiating bereavement support can be difficult in these circumstances and the ABC'S approach is a good starting point in building the relationship (Figure 39.2). Amy's parents decided she should die at home and the community children's nursing (CCN) team and the specialist hospice community nurse worked together to facilitate this with support from the wider team. Making memories, taking photos, hand and footprints, and encouraging parents to hold and wash their child after death may help in the grieving process. Amy's parents had been able to plan and express their wishes for Amy's funeral and this had been discussed with their chaplain at an early stage. Funeral rituals may be subjectively perceived as helpful in dealing with loss (Mitima-Verloop et al. 2019). Mourning processes give the family a focus and a structure to get them through the initial phase in the bereavement process. In supporting bereaved parents, we must be mindful of their wishes, their individuality, and culture. The family must make the decisions which feel right for them (Sim et al. 2020). Faith and cultural customs can provide much support for the family at this time; however, this may not always be the case. For example, Kim et al. (2021) state that, traditional views in Korean culture can put the blame on parents for a child's death. It is important to consider family background and culture when providing bereavement support, there is no universal 'right' way to grieve.

Most parents appreciate ongoing support from healthcare staff and peers after their child's death (Snaman et al. 2017). Planning bereavement visits is important and requires coordination, especially when many different disciplines have been involved, for example, hospital, hospice, community, and bereavement teams, along with the multidisciplinary team. At the joint visit after the funeral, Helen expressed how much it meant to her to see the various staff who made contact, visited, or attended the funeral. She was very emotional, talking about Amy, and expressing how she felt lost and could not focus when she did not have the routine of caring for Amy. The CCN and hospice nurse listened to Helen, comforted her, answered any questions she had and offered support. Helen was concerned about the children's behaviours. She was reassured by the CCN that changes in behaviour and regression were very common in young children when someone close to them dies and was offered strategies for coping with their behaviours. The hospice nurse was able to offer advice and details of local resources and support groups to help the family to come to terms with Amy's death. Peer support and meeting others in a similar position can be very beneficial (Aho et al. 2018). Information about online resources was also provided (see Figure 39.4). Helen also had the opportunity to discuss her feelings about her husband returning to work, Stroebe and Schut's (2016) DPM suggests men often use work as a distraction from grief.

The second visit, when Ian was at home, allowed him to express his concerns; he revealed the huge pressure he was under to support the family financially and also that he needed to appear to be strong and protect Helen. The visit provided the couple with a chance to understand each other's difficulties. On subsequent visits over the next year the CCN witnessed the family becoming stronger and supporting each other. There were emotional ups and downs but Helen felt comfortable phoning the CCN to discuss issues when she needed to. Helen expressed relief that Amy's suffering was over, but also felt guilty for feeling this; the CCN was able to reassure her this was a normal reaction, (Kim et al. 2021; Worden 2018). The hospice nurse specialist also made contact over the two-year period following Amy s death. Healthcare professionals can encourage families to continue the bond with their child to provide solace (Kim et al. 2021; Klass 2017). Nurses acknowledging the difficult days like birthdays and holidays and helping families to build new traditions to remember the child may be comforting (Jonas et al. 2018). Listening to the family, giving them information at the pace they required, guiding them when they are overwhelmed, but also having the perception and understanding of the family to step back and allow the family to take the lead again was important for the success of the bereavement care. Helen and Ian raised money for the CCN team and the Hospice in Amy's memory. They both expressed their gratitude for the support they had received and the fact that other people outside the family remembered Amy.

There can be a theory/practice gap in bereavement care (Hay et al. 2021). The increased awareness of bereavement support, provision of specialist bereavement education, and bereavement coordinator roles aim to bridge this gap in to improve the lives of those who have been bereaved. Professionals have an important role in providing care and support in the period leading up to and after the death of a child and beyond (McConnell et al. 2016). The nurse's role in bereavement support is varied and individualized and must be child and family centred. It is a challenging role, and many nurses feel ill-equipped (Raymond et al. 2017). Specialist nurses have a very important role to play in supporting the family and advising staff at this time, however expertise in bereavement care is not a prerequisite to making a difference for a bereaved family. Figure 39.3 includes key actions to consider.

1. If you are not already aware, familiarise yourself with the medical history and details of the child's death.
2. Liaise with the team who provided end-of-life care, if you have not been involved.
3. Contact parents and arrange a visit and give them contact details.
4. Manage each situation individually; be aware that some parents may wish to deal with the death of their child within their own circle of family and friends and may not want involvement from professionals.
5. Respect cultural and religious customs.
6. Use the child's name when discussing them.
7. Listen to parents and/or siblings, be sensitive and show compassion.
8. Reassure parents that the rollercoaster of emotions they are feeling is normal, there is not right or wrong way to grieve.
9. Offer practical support and advice if needed, for example registering the death, how to make funeral arrangements, etc.
10. Give information at the pace the family is ready to receive it.
11. Be sensitive when removing healthcare equipment from the home (if the child has had home care) in terms of when the parents want it done. Some parents may want it removed immediately on the child's death; others may need time before it is removed from their home.
12. Always tell the truth; admit if you do not know something but offer to try to find out the information they are seeking.
13. Try to involve both parents and siblings, at times fathers can be reluctant to participate or can be forgotten about.
14. Allow siblings space to vent their feelings; they may feel neglected. Bereaved parents may not be able to cope with their children's grief as well as their own. Offer a meeting specifically focusing on the children and be familiar with resources that professionals or parents may use with their children.
15. Refer parents for further professional help if there are signs of complicated grief.
16. Bring parents any written documentation about bereavement and support available in your locality and information about local support groups, if appropriate.
17. Be up-to-date with remembrance service details.
18. Document all care in a bereavement care plan.
19. Attend bereavement training and liaise with the bereavement coordinator.

FIGURE 39.3 Key Actions to Support a Bereaved Family.

WHY IS SELF-CARE IMPORTANT FOR STAFF WHEN SUPPORTING BEREAVED FAMILIES?

Caring for families with a child at the end of life and beyond is particularly stressful and challenging for practitioners (Bergsträsser et al. 2017). As such it is really important that those caring for families look after themselves. Self-care, for example, social support and spending time with friends and family, relaxation techniques such as mindfulness, good working relationships, and team working can all help to reduce stress and prevent compassion fatigue and burnout (Hospice, UK, 2015). Multi-disciplinary, multi-agency reflective debriefing after the death of a child can also be cathartic and contribute to practice development by identifying learning and actions that can be taken forward. Using a specific reflective model for children's palliative care (see McNeilly et al. 2022) can help to focus discussions and actively address and improve issues both for families and practitioners working in this area.

CONCLUSION

After the death of a child, bereaved families face a difficult journey to try to adjust to their new reality. Healthcare professionals offer help by providing bereavement support which is underpinned by modern theories of bereavement. Consideration of the uniqueness of the family's cultures and beliefs, and recognition that members of the family may grieve differently are essential to tailor the

> - Winston's Wish – giving hope to grieving children (winstonswish.org)
> - Together for Short Lives: Children's Charities – Children Hospices
> - Children and Young People – The Palliative Hub | (childrenspalliativehub.com)
> - Childhood Bereavement Network
> - Child Bereavement UK
> - CYPACP – Child & Young Persons Advance Care Plan

FIGURE 39.4 Resources.

support to meet their individual needs. Family involvement in advance care planning where possible, gives the family a platform for their preferences and promotes communication of these with healthcare professionals. Good communication, compassion, professionalism, and a willingness to listen and be led by the family's wishes are important qualities and skills for healthcare professionals. Bereavement specialists and palliative care nurse specialists provide support for staff and parents, and have a wealth of knowledge and experience but when healthcare professionals feel unsure dealing with bereaved families the ABC'S model (Figure 39.2) offers a simple mnemonic to help them begin the process and keep it family centred. Providing such care and support can be stressful and those working with families need to be mindful to look after themselves to prevent compassion fatigue. Clearly ongoing training around bereavement care is essential.

REFERENCES

Aho, A.L., Malmisuo, J. & Kaunonen, M. (2018) The effects of peer support on post-traumatic stress reactions in bereaved parents. *Scandinavian Journal of Caring Sciences*, **32**(1), 326–334. doi:10.1111/scs.12465.

Baumann, I., Künzel, J., Goldbeck, L., Tutus, D. & Niemitz, M. (2020) Prolonged grief, posttraumatic stress and depression among bereaved parents: prevalence and response to an intervention program. *Journal of Death and Dying*, **0**(0), 1–19. doi:10.1177/0030222820918674.

Bergsträsser, E., Cignacco, E. & Luck, P. (2017) Health care professionals' experiences and needs when delivering end-of-life care to children: a qualitative study. *Palliative Care: Research and Treatment*, **10**, 1–10. doi:10.1177/1178224217724770.

Bogetz, J.F., Revette, A., Rosenberg, A.R. & DeCourcey, D. (2020) "I could never prepare for something like the death of my own child": parental perspectives on preparedness at end of life for children with complex chronic conditions. *Journal of Pain and Symptom Management*, **60**(6), 1154–1162.e1. https://doi.org/10.1016/j.jpainsymman.2020.06.035.

Bregman, L. (2019) Kübler-ross and the re-visioning of death as loss: religious appropriation and responses. *Journal of Pastoral Care & Counseling*, **73**(1), 4–8. doi:10.1177/1542305019831943.

Brooten, D. & Youngblut, J.M. (2017) School aged children's experiences 7 and 13 months following a sibling's death. *Journal of Child and Family Studies*, **26**, 1112–1123. doi: 10.1007/s10826-016-0647-7.

Cacciatore, J., Thieleman, K., Lieber, A.S., Blood, C. & Goldman, R. (2019) The long road to farewell: the needs of families with dying children. *Journal of Death and Dying*, **78**(4), 404–420. doi: 10.1177/0030222817697418.

Denhup, C. (2019) Bereavement care to minimize bereaved parents' suffering in their lifelong journey towards healing. *Applied Nursing Research*, **50**(2019), 151205. https://doi.org/10.1016/j.apnr.2019.151205.

Devine, M. (2017) *It's OK that You're Not OK: Meeting Grief and Loss in a Culture that Doesn't Understand*. Colorado: Sounds True Inc. ISBN: 9781622039081.

Edelman, H. (2021) *The AfterGrief: Finding Your Way on the Long Path of Loss*. London: Michael Joseph; Penguin Books. ISBN: 9780241492895.

Gill, F.J., Hashem, Z., Stegmann, R. & Aoun, S.M. (2021) The support needs of parent caregivers of children with a life-limiting illness and approaches used to meet their needs: A scoping review. *Palliative Medicine*, **35**(1), 76–96. doi: 10.1177/0269216320967593.

Hay, A., Hall, C.W., Sealey, M., Lobb, E.A. & Breen, L.J. (2021) Developing a practice-based research agenda for grief and bereavement care. *Death Studies*, **45**(5), 331–341. doi: 10.1080/07481187.2019.1636897.

Jonas, D., Scanlon, C., Rusch, R., Ito, J. & Joselow, M. (2018) Bereavement after a child's death. *Child and Adolescent Psychiatric Clinics of North America*, **27**, 579–590.

Klass, D. and Steffen, E. (2017) *Continuing Bonds in Bereavement. New Directions for Research and Practice*. New York: Routledge.

Kenny, K., Darcy-Bewick, S., Martin, A., Eustace-Cook, J., Hilliard, C., Clinton, F., Storey, L., Coyne, I., Murray, K., Duffy, K., Fortune, G., Smith, O., Higgins, A. &

Hynes, G. (2020) You are at rock bottom: a qualitative systematic review of the needs of bereaved parents as they journey through the death of their child to cancer. *Journal of Psychosocial Oncology*, **38**(6), 761–781. doi:10.1080/07347332.2020.1762822.

Kim, M.A., Yi, J., Sang, J. & Jung, D. (2021) A photovoice study on the bereavement experience of mothers after the death of a child. *Death Studies*, **45**(5), 390–404. doi: 10.1080/07481187.2019.1648333.

Kochen, E.M., Jenken, F., Boelen, P.A., Deben, L.M.A., Fahner, J.C., van den Hoogen, A., Teunissen, S.C.C.M., Geleijns, K. & Kars, M.C. (2020) When a child dies: a systematic review of well-defined parent-focused bereavement interventions and their alignment with grief- and loss theories. *BMC Palliative Care*, **19**, 28. https://doi.org/10.1186/s12904-020-0529-z.

Kübler-Ross, E. (1969) *On Death and Dying*. New York: Macmillan.

McConnell, T., Scott, D. & Porter, S. (2016) Healthcare staff's experience of providing end-of-life care to children: a mixed method review. *Palliative Medicine*, **30**(10), 905–919. https://pubmed.ncbi.nlm.nih.gov/27129677/ [Accessed 6 March 2023].

McNeil, M.J., Baker, J.N., Snyder, I., Rosenberg, A.R. & Kaye, E.C. (2022) Grief and bereavement in fathers after the death of a child: a systematic review. *Pediatrics*, **147**(4), e2020040386.

Mitima-Verloop, H.B., Mooren, T.T.M. & Boelen, P.A. (2019) Facilitating grief: An exploration of the function of funerals and rituals in relation to grief reactions 11 Nov 2019 https://doi.org/10.1080/07481187.2019.1686090

Raymond, A., Lee, S.F. & Bloomer, M.J. (2017) Understanding the bereavement care roles of nurses within acute care: a systematic review. *Journal of Clinical Nursing*, **26**, 1787–1800.

Sim, C.W., Heuse, S., Weigel, D. & Kendel, F. (2020) If only I could turn back time—Regret in bereaved parents. *Pediatric Blood & Cancer; Psychosocial and Supportive Care*: Research Article; the American Society of Pediatric Hematology/Oncology. doi: 10.1002/pbc.28265 https://pubmed.ncbi.nlm.nih.gov/32196890/ [Accessed 6 March 2023].

Snaman, J.M., Kaye, E.C., Levine, D.R., Cochran, B., Wilcox, R., Sparrow, C.K., Noyes, N., Clark, L., Avery, W. & Baker, J.N. (2017) Empowering bereaved parents through the development of a comprehensive bereavement program. *Journal of Pain and Symptom Management*, **53**(4), 767–775. ISSN 0885-3924. https://doi.org/10.1016/j.jpainsymman.2016.10.359 [Accessed 6 March 2023].

Stroebe, M. & Schut, H. (2016) Overload: a missing link in the dual process model? *OMEGA - Journal of Death and Dying*, **74**(1), 96–109. doi: 10.1177/0030222816666540.

Tatterton, M.J. & Walshe, C. (2019) How grandparents experience the death of a grandchild with a life-limiting condition. *Journal of Family Nursing*, **25**(1), 109–127.

Together for Short Lives (2019) *Caring for a child at end of life (2019) A guide for professionals on the care of children and young people*. Bristol: Together for Short Lives

Worden, J.W. (2018) *Grief Counseling and Grief Therapy, 5th Edition A Handbook for the Mental Health Practitioner*. New York: Springer Publishing.

Index

Page locators in **bold** indicate tables. Page locators in *italics* indicate figures. This index uses letter-by-letter alphabetization.

A

AA *see* academic assessors
ABCDE assessment
    acute kidney injury, 276–277
    closed head injury, 139–140
    complex needs, 302–303, *304*
    critical care, 65–69
    neonatal respiratory distress syndrome, 161–166, **162**, *163*
    nut allergy, 133–135
    principles of care planning, 4–5
    ABC'S model, 325, 328
absence seizures, 126
abuse *see* safeguarding
academic assessors (AA), 72, 73
accountability, 35–38
ACE *see* adverse childhood experience
ACS *see* acute chest syndrome
Action for Sick Children (ASC), 37
active listening, 314
acute chest syndrome (ACS), 311
acute kidney injury (AKI), 273–279
    aetiology and presentation, 274
    assessment of renal function recovery, 279
    care planning, 274–277
    case study, 273
    definitions, **273**
    nephrotic syndrome, 260
    rationale for dialysis modality, 278
    renal replacement therapy (RRT), 274, 277
    types of dialysis, 277, *278*
acute limb compartment syndrome, 18–19
adrenaline, 133, 135–136, *135*, 141
advanced care planning, 13
adverse childhood experience (ACE), 23, **24**
advocacy, care planning, 36–38
AED *see* anti-epileptic drugs
affective touch, 305–306
airway obstruction, 65–67
albumin, 259, 264
albuminuria, 259
alcohol use, 54, 127
allergens, 177
altruism, 82
anaesthesia, 201–202
analgesic corridor, *311*
anaphylaxis, 133–136
angioedema, 133–134
ankyloglossia, 236
antibiotics
    cystic fibrosis, 168, 169, 172, 173
    infected eczema, 287–288
    nephrotic syndrome, 260, 262, 264
    sickle cell disease, 313

anti-epileptic drugs (AED), 127–129
antihistamines, 133
antipyretics, 228
anxiety *see* stress and anxiety
apnoea of prematurity, 166
appendicectomy, 208–213
    case study, 208
    pathophysiology of appendicitis, 208–209
    personal cleansing/dressing, 210–211
    postoperative care, 211–213, *212*
    wound healing and dressings, 209–210, **209**
appetite, 94
APVU score, 69
ASC *see* Action for Sick Children
aseptic non-touch technique, 210
assent, 38–39
assessment
    acute kidney injury, 279
    burns injury, 293–295, **294**
    cerebral palsy, 242
    closed head injury, 139–141, **139**, 143–145, *144–145*
    congestive cardiac failure, 190–193
    continuous analgesia, 112
    critical care, 62–65, **62–64**
    epidural analgesia, 117
    epilepsy, 126–127
    family-centred care, 79
    infected eczema, 284–285
    mental health and wellbeing, 94–95, **95**
    neonatal respiratory distress syndrome, 161–163, **162**, *163*
    nephrotic syndrome, 260–261
    nut allergy, 133–135
    pain management in neonates, 101–103, **102**
    principles of care planning, 4–5
    sickle cell disease, 310
    truth telling, 45, **46**
    see also risk assessment and management
asthma, 175–181
    aetiology and presentation, 175–176
    case study, 175
    discharge planning, 179–180
    importance of medication and education, 177–179, *178–179*
    monitoring vital signs, 176–177
    nut allergy, 131–132
    risk and trigger factors, 177
    tonsillectomy, 201
atonic seizures, 126
atopic march, 283
atracurium, 141, 143
atropine, 141

auditory exposure, 105–106
auras, 126, 127
autonomy, 44

B

balloon pulmonary valvuloplasty, 185
behavioural cues, 102–103, **102–103**
bereavement support, 323–329
    case study, 325
    concepts and definitions, 323–324, *323*
    families' experiences, 324
    resources, *328*
    self-care for staff, 327
    supporting the family, 325–326, *327*
    theory/practice gap, 326
bi-level positive airway pressure (BiPAP), 302–303, *303*
biopsychosocial model, 94
BiPAP *see* bi-level positive airway pressure
blisters, 292, 293
blood glucose monitoring, 268–269
blood transfusion/blood products
    appendicectomy, 209
    sickle cell disease, 314
    tonsillectomy, 204–206
BMI *see* body mass index
body image, 297
body mass index (BMI), 150–151, *151*, 155
bone marrow transplant, 314
bottle-feeding, 235, 236–237
brain injury, 138, *139*
brain stem assessment, 145
breastfeeding *see* lactation and breastfeeding
bronchiolitis, 57–58
bronchodilators, 175–180
burns injury, 292–299
    care of blisters, 293
    case study, 292
    classification in children, 293
    first aid, 292
    fluid resuscitation, 292, 294–295, **295–297**
    immediate assessment, 293–295, **294**
button gastrostomy, 249–250, *250*

C

caffeine, 166
CAMHS *see* Child and Adolescent Mental Health Services
capillary refill time, 191
cardiac catheterisation, 185–189
    assessing and planning care, 187–188
    case study, 185
    congenital heart disease, 185–186
    congestive cardiac failure, 197

Orem's self-care model, 187–189
procedure, 186
transitional care, 186, 189
treatment of pulmonary stenosis, 186
cardiopulmonary resuscitation (CPR), 166
cardiovascular assessment, 139–140
care planning
    acute kidney injury, 274–277
    appendicectomy, 210–211
    assent, consent, and refusal of consent, 38–39
    burns injury, **295–297**
    cardiac catheterisation, 187–188
    cerebral palsy, 243
    challenges to healthcare decisions and actions, 40
    closed head injury, 140
    complex needs, 305–306
    concepts and definitions, 6–7, 33–34
    congestive cardiac failure, 194–196
    cystic fibrosis, 172–173
    decision-making, 34–35
    developmental dysplasia of the hip, 226, *227*, **229–230**
    diabetes mellitus, 269
    documentation and record-keeping, 40–41
    duty of care, duty of candour, accountability, negligence, 35–38
    epilepsy, 128
    ethical, legal, and professional implications, 33–43
    evidence-based practice, 40
    gastro-oesophageal reflux, 237–239, **238**
    infected eczema, 285
    mental health and wellbeing, **95**
    neonatal respiratory distress syndrome, 163–164, *164*
    nut allergy, 132
    obesity, 153, **154**, 155, **156**
    professional standard of care, 35
    reflective account, 86–87, *86*
    sickle cell disease, 310–311, *311–312*
    student/staff nurse perspective, 13, *14*
    transitional care, 319, *319–320*
    UN Convention on the Rights of the Child, 38
    United Nations Convention on the Rights of the Child, 38
Care Quality Commission (CQC), 317
casein-based milk, 235
Casey's model of nursing, 228, 285
CBT *see* cognitive behavioural therapy
CCF *see* congestive cardiac failure
Cerebral Function Analysing Monitoring (CFAM), 146
cerebral hypoxia, 142
cerebral palsy (CP), 241–247
    aetiology and presentation, 241–242
    assessment of needs, 242
    care planning, 243
    case study, 241
    gastrostomy care, 248–255
    pre-procedural care, 243–244
    procedure for passing a nasogastric tube, **245–246**
    rationale for enteral feeding, 242

    routes of administration, 242–243
    transitional care, 316, 321
cerebral perfusion pressure (CPP), 142, 146
CF *see* cystic fibrosis
CFAM *see* Cerebral Function Analysing Monitoring
CHD *see* congenital heart disease
chest infection, 85–88
chest X-ray
    congestive cardiac failure, 197
    neonatal respiratory distress syndrome, 163, *163*
CHI *see* closed head injury
Child and Adolescent Mental Health Services (CAMHS), 94, 96
child-centred care, 9–11, *10*
child exploitation, 26
child protection *see* safeguarding
Children Act (2003), 28
Children's Commissioners, 37–38
child sexual exploitation (CSE), 25
chloral hydrate, 142
chronic lung disease (CLD), 164
chronic osteomyelitis, 218
CLD *see* chronic lung disease
Climbié, Victoria, 27–28
clonic seizures, 126
closed head injury (CHI), 138–148
    assessment and interventions, 139–141, **139**
    brain stem, 145
    case study, 138
    common drugs used for intubation, **141**
    concepts and definitions, 138, *139*
    cortical response, 144–145, *145*
    emergency procedures, **140**
    further observations and monitoring, 145–146
    maintaining adequate fluid balance, 147
    neurological status assessment, 143–145, *144–145*
    pain relief and sedation, 143
    risk management, 147
Code of Professional Conduct (NMC 2018), 45
cognitive behavioural therapy (CBT), 96
cognitive development, 235–236
colostomy, 109
comfort holding, 104, *105*
communication
    appendicectomy, 211, *212*
    cerebral palsy, 243–244
    complex needs, 303–304, *304*
    congestive cardiac failure, 192, 195
    critical care, 69
    family-centred care, 81–82
    nephrotic syndrome, 263
    principles of care planning, 3, 4
    sexual health, 53–54
    truth telling, 44–50
community nursing
    bereavement support, 325–326
    complex needs, 300, 304–306, *305*
    cystic fibrosis, 173
    see also family-centred care
compartment syndrome, 294–295
compensated shock, 66

complex needs, 300–307
    breathing difficulties, 301–302, *303*
    case studies, 300
    communication, 304–305, *305*
    holorosencephaly, 300–302, *302*
    infantile onset pome disease, 300–302
    non-invasive ventilation, 301–302
    participation of children and young people, 306
    touch and mouth care, 305–306
complex partial seizures, 125
concussion, 123
confidentiality, 53–54
congenital heart disease (CHD), 185–186
congestive cardiac failure (CCF), 190–197
    aetiology, 193, **193**
    assessment, 190–193
    care plan, 194–196
    case study, 190
    cyanosis, 193–194
    immediate investigations, 196–197
    Roper-Logan-Tierney Model, 191–193
consciousness
    closed head injury, 139–141, **139**, 143–144, *144*
    diabetes mellitus, 271
    epilepsy, 125
    nut allergy, 133
consent *see* informed consent
continuous analgesia, 109–115
    case study, 109
    common opiates and cautions, 111
    ketamine infusion, 111
    nurse-controlled analgesia, 110
    nursing management, 112–113
    nursing process and model of care, 111–112
    patient-controlled analgesia, 110–113, **113–114**
    postoperative nursing care, **113–114**
continuous positive airway pressure (CPAP), 101, 161, 163–165
contraception, 51, 53
contre-coup injury, 138, *139*
co-production, 80
cortical response, 144–145, *145*
corticosteroids, 263–264, 286
cough reflex, 145
counselling, 53
coup injury, 138, *139*
COVID-19/SARS-CoV-2
    complex needs, 306
    mental health and wellbeing, 92–94
    principles of care planning, 3
CP *see* cerebral palsy
CPAP *see* continuous positive airway pressure
CPP *see* cerebral perfusion pressure
CPR *see* cardiopulmonary resuscitation
CQC *see* Care Quality Commission
CRIES tool, 102
critical care
    ABCDE assessment, 65–69
    airway, 65–67, **67**
    breathing and ventilation, 67–68
    case study, 60–61
    challenges, 69
    circulation, 68
    concepts and definitions, 60

debriefing, 69
disability, 68–69
exposure, 69
hyponatremia, 68
immediate assessment, 63–65
interprofessional assessment and care planning, 60–71
interprofessional working, 61–65, **62–64**
crizanlizumab, 314
Crohn's disease
continuous analgesia, 109–115
epidural analgesia, 116–120
cryptogenic epilepsy, 124
cyanosis, 193–194
cystic fibrosis (CF), 168–174
care planning, 172–173
case study, 168
community nurse specialist, 173
diagnostic approach, 168–169
medical treatment, 169
totally implantable venous access device, 168, 169–171, *170*, **171**

D

DDH *see* developmental dysplasia of the hip
death and dying
bereavement support, 323–329
complex needs, 300–307
congestive cardiac failure, 192–193
end-of-life care, 13, 78
family-centred care, 78–82
debriefing, 69
DECIDE model, 44
decompensated shock, 66
dehydration, 313
depression, 96
developmental dysplasia of the hip (DDH), 225–231
aetiology and presentation, 225–226
care planning, 226, *227*, **229–230**
case study, 225
hip spica cast, 226, *226*, **227**, **229–230**
thermoregulation, 228
diabetes mellitus type 1 (DMT1)
administration of insulin injection, 269–270
blood glucose monitoring, 268–269
calculation of insulin dose, 270
care plan, 269
case study, 266
categorisation, 266
discharge planning, 270–271
impact on patient and family, 267–268
newly diagnosed diabetic, 266–272
pathophysiology, 267
storage of drugs, 270
types of insulin, 270
dialysis, 277–278, *278*
disability, 68–69
discharge planning
asthma, 179–180
diabetes mellitus, 270–271
gastrostomy care, 252–253, *254*
Ilizarov frame/technique, 223–224
tonsillectomy, 204
disclosure/non-disclosure *see* truth telling
disease modification, 314

dissociative seizures, 124
diuretics, 264
DMT1 *see* diabetes mellitus type 1
documentation and record-keeping
care planning, 40–41
reflective account, 87
safeguarding, 31
donor wounds, 298
dopamine, 142
dual process model (DPM), 324, 326
duty of candour *see* truth telling
duty of care, 35–38

E

early intervention and prevention
mental health and wellbeing, 92, 93
obesity, 153
eating disorders, 92
EBP *see* evidence-based practice
ECG *see* electrocardiography
echocardiography, 197
eczema
aetiology and presentation, 283–284
assessment, 284–285
care planning, 285
case study, 283
evidence-based practice, 285–289
infected eczema, 283–291
nut allergy, 131–132
EDI *see* equality, diversity, and inclusion
education and schools
asthma, 180
cystic fibrosis, 173
diabetes mellitus, 270, 271
Ilizarov frame/technique, 224
mental health and wellbeing, 95
obesity, 149–155
reflective account, 90–91
support and supervision, 74
electrocardiography (ECG), 141, 197
elimination
acute kidney injury, 275
congestive cardiac failure, 192
developmental dysplasia of the hip, 229
emergency care
asthma, 175
burns injury, 292
closed head injury, **140**
epilepsy, 123
nut allergy, 135–136, *135*
sickle cell disease, 308
emollients, 286, 288
emotional abuse and exploitation, 26
end-of-life care, 13, 78
endotracheal (ET) intubation
closed head injury, 141–142
neonatal respiratory distress syndrome, 161, 164–165
enteral feeding
cerebral palsy, 242–244, **245–246**
gastrostomy care, 248–255
pre-procedural care, 243–244
procedure for passing a nasogastric tube, **245–246**
routes of administration, 242–243
environmental allergens, 177

environmental stimulants, 128
enzyme replacement therapy (ERT), 301
epidural analgesia, 116–120
case study, 116
concepts and definitions, 116–117
nursing management, 118
nursing process and model of care, 117
postoperative nursing care, **118–120**
pre-operative interventions, 117
epilepsy, 123–130
assessment, 126–127
care plan, 128
case study, 123
classification of seizures, 125–126, **125–126**
concepts and definitions, 123–124
impacts of diagnosis, 129–130
nursing process, 127
phases, 124
triggers, 127–128
epinephrine, 133, 135–136, *135*, 141
equality, diversity, and inclusion (EDI), 3, 33
ERT *see* enzyme replacement therapy
ET *see* endotracheal
ethics
assent, consent, and refusal of consent, 38–39
care planning, 35–39
truth telling, 35–38, 44–47, **46**
ethnicity, 53
evidence-based practice (EBP)
care planning, 40
infected eczema, 285–289
integrated care pathways, 55–56, 58
principles of care planning, 3, 7
eye opening, 144

F

fabricated induced illness (FII), 24, 27
family-centred care (FCC), 78–84
adaptation to child's illness, 79–81
altruism, 82
appendicectomy, 211–213, *212*
asthma, 180
bereavement support, 323–329
care planning, 86–87, *86*
cerebral palsy, 242–244, **245–246**
complex needs, 300, 303–306, *304*
concepts and definitions, 78, 79
continuous analgesia, 111–112
coping with the diagnosis, 78, 80
co-production, 80
cystic fibrosis, 171, 173
developmental dysplasia of the hip, 228
diabetes mellitus, 267–271
empowering parents, 80, 81–82, *81*
epilepsy, 129–130
experience at home, 88
gastrostomy care, 249–250, 252–253
hospital to home, 87
Ilizarov frame/technique, 223–224
impacts on education and family life, 90–91
infected eczema, 285–289
information about their child, 81–82
involving parents in child's care, 82
mental health and wellbeing, 95–96
neonatal respiratory distress syndrome, 166

nephrotic syndrome, 260–263
nursing models, 9–11, *10*
nursing process, 4–6, *4*
nut allergy, 132–133
obesity, 152–153, **154**
opportunities to learn new skills, 82
origins and development, 78–79
pain management in neonates, 103–106, *103*, *105*
parents as carers, 88–89
reflective account, 85–91
siblings and extended family, 89–90
sickle cell disease, 309, 313–314
tonsillectomy, 202
transitional care, 318–321
truth telling, 44–50
family history, 177, 193
FCC *see* family-centred care
fentanyl, 111, 142
fever
appendicectomy, 209
congestive cardiac failure, 194
developmental dysplasia of the hip, 228
sickle cell disease, 313
FII *see* fabricated induced illness
first aid, 292
flucloxacillin, 169
fluid resuscitation
burns injury, 292, 294–295, **295–297**
closed head injury, 146–147
critical care, 66, **67**, 68
cystic fibrosis, 172
sickle cell disease, 313
focal segmental glomerulosclerosis (FSGS), 260
Francis Report (2013), 35
FSGS *see* focal segmental glomerulosclerosis
full-thickness burns, 293
fundoplication, 85–87, 237

G

gag reflex, 145
gastrografin, 169
gastro-oesophageal reflux, 235–240
administration of oral medication, 237–239, **238**
aetiology and presentation, 236
case study, 235
identification of tongue-tie, 236
nursing and medical investigations, 236
reflective account, 85
sensorimotor stage in cognitive development, 235–236
treatment and management, 236–237
gastrostomy care, 248–255
case study, 248
discharge planning, 252–253, *254*
enteral feed pump, *252*
post-procedural care, 251–252
technique and types of tube, 249–250, *249–250*
GCS *see* Glasgow Coma Scale
generalised seizures, 125–126, **126**
general practitioners (GP), 317
genetic screening, 308–309
Glasgow Coma Scale (GCS), 139–141, **139**, 143–145, *144–145*

Glasgow Meningococcal Septicaemia Prognostic Scoring Tool, 62, **63**, 69
glycogen storage disorders (GSD), 301
Gosport War Memorial Hospital Inquiry (2018), 35
GP *see* general practitioners
grafting surgery, 292, 298
grief, 323–324
GSD *see* glycogen storage disorders

H

haemodiafiltration, 277–278
haemodialysis, 277–278, *278*
haemorrhage
burns injury, 298
intraventricular haemorrhage, 248
tonsillectomy, 201, 204
health promotion, 52, 53
heated, humidified high-flow nasal cannula (HHFNC), 101
High Flow Nasal Cannula (HNFC), 166
hip spica cast, 226, *226*, **227**, **229–230**
HNFC *see* High Flow Nasal Cannula
holorosencaphaly (HPE), 300–302, *302*
hormone changes, 128
HPE *see* holorosencaphaly
hydrocortisone, 286
hydroxycarbamide, 314
hygiene hypothesis, 131–132
hyperglycaemia, 270–271
hyperlipidaemia, 259–260
hypertension, 260
hyperventilation, 295
hypoglycaemia, 69, 270–271
hyponatraemia, 147
hyponatremia, 68
hypothermia, 297
hypovolaemia/hypovolaemic shock, 260, 261, 293–294
hypoxia, 65–66

I

ibuprofen, 201, 202, 228
ICP *see* integrated care pathways; intracranial pressure
ictal phase, 124, 127
ICU *see* intensive care unit
idiopathic epilepsy, 124
IgE *see* immunoglobulin E
Ilizarov frame/technique, 217–224
best practice, **221**
case study, 217
discharge planning, 223–224
phases of treatment, **219**
pin site care/management, 221, **221–223**
postoperative care, 220–221
preoperative care, 218–220
principles and procedures, 217–218, *218*, **218**
immune reactive trypsin (IRT), 169
immunisation
congestive cardiac failure, 192
nephrotic syndrome, 264
immunoglobulin E (IgE), 132
infantile onset pompe disease (IOPD), 300–302

infected eczema, 283–291
aetiology and presentation, 283–284
assessment, 284–285
care planning, 285
case study, 283
evidence-based practice, 285–289
infection
appendicectomy, 209–210, **209**
cystic fibrosis, 168
epilepsy, 128
gastrostomy care, 252
Ilizarov frame/technique, 221, **221–223**
neonatal respiratory distress syndrome, 166
nephrotic syndrome, 260, 262
reflective account, 85–88
inflammation
burns injury, 293–294
infected eczema, 285–286
informed consent
administration of oral medication, 238
cerebral palsy, 243–244
ethical, legal, and professional implications, 39
inhalers
asthma, 175–180, *178–179*
reflective account, 91
integrated care pathways (ICP), 55–59
best practice, 55–56
clinical scenario, 57–58
concepts and definitions, 55
elements, 57
evidence-based practice, 55–56, 58
origins and development, 55–56
rationale and application, 56
intensive care unit (ICU), 101–108
assessment of neonatal pain, 101–103, **102**
closed head injury, 141–147
complex needs, 300
consequences of poor pain management, 106
neonatal respiratory distress syndrome, 161–167
preparing for invasive diagnostic procedures, 103–104, **103**
reflective account, 85, *86*
support during invasive diagnostic procedures, 104–106, *105*
inter-ictal phase, 124
interprofessional team *see* multidisciplinary team
intracranial pressure (ICP), 142–143, 145–146
intraventricular haemorrhage, 248
IOPD *see* infantile onset pompe disease
IRT *see* immune reactive trypsin

K

Kaftrio, 173
kangaroo care, 104–105, *105*
ketamine infusion, 111
kidney failure, 295

L

lactation and breastfeeding
congestive cardiac failure, 191–192
gastro-oesophageal reflux, 235, 236–237
pain management in neonates, 106
Laming Report (2003), 27–28, 30

laparoscopic colostomy, 109
leg length discrepancy (LLD), 217
less-invasive surfactant administration (LISA), 163
LGBTQIA+, 53
link lecturers, 74–75
LISA *see* less-invasive surfactant administration
LLD *see* leg length discrepancy
local anaesthesia, 116–120
Local Safeguarding Children Boards (LSCB), 29
low-profile skin-level gastrostomy, 249–250, *250*
LSCB *see* Local Safeguarding Children Boards
Lund and Browder Chart, 294, **294**

M

maltreatment *see* safeguarding
Markwell, Ryan, 85–91
MCD *see* minimal change disease
MCGN *see* mesangiocapillary glomerulosclerosis
MDI *see* metered dose inhalers
MDT *see* multidisciplinary team
Mead model of nursing, 11, **11**
    closed head injury, 139–141, **139**, 143
meningococcal disease/meningitis, 60–69
Mental Capacity Act (2005), 39
mental health and wellbeing, 92–97
    assessment and formulation, 94–95, **95**
    care planning, **95**
    case study, 93–96
    COVID-19/SARS-CoV-2, 92–94
    early intervention and prevention, 92, 93
    global burden of disease, 92–93
    interventions and rationale, 96, **96**
mesangiocapillary glomerulosclerosis (MCGN), 260
metered dose inhalers (MDI), 175, 178–179, *178–179*
midazalam, 141
minimal change disease (MCD), 260
mobility
    burns injury, 297
    congestive cardiac failure, 192
    developmental dysplasia of the hip, 229
moisturisation, 285–286
mood, 95
morphine, 111, 141
motor responses, 144–145
mourning, 323–324
multidisciplinary team (MDT)
    assessment and care planning in critical care, 60–71
    asthma, 180
    care planning, 40
    complex needs, 303–304, *304*
    integrated care pathways, 56
    principles of care planning, 3, 7
    support and supervision, 72
multi-organ failure, 295
myelodysplastic syndrome, 44
myoclonic seizures, 126

N

NANDA International *see* North American Nursing Diagnosis Association
nasogastric (NG) intubation
    cerebral palsy, 242–244, **245–246**
    closed head injury, 141–142
    pre-procedural care, 243–244
    procedure for passing a nasogastric tube, **245–246**
    routes of administration, 242–243
National Association for the Welfare of Sick Children in Hospital (NAWCH), 9, 37
National Child Measurement Programme (NCMP), 150
National Confidential Enquiry into Patient Outcome and Death (NCEPOD), 317
National Council for the Professional Development of Nursing and Midwifery (NCNM), 55–56
National Institute for Health and Care Excellence (NICE)
    cerebral palsy, 243
    critical care, 62, **63**, 66–67
    developmental dysplasia of the hip, 228
    gastro-oesophageal reflux, 236
    integrated care pathways, 55, 57–58
    nut allergy, 131–132
    obesity, 151
    risk assessment and management, 17–18
    safeguarding, 24, 27
    transitional care, 186, 316, 318–321
National Society for Prevention of Cruelty to Children (NSPCC), 30
NAWCH *see* National Association for the Welfare of Sick Children in Hospital
NCA *see* nurse-controlled analgesia
NCEPOD *see* National Confidential Enquiry into Patient Outcome and Death
NCMP *see* National Child Measurement Programme
NCNM *see* National Council for the Professional Development of Nursing and Midwifery
neglect, 26–27
negligence, 36
neonatal infant pain score (NIPS), 102
neonatal intensive care unit (NICU), 101–108
    assessment of neonatal pain, 101–103, **102**
    complex needs, 300
    consequences of poor pain management, 106
    preparing for invasive diagnostic procedures, 103–104, **103**
    reflective account, 85, *86*
    respiratory distress syndrome, 161–167
    support during invasive diagnostic procedures, 104–106, *105*
nephrotic syndrome (NS), 259–265
    aetiology and presentation, 259–260
    assessment and early management, 260–263
    case study, 259
    maintaining tissue fluid balance, 263
    pharmaceutical management, 263–264
Neuman systems model, 13
    obesity, 150, 152–153
neuroimaging, 318
neurological assessment
    burns injury, 294
    closed head injury, 143–144, *144*
    critical care, 67, 68–69

neurology continuum, Mead model, 11, **11**
neuromuscular blockade, 146
neurovascular assessment, 294
neurovascular monitoring, 18–19
Newborn Blood Spot Programme, 309
NG *see* nasogastric
NICE *see* National Institute for Health and Care Excellence
NICPR *see* Northern Ireland Cerebral Palsy Register
NICU *see* neonatal intensive care unit
NIPEC *see* Northern Ireland Practice Education Committee
NIPS *see* neonatal infant pain score
NMC *see* Nursing and Midwifery Council; Nursing Midwifery Council
non-invasive ventilation, 302
non-nutritive sucking, 106
nonsteroidal anti-inflammatory drugs (NSAID), 109, 116
North American Nursing Diagnosis Association (NANDA International), 6
Northern Ireland Cerebral Palsy Register (NICPR), 316
Northern Ireland Practice Education Committee (NIPEC), 33
NS *see* nephrotic syndrome
NSAID *see* nonsteroidal anti-inflammatory drugs
NSPCC *see* National Society for Prevention of Cruelty to Children
nurse-controlled analgesia (NCA), 110
Nursing and Midwifery Council (NMC)
    ethical, legal, and professional implications, 33–35
    gastro-oesophageal reflux, 237–238
    nut allergy, 136
    support and supervision, 72–75
nursing models, 8–13
    acute kidney injury, 274–275
    advanced care planning, 13
    asthma, 176
    cardiac catheterisation, 187–188
    child- and family-centred care, 9–11, *10*
    closed head injury, 139–141, **139**, 143
    complex needs, 304–305
    congestive cardiac failure, 191–193
    continuous analgesia, 111–112
    developmental dysplasia of the hip, 228
    diabetes mellitus, 267–268
    epidural analgesia, 117
    infected eczema, 285
    Mead model, 11, **11**
    Neuman's systems model, 13
    obesity, 150, 152–153
    Orem's self-care model, 12–13, **12**
    Roper, Logan, and Tierney model, 8, **9**
    sickle cell disease, 313
nursing process
    administration of oral medication, 237–239, **238**
    calculation of drugs, 239
    cardiac catheterisation, 187–188
    cerebral palsy, 243–244
    continuous analgesia, 111–112
    epidural analgesia, 117

epilepsy, 127
nephrotic syndrome, 260–263
nursing diagnosis, 6
practical aspects, 6
sickle cell disease, 310–311, *311–312*
stages of family-centred care, 4–6, *4*, 45–48, **46–47**, *49*
storage and transportation of drugs, 239
nut allergy, 131–137
anaphylaxis, 133–136
case study, 131
diagnostic approaches, 132
emergency procedures, 135–136, *135*
management at home/school, 132–133
prevalence and possible causes, 131–132
nutrition
acute kidney injury, 275–276
cerebral palsy, 242–244, **245–246**
congestive cardiac failure, 191–192, 196
developmental dysplasia of the hip, 230
diabetes mellitus, 271
gastrostomy care, 251–252, 253
nephrotic syndrome, 261

O

obesity, 149–158
case study, 149
concepts and definitions, 150–151
consequences of childhood obesity, 152
healthy weight care plan, 153, **154**, 155, **156**
nursing models, 150, 152–153
RCPCH UK-WHO growth charts, 151, *151*, 157
risk factors for childhood obesity, 151
stressors and lines of defence/resistance, 152–153, 155
oedema
burns injury, 295
nephrotic syndrome, 259–261, 263–264
omeprazole, 237–239, **238**
opioids
continuous analgesia, 109–115
epidural analgesia, 116–117
sickle cell disease, 310–311, *312*
oral care, 305–306
oral sucrose/glucose, 106
Orem's self-care model, 12–13, **12**
cardiac catheterisation, 187–189
orthopaedic surgery, 18–19
overgranulation tissue, 253, *254*
oxygen saturation, 176–177, 191
oxygen therapy
congestive cardiac failure, 194
critical care, 66
reflective account, 85–86

P

PA *see* practice assessors
PACE framework, 11
pacifiers, 106
Paediatric Early Warning Score (PEWS), 19, 251
paediatric intensive care unit (PICU), 141–147, 300
Paediatric Yorkhill Malnutrition Score (PYMS), 251

pain management
appendicectomy, 209, 210, 213
burns injury, 295, 298
closed head injury, 141–143, **142**
continuous analgesia, 109–115
epidural analgesia, 116–120
gastrostomy care, 251
neonatal pain in the ICU, 101–108
sickle cell disease, 310–312, *311–312*
palliative care, 78, 80
pancreatic enzyme supplementation, 169
paracetamol
closed head injury, 142
continuous analgesia, 112
developmental dysplasia of the hip, 228
epidural analgesia, 116, 120
partial seizures, 125, **125**
partial-thickness burns, 292, 293–294
paternalism, 46
patient-controlled analgesia (PCA), 110–113, **113–114**
sickle cell disease, 311, *312*
patient positioning
burns injury, 297, 298
congestive cardiac failure, 194
developmental dysplasia of the hip, 229
PCA *see* patient-controlled analgesia
peak expiratory flow, 177
PEEP *see* positive end expiratory pressure
peer group, 51, 53
PEG *see* percutaneous endoscopic gastrostomy
percutaneous endoscopic gastrostomy (PEG) tube, 249–250, *249–250*
peritoneal dialysis, 277, *278*
peritonitis, 209
personal cleansing/dressing
appendicectomy, 210–211
congestive cardiac failure, 192, 196
gastrostomy care, 252, 253
infected eczema, 288
personal tutors, 74
person-centred transition support, 319, 321
PEWS *see* Paediatric Early Warning Score
PGD *see* prolonged grief disorder
philosophy of care, 8
physical abuse, 24–25
PICU *see* paediatric intensive care unit
PIPP *see* premature infant pain profile
play
congestive cardiac failure, 192
developmental dysplasia of the hip, 229–230
nephrotic syndrome, 262–263
positive end expiratory pressure (PEEP), 164
positive touch, 104
post-ictal phase, 124, 127
practice assessors (PA), 72, 73
practice education facilitator, 74
practice supervisors (PS), 72
pregnancy, 51–52
pre-ictal phase, 124
premature birth, 101–103
premature infant pain profile (PIPP), 102
primary prevention, obesity, 153
prodromal period, 125–126, 127
prolonged grief disorder (PGD), 324

propofol, 141
proteinuria, 259, 261
PS *see* practice supervisors
psychological interventions, 96
pulmonary oedema, 295
pulmonary stenosis, 185, 186
PYMS *see* Paediatric Yorkhill Malnutrition Score
pyrexia *see* fever

R

RCN *see* Royal College of Nursing
RCPCH UK-WHO growth charts, 151, *151*, 157
RDS *see* respiratory distress syndrome
record-keeping *see* documentation and record-keeping
referral, 28–31, **29**
refusal of consent, 39
Registered Nurse (RN Child), 33
religion, 53
renal replacement therapy (RRT), 274, 277
resource allocation, 82
respiratory assessment
burns injury, 295
complex needs, 301–302, *302*
respiratory distress syndrome (RDS), 161–167
assessment of respiratory needs, 161–163, **162**, *163*
care planning, 163–164, *164*
case study, 161
evaluation and discontinuation, 166
optimising respiratory function, 164–166
respiratory syncytial virus (RSV), 166
retinopathy of prematurity (ROP), 164
RIFLE criteria, 274
risk assessment and management, 17–21
categories of risk, 18–19
closed head injury, 147
examples of risk, 19–20
following an incident, 20
risk assessment, 17–19
risk management, 19
sources of risk, 17–18
RN Child *see* Registered Nurse
rooming-in, 104–105
ROP *see* retinopathy of prematurity
Roper-Logan-Tierney Model, 8, **9**
asthma, 176
complex needs, 305–306
congestive cardiac failure, 191–193
continuous analgesia, 112
developmental dysplasia of the hip, 228
diabetes mellitus, 267–268
sickle cell disease, 313
Royal College of Nursing (RCN), 17, 18–19
RRT *see* renal replacement therapy
RSV *see* respiratory syncytial virus
Rule of Nines method, 294, **294**
Russian pin site care/management, **222–223**

S

safeguarding, 22–32
adverse childhood experience and risk factors, 23, **24**

categories of maltreatment, 24
concepts and definitions, 22
documentation and record-keeping, 31
emotional abuse and child exploitation, 26
escalation of concern/referral services, 28–31, **29**
fabricated induced illness, 24, 27
inquiry into Victoria Climbié, 27–28
maltreatment, abuse, and neglect, 22–23
neglect, 26–27
physical abuse, 24–25
policies and procedures, 28–30, **29**
recognition of child maltreatment, 24
sexual abuse and exploitation, 25
Safeguarding Board Northern Ireland (SBNI), 23, 29
safety/safe environment
    acute kidney injury, 275, 276
    complex needs, 303, *304*
    congestive cardiac failure, 192
    developmental dysplasia of the hip, 230
    gastro-oesophageal reflux, 237–239
    gastrostomy care, 251, 253
    nephrotic syndrome, 262
salbutamol, 176, 178
SBAR model/tool, 62–64
SBNI *see* Safeguarding Board Northern Ireland
SCD *see* sickle cell disease
Scottish Intercollegiate Guidelines Network (SIGN), 58
secondary prevention, 153
sedation, 141–143, **142**
seizures *see* epilepsy
self-care for staff, 327
self-care model, 12–13, **12**
    cardiac catheterisation, 187–189
self-harm, 93–96, **93**
sensorimotor stage, 235–236
sepsis/septicaemia, 60–69, 313
SES *see* socioeconomic status
sexual abuse, 25
sexual health, 51–54
    problems with maintaining sexual health, 53–54
    self-promotion of sexual health, 52–53
    what constitutes good sexual health, 51–52
sexually transmissible infections, 51–52
sexual violence, 52–54
Shipman Inquiry (2003–2005), 35
sickle cell disease (SCD), 308–315
    aetiology and presentation, 308
    care planning, 310–311, *311–312*
    case study, 308
    diagnosis, treatment and long-term management, 309
    fever, 313
    fluid resuscitation, 313
    future directions, 313–314
    genetic inheritance, carrier, and screening, 308–309
SIGN *see* Scottish Intercollegiate Guidelines Network
simple partial seizures, 125
skin grafts, 292, 298
skin prick tests, 132
sleep
    congestive cardiac failure, 190, 191, 196
    epilepsy, 124, 127
    mental health and wellbeing, 94
SMART goals, 5, 310
smoking, 177
socioeconomic status (SES), 149
spirometry testing, 177
spontaneous breathing, 145
SSNS *see* steroid-sensitive nephrotic syndrome
Standards for Student Supervision and Assessment (SSSA), 72
status epilepticus, 129
steroids
    asthma, 180
    infected eczema, 286
    nephrotic syndrome, 263–264
steroid-sensitive nephrotic syndrome (SSNS), 260
strengths-based transition support, 318, 321
stress and anxiety
    cardiac catheterisation, 187–188
    cystic fibrosis, 170–171
    epilepsy, 127
    family-centred care, 80
    reflective account, 89
substance use, 54, 128
sudden unexpected death in epilepsy (SUDEP), 129
sudden unexpected death in infancy (SUDI), 166
SUDEP *see* sudden unexpected death in epilepsy
SUDI *see* sudden unexpected death in infancy
suicidality, 93–94, **93**
superficial burns, 292, 293
support and supervision, 72–77
    academic assessors, 72, 73
    case study, 75–76
    critical analysis, 76
    link lecturers, 74–75
    personal tutors, 74
    practice assessors, 72, 73
    practice education facilitator, 74
    practice supervisors, 72
surfactant deficiency, 163
suxamethonium, 141
symptomatic epilepsy, 124

T

TBSA *see* total body surface area
TCI *see* topical calcineurin inhibitors
tertiary prevention, 153
theory/practice gap, 326
thermoregulation
    burns injury, 297
    congestive cardiac failure, 191, 194
    developmental dysplasia of the hip, 228
thiopentone sodium, 141
thrombosis, 260
tissue fluid balance, 263
TIVAD *see* totally implantable venous access device
Together for Short Lives (2018), 79, 80
tongue-tie, 236
tonic-clonic seizures, 126
tonic seizures, 126
tonsillectomy, 201–207
    blood transfusion, 204–206
    case study, 201
    discharge planning, 204
    haemorrhage, 201, 204
    postoperative care, 203
    preoperative care, 202–203
    procedure, 202
topical calcineurin inhibitors (TCI), 287
total body surface area (TBSA), 293, 294–295
totally implantable venous access device (TIVAD), 168, 169–171, *170*, **171**
total parenteral nutrition (TPN), 101
touch and mouth care, 305–306
TPN *see* total parenteral nutrition
tracheostomy, 85–91
transitional care, 316–322
    cardiac catheterisation, 186, 189
    cerebral palsy, 316, 321
    concepts and definitions, 316
    context, 317–318
    guidelines, 318–321
    overarching principles, 318–319
    support after transfer, 320
    support before transfer, 320
    supporting infrastructure, 320–321
    transition planning, 319, *319–320*
truth telling, 44–50
    assessment stage, 45, **46**
    care planning, 35–38
    concepts and definitions, 44
    critical care, 69
    evaluation stage, 48, **49**
    implementation stage, 47–48
    planning stage, 45–47, **47**
twelve activities of living model, 8, **9**

U

UAC *see* umbilical arterial catheter
UK Sepsis Trust Screening Tool, 62, **64**
umbilical arterial catheter (UAC), 161
umbilical venous catheter (UVC), 161
UN Convention on the Rights of the Child (UNCRC), 38
UNCRC *see* United Nations Convention on the Rights of the Child
underfill theory, 260
Understanding the Needs of Children in Northern Ireland (UNOCINI), 28
UNICEF, 93
United Nations Convention on the Rights of the Child (UNCRC), 38, 92
UNOCINI *see* Understanding the Needs of Children in Northern Ireland
urinalysis, 147
urticaria, 133–134
UVC *see* umbilical venous catheter

V

vaccines *see* immunisation
vecuronium bromide, 146
venepuncture, 132

ventilation
  closed head injury, 142
  complex needs, 302–303, *303*
  critical care, 65, 67–68
  neonatal respiratory distress syndrome, 161, 163–164, *164*
  reflective account, 85
verbal responses, 145
visual exposure, 105–106
Visual Infusion Phlebitis scoring chart, 206

vital signs
  asthma, 176–177
  congestive cardiac failure, 191
vitamin supplementation, 169
volume-targeted ventilation (VTV), 161

W
WETFLAG values, 64–65
wet wrap therapy (WWT), 287
World Health Organisation (WHO)
  mental health and wellbeing, 92, 93
  obesity, 150–151
  safeguarding, 22
  sexual health, 51
  sickle cell disease, 310
wound care
  appendicectomy, 209–210, **209**
  burns injury, 298
  Ilizarov frame/technique, 221, **221–223**
WWT *see* wet wrap therapy